Manual of
Rational Skin Therapy and Dermatological Drugs

Disclaimer and Conflict of Interest

Medicine, being a dynamic and rapidly changing science, is continuously gaining knowledge everyday by newer clinical experience and research from all over the globe. The authors and publisher have left no stone unturned to provide updated and complete information from authentic and reliable sources. Still there could be some lacunae due to human error and constant changes in the subject. Thus, neither the authors nor the publisher warrants that the information provided in this book is in every respect correct or complete, and they disclaim all responsibilities for any errors or omissions or for the outcome happened from use of information contained in this book.

The authors and publisher also declare that they had no conflict of interest while writing or publishing this book.

Books by the same author (from Jaypee Brothers Medical Publishers)

1. Recent Advances in Dermatology Vol 1
2. Recent Advances in Dermatology Vol 2
3. Recent Advances in Dermatology Vol 3
4. 201 Skin Diseases: Diagnosis and Treatment
5. Atlas and Synopsis of Contact and Occupational Dermatology
6. Step-by-Step Management of Urticaria

Manual of Rational Skin Therapy and Dermatological Drugs

Second Edition

Sanjay Ghosh MD(Dermatology and Venerology) (California)
Professor
Department of Dermatology
Santiniketan Medical College
Bolpur, West Bengal, India
Former Professor and Head
Department of Dermatology
MGM Medical College and LSK Hospital
Kishanganj, Bihar, India

Partha Mukherjee MD(DVL)
Clinical Tutor
Department of Dermatology
College of Medicine and JNM Hospital
Kalyani, West Bengal, India

Sanjib Chowdhuri DVD(Kolkata)
Senior Consultant Dermatologist
Fortis Hospital, Anandapur
Kolkata, West Bengal, India

Subhadeep Mallick MD(DVL)
Senior Resident
Department of Dermatology
College of Medicine and JNM Hospital
Kalyani, West Bengal, India

Sujata DVDL DNB(DVL)
Senior Resident
SNM Medical College and Hospital
Dhanbad, Jharkhand, India

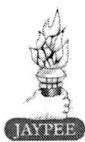

JAYPEE BROTHERS MEDICAL PUBLISHERS
The Health Sciences Publisher
New Delhi | London

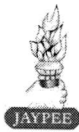 **Jaypee Brothers Medical Publishers (P) Ltd**

Headquarters
EMCA House
23/23-B, Ansari Road, Daryaganj
New Delhi 110 002, India
Landline: +91-11-23272143, +91-11-23272703
+91-11-23282021, +91-11-23245672
E-mail: jaypee@jaypeebrothers.com

Corporate Office
Jaypee Brothers Medical Publishers (P) Ltd.
4838/24, Ansari Road, Daryaganj
New Delhi 110 002, India
Phone: +91-11-43574357
Fax: +91-11-43574314
E-mail: jaypee@jaypeebrothers.com

Overseas Office
JP Medical Ltd.
83, Victoria Street, London
SW1H 0HW (UK)
Phone: +44-20 3170 8910
Fax: +44(0)20 3008 6180
E-mail: info@jpmedpub.com

Website: www.jaypeebrothers.com
Website: www.jaypeedigital.com

© 2025, Jaypee Brothers Medical Publishers

The views and opinions expressed in this book are solely those of the original contributor(s)/author(s) and do not necessarily represent those of editor(s) or publisher of the book.

All rights reserved. No part of this publication may be reproduced, stored or transmitted in any form or by any means, electronic, mechanical, photocopying, recording or otherwise, without the prior permission in writing of the publishers.

All brand names and product names used in this book are trade names, service marks, trademarks or registered trademarks of their respective owners. The publisher is not associated with any product or vendor mentioned in this book.

Medical knowledge and practice change constantly. This book is designed to provide accurate, authoritative information about the subject matter in question. However, readers are advised to check the most current information available on procedures included and check information from the manufacturer of each product to be administered, to verify the recommended dose, formula, method and duration of administration, adverse effects and contraindications. It is the responsibility of the practitioner to take all appropriate safety precautions. Neither the publisher nor the author(s)/editor(s) assume any liability for any injury and/or damage to persons or property arising from or related to use of material in this book.

This book is sold on the understanding that the publisher is not engaged in providing professional medical services. If such advice or services are required, the services of a competent medical professional should be sought.

Every effort has been made where necessary to contact holders of copyright to obtain permission to reproduce copyright material. If any have been inadvertently overlooked, the publisher will be pleased to make the necessary arrangements at the first opportunity.

Inquiries for bulk sales may be solicited at: jaypee@jaypeebrothers.com

Manual of Rational Skin Therapy and Dermatological Drugs / Sanjay Ghosh, Partha Mukherjee, Sanjib Chowdhuri, Subhadeep Mallick, Sujata

First Edition: 2010
Second Edition: **2025**
ISBN: 978-93-6616-275-1
Printed in India

DEDICATED

*To
our patients
from whom we learnt a lot*

Preface to the Second Edition

In spite of repeated requests from the publisher and dear readers, who liked the first edition very much, I could not make out time for the second edition, which was pending for a long time, due to my hectic professional and personal schedules. Finally, I could make it possible now! For this, I am thankful to all my coauthors Drs Partha Mukherjee, Sanjib Chowdhuri, Subhadeep Mallick, and Sujata for their sincere and earnest effort.

I am also grateful to the whole team of Jaypee Brothers Medical Publishers (P) Ltd, New Delhi, India, for wholehearted support and cooperation while preparing the book.

I hope that this time also, similar to the previous edition, the book would be warmly accepted by readers of all sectors, from postgraduate students to practicing dermatologists. Our labor and attempt would only be fruitful if they find the book useful in their daily practice.

Sanjay Ghosh

Preface to the First Edition

When Jaypee Brothers approached me for writing this book, I was a bit reluctant thinking another derma book is really needed or not and also for my time constraint. Later, after analyzing the pros and cons of the projects, I ultimately took the responsibility mainly for two reasons: (a) These would be our recapitulations and updating ourselves as well as intermingling of available information with our day-to-day experience; (b) This book may be a ready reference in our busy hospital or chamber practice where a bigger book consultation becomes almost next to impossible.

However, this concise book is never a replacement for larger books on this subject. We have indeed freely consulted these books for recent information and also to erase different therapeutic dilemma. We must confess here our indebtedness to them and hence we have included all their names at the end as *Further Reading* for interested readers to get the source.

Though I started the job in single hand, but due to my hectic schedule and various academic commitments, I was a bit slow in the journey. So I decided to involve almost whole of my department and they agreed enthusiastically. My heartiest congratulations should go to Dr Kishalay Ghosh, Dr Saurav Kundu, and Dr Vikas Shankar for the excellent contributions they have made for the birth of this book.

I must also acknowledge the sincere help I got from the other members of my Department, namely Dr Pranab Kumar Saha, Associate Professor; Dr Jyoti, Assistant Professor; Dr Jayoti Nandy, Junior Resident; Dr Rajib Roy, Junior Resident; Department of Dermatology, MGM Medical College and LSK Hospital, Kishanganj, Bihar, India.

I also convey here my deep regards and gratitude to Professor Prasanta Kumar Mukherjee, Academic Director, and Dr Dilip Kumar Jaisawal, Director, MGM Medical College and LSK Hospital, Kishanganj, Bihar, India, for constant support and inspiration for such an academic project.

I should also pay my earnest thanks to the whole team of Jaypee Brothers Medical Publishers (P) Ltd, from both Delhi and Kolkata for cooperating with me wholeheartedly for making this project successful.

Last but not the least we, we must express gratefulness to our family members for constantly bearing us and providing constant enthusiasm for this obsessive effort.

Sanjay Ghosh
E-mail: *drsanjayghosh1@gmail.com*

Contents

1. RATIONAL SKIN THERAPY 1

- Acanthosis Nigricans *2*
- Acne Vulgaris *2*
- Acrodermatitis Enteropathica *4*
- Actinic Keratoses *4*
- Actinic Prurigo *5*
- Actinomycosis *5*
- Acute Generalized Exanthematous Pustulosis *6*
- Allergic/Irritant Contact Dermatitis *6*
- Alopecia Areata *7*
- Androgenetic Alopecia *8*
- Angular Cheilitis *8*
- Recurrent Aphthous Stomatitis *9*
- Atopic Dermatitis *9*
- Non-tuberculous Mycobacterial/Atypical Mycobacterial Skin Infection *10*
- Basal Cell Carcinoma *11*
- Behçet's Disease *11*
- Bullous Pemphigoid *12*
- Candidiasis *13*
- Cellulitis/Erysipelas *13*
- Chancroid *14*
- Chilblains *14*
- Chronic Actinic Dermatitis *15*
- Condyloma Acuminata *15*
- Cutaneous Amyloidosis *16*
- Cutaneous Larva Migrans (Creeping Eruption) *16*
- Cutaneous Leishmaniasis *17*
- Darier's Disease *17*
- Decubitus Ulcer *17*
- Dermatitis Herpetiformis *18*
- Dermatomyositis *18*
- Diaper Dermatitis *19*
- Discoid Eczema (Nummular Eczema) *19*
- Discoid Lupus Erythematosus *20*

- Drug Eruption 20
- Erythema Multiforme 21
- Erythema Nodosum 21
- Erythrasma 22
- Erythroderma (Exfoliative Dermatitis Syndrome) 22
- Furunculosis 23
- Gonorrhea 23
- Granuloma Inguinale 24
- Herpes Simplex (Including Herpes Genitalis) 24
- Herpes Zoster 24
- Hidradenitis Suppurativa 25
- Hirsutism 25
- Hyperhidrosis 27
- Ichthyosis 27
- Impetigo 28
- Infantile Hemangiomas 28
- Insect Bite Hypersensitivity 29
- Keloid 29
- Keratosis Pilaris 30
- Leg Ulcers 30
- Leprosy and Its Reaction 31
- Lupus Erythematosus: Specific Skin Lesion 31
- Lichen Nitidus 32
- Lichen Planus 32
- Lichen Sclerosus 33
- Lichen Simplex Chronicus 33
- Lymphogranuloma Venereum 34
- Melasma 34
- Miliaria 35
- Molluscum Contagiosum 35
- Morphea 36
- Mycetoma 36
- Mycosis Fungoides 36
- Palmoplantar Pustulosis 37
- Parapsoriasis 37
- Paronychia 38
- Pediculosis 38
- Pemphigus Vulgaris and Foliaceous 39
- Pityriasis Lichenoides Chronica 40
- Pityriasis Lichenoides Et Varioliformis Acuta 40
- Pityriasis Rosea 40

- Pityriasis Rubra Pilaris 40
- Pityriasis Versicolor 41
- Polymorphous Light Eruption 41
- Pompholyx 42
- Pregnancy Dermatoses 42
- Prurigo Nodularis 43
- Psoriasis 44
- Pseudofolliculitis Barbae 45
- Pyoderma Gangrenosum 46
- Rosacea 47
- Sarcoidosis 48
- Scabies 48
- Systemic Sclerosis: Cutaneous Management 48
- Seborrheic Dermatitis 49
- Stevens–Johnson Syndrome/Toxic Epidermal Necrolysis 50
- Sporotrichosis 51
- Syphilis 52
- Tinea Infection 52
- Tuberculosis 54
- Urticaria 54
- Vasculitis 57
- Viral Warts 57
- Vitiligo 58

2. SYSTEMIC DRUGS 61

- Systemic Corticosteroids 62
- Systemic Immunosuppressive and Immunomodulatory Agents 67
- Cyclosporine 71
- Azathioprine 73
- Mycophenolate Mofetil 75
- Cyclophosphamide 77
- Bleomycin 79
- Antihistamines 81
- Antileukotrienes 85
- Systemic Antibacterial Agents 87
- Fluoroquinolones 91
- Oxazolidinones 95
- Systemic Antifungal 96
- Terbinafine 96
- Itraconazole 97
- Griseofulvin 99

- Voriconazole 99
- Posaconazole 100
- Systemic Antiviral Agents 100
- Famcilovir 102
- Foscarnet 103
- Antiparasitic 103
- Albendazole 104
- Thiabandazole 105
- Ivermectin 106
- Antileprotics 107
- Rifampin and Other Rifamycins 108
- Clofazimine 110
- Antitubercular Drugs 111
- Pyrazinamide 112
- Ethambutol 113
- Antiretroviral Drugs 114
- Maraviroc 116
- Nucleoside and Nucleotide Reverse Transcriptase Inhibitors 116
- Nonnucleoside Reverse Transcriptase Inhibitors 118
- Protease Inhibitors 120
- Integrase Inhibitors/Integrase Strand Transfer Inhibitors 123
- Post-exposure Prophylaxis 125
- Antimalarials 126
- Systemic Retinoids 128
- Colchicine 134
- Biological Therapy/Immunobiologics 135
- Etanercept 136
- Infliximab 137
- Adalimumab 137
- Golimumab 138
- Certolizumab Pegol 139
- Interleukin 17 Inhibitors 140
- Ixekizumab 141
- Brodalumab 141
- Guselkumab 144
- Tildrakizumab 145
- Risankizumab 145
- Rituximab 146
- Dupilumab 148
- IL-13 Inhibitors 149
- Lebrikizumab 149

- Tralokinumab *150*
- IL-31 Receptor Antagonist *150*
- IL-36 Receptor Antagonist *151*
- IL-1 Antagonists *152*
- Anti-IgE Antibodies *153*
- B Lymphocyte Stimulator Specific Inhibitor *154*
- PDE4 Inhibitor *155*
- JAK Inhibitors *156*
- Oral JAK inhibitors *157*
- Baricitinib *159*
- Abrocitinib *160*
- Upadacitinib *161*
- Ritlecitinib *162*
- Deucravacitinib *163*
- Anti-androgen *164*
- Spironolactone *166*
- Hedgehog Pathway Inhibitors *172*
- Beta-blockers *174*
- Oral Minoxidil *175*
- Oral Vitamins *176*
- Thalidomide *176*
- Lenalidomide *179*
- Systemic Psoralen plus Ultraviolet A Photochemotherapy *179*
- Botulinum Toxin *181*
- Vaccines in Dermatology *182*

3. TOPICAL DRUGS 185

- Topical Drugs *186*
- Fusidic Acid *186*
- Retapamulin *187*
- Ozenoxacin *187*
- Neomycin *188*
- Nadifloxacin *189*
- Silver Sulfadiazine *189*
- Antiseptics *189*
- Hydrogen Peroxide *190*
- Chlorhexidine *190*
- Povidone-iodine *190*
- Topical Antiacne Drugs *191*
- Clindamycin *191*
- Azelaic Acid *192*

- Metronidazole *193*
- Dapsone *193*
- Topical Antifungal Agents *194*
- Azoles *195*
- Amorolfine *200*
- Topical Antivirals *200*
- Cidofovir *202*
- Immune-Enhancing Drugs *202*
- Topical Antiparasitic Agents *205*
- Topical Glucocorticoids *207*
- Topical Retinoids *211*
- Bexarotene *214*
- Trifarotene *215*
- Topical Immunomodulators *215*
- Calcipotriene *218*
- Contact Sensitizer *219*
- Squaric Acid Dibutyl Ester *220*
- Topical Phosphodiasterase-4 Inhibitors *221*
- Topial Minoxidil *224*
- Sunscreen *224*
- Depigmenting Agents *229*
- Azelaic Acid *230*
- Kojic Acid *230*
- Monobenzyl Ether of Hydroquinone *230*
- Moisturizers *231*
- Keratolytics *232*
- Urea *233*
- Ammonium Lactate *233*
- Topical Antipruritic Agents *233*
- Phenol *234*
- Camphor *234*
- Hypohidrotic Agents *235*
- Barrier Cream *236*
- Local Anesthetic Agent *236*
- EMLA *236*
- Vitamin B Complex *238*
- Suggested Readings *240*

Index **241**

CHAPTER

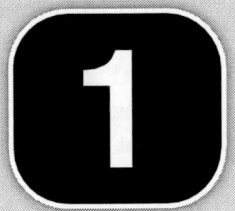

Rational Skin Therapy

ACANTHOSIS NIGRICANS

1. To search and manage background etiological factors, if any
2. Topical tretinoin 0.025 to 0.05% once daily at evening or night
3. 12% ammonium lactate twice daily may added alongwith once daily tretinoin
4. Topical adapalene 0.1% for pediatric age group
5. Topical tazarotene 0.05% once daily at evening or night
6. Topical vitamin D analogs (calcipotriene 0.005%) twice daily for 3 months

> **PRACTICAL HINTS**
>
> 1. Proper methods of application should be explained to patients while prescribing topical retinoids to avoid irritation and poor patient's compliance.
> 2. It is better to start topical tretinoin at lower strength (0.025%) for minimum duration (1 hour) very gently in thin layer only over the affected area. Then the strength and time duration can be gradually escalated as per patient's tolerance and response.
> 3. Topical tazarotene can be started as short contact therapy (10–15 minutes) on alternate day and gradually the timespan can be increased to daily and longer regimen when patient can get experienced and convinced about its use.
> 4. Referral to endocrinologist is mandatory if insulin resistance detected

ACNE VULGARIS

Milder Form

Comedonal

- *Topical retinoids:* Adapalene, trifarotene, tretinoin, or tazarotene (short contact)
- *Alternatives:* Azelaic acid or salicylic acid.

Mild Papulopustular or Mixed Comedonal/Papulopustular

Combination treatment of topical retinoids and topical antimicrobials. Preferred antimicrobials are benzoyl peroxide or benzoyl peroxide plus topical clindamycin.

Moderate Form

Mixed and Papular/Pustular

1. Oral antibiotic and topical retinoids with benzoyl peroxide
2. *Alternative:* Oral antibiotic and azelaic acid with benzoyl peroxide
3. *In females:* Oral antiandrogens and topical retinoids/azelaic acid with benzoyl peroxide.

Nodular

1. Oral antibiotic and topical retinoids with benzoyl peroxide
2. *Alternative:* Oral isotretinoin or oral antibiotic and azelaic acid with benzoyl peroxide
3. *In females:* Oral antiandrogens and topical retinoids/azelaic acid with benzoyl peroxide

Severe Form

Nodular/Conglobate

1. Oral isotretinoin
2. *Alternatives:* High dose oral antibiotics and topical retinoids and benzoyl peroxide
3. *In females:* High dose oral antiandrogens and topical retinoids with topical antimicrobials.

Maintenance Therapy

Topical retinoids with benzoic acid.

Postinflammatory Hyperpigmentation

Photoprotection, topical retinoids, azelaic acid, superficial chemical peels

Acne Scar

Early and effective treatment of active acne 2 weeks prior with topical retinoids.
As monotherapy: Adapalene 0.3%, tazarotene 0.1%, trifarotene 0.005% and in combination—adapalene 0.1% + BPO 2.5%, BPO 2.5% + adapalene 0.3%, retinoic acid 0.025% + glycolic acid 12%

Noncomedogenic sunscreen and moisturizers to be advised.

Procedures for atrophic post acne scars:
- Vascular lasers or light: Pulse dye laser, potassium titanyl phosphate, intense pulse light, erbium doped fractional laser helps in improving scar associated erythema and may induce collagen induction.
- Ablative lasers CO_2 and Er:YAG: Removes epidermis and part of the dermis leading to collagen remodelling
- Fractional ablative laser CO_2, 2,940 nm Er:YAG, 1,540 nm Erglass leads to faster recovery, safer in darker phototypes and less dyschromia
- Non ablative lasers: Q switched NdYAG, diode and picosecond 755 nm alexandrite leads to dermal thermal injury while preserving epidermis with lesser downtime
- Fractional radiofrequency +/- needling offers best results for ice-pick and boxscars with no PIH
- Needling device rolled over skin is low cost where the deposition of new collagen is slow and the final result takes 8 to 12 months
- Chemical peeling and microdermabrasion: Spot TCA for ice pick scars and deep spot TCA and microdermabrasion for rolling scars
- Fillers (hyaluronic acid, poly-l-lactic acid, calcium hydroxylapatite) address the volume loss resulting from atrophic acne scars
- PRP and stem cell therapy enhances wound healing and better in combination with fractional laser or skin needling

Surgical management:
- Punch excision suitable for ice pick scars and small <3 mm boxcars
- Elliptical excision more favourable in larger scars
- Punch elevation for boxcars

Hypertrophic and keloidal scars:
- Initially silicon gels under occlusion or silicon sheets to be given
- For early red lesions, pulsed dye laser 585 nm or intense pulsed light (IPL) may be used
- If lesions are significantly raised intralesional triamcinolone acetonide with or without 5-FU/bleomycin to be given
- Intralesional radiofrequency or cryotherapy can be used to debulk if there are multiple or larger lesions.

PRACTICAL HINTS

1. Oral antibiotics lead to resistance in commensal flora at all body sites while topical antibiotics lead to resistance largely confined to skin of treated sites.
2. Combining topical or oral antibiotic therapy with topical benzoyl peroxide will decrease risk of development of antibiotic-resistant strains of *Cutibacterium acnes*.
3. Oral antibiotics are recommended only for moderate to severe acne.
4. Topical antibiotics can be used in mild-to-moderate acne always by combining with benzoyl peroxide and a topical retinoids.
5. Use of antibiotic is to be limited; response and continuing need of antibiotic has to be assessed at 6 to 12 weeks.
6. Antibiotics either topical or oral as monotherapy should not be used. Benzoyl peroxide is to be added in regimen containing simultaneous oral and topical antibiotics, particularly if chemically different.
7. Antibiotics should not be used as maintenance therapy.
8. Topical retinoids can be used in both noninflammatory and inflammatory acne. Adapalene is less irritant than other retinoids.
9. Higher strength of benzoyl peroxide is not more effective than its lower strength but can lead to more irritation.

ACRODERMATITIS ENTEROPATHICA

1. *Oral zinc supplementation:* Higher replacement dose are recommended—approximately 3 mg/kg/day of elemental zinc (13.2 mg/kg/day of zinc sulfate or 10.1 mg/kg/day of zinc acetate) [2 to 3 times of normal recommended recommended daily allowance (RDA)] until all symptoms and signs disappear.
2. Further monitoring of the dose is to be done by follow-up blood zinc levels at every 3 to 6 months and adjusting the dose up or down as required.

PRACTICAL HINTS

1. Patients with acrodermatitis enteropathica require higher doses of zinc to combat the defect in abdominal zinc absorption.
2. Various zinc preparation may be available in the form of its different salts: Zinc sulfate, zinc acetate, zinc gluconate, etc. Prescribers should verify the amount of elemental zinc in each preparation (e.g., 220 mg zinc sulfate contains only 55 mg of elemental zinc).
3. Toxicity from zinc supplementation is rare, however, long-continued higher doses may induce deficiencies of other minerals like iron and copper.

ACTINIC KERATOSES

1. Sunscreen
2. Topical 5-fluorouracil (5-FU)
3. Topical imiquimod 5%
4. Photodynamic therapy (PDT);
5. Topical adapalene gel
6. Topical diclofenac gel 3.0% (in 2.5% hyaluronan gel)
7. Cryosurgery
8. Curettage
9. Excision

PRACTICAL HINTS

1. *Single/few lesions (thin or hyperkeratotic)*: Liquid nitrogen cryotherapy preferable
2. *Multiple thin lesions*: 5-FU/imiquimod/PDT; multiple hyperkeratotic

lesions—liquid nitrogen therapy followed by 5-FU preferable
3. Evidence failed to show that any treatment form is beneficial in reducing the incidence of invasive squamous cell carcinoma.
4. As there are high rate of spontaneous resolution of actinic keratoses the issue whether all patients required treatment or not has not yet been settled.

ACTINIC PRURIGO

1. Sunscreens
2. Class II or I topical corticosteroids
3. Topical tacrolimus (in milder lesions or maintenance)
4. Thalidomide 50–100 mg/daily (with subsequent tapering and lowest dose maintenance)
5. Narrow-band UVB phototherapy
6. PUVA photochemotherapy

> **PRACTICAL HINTS**
> 1. Counseling of the patients regarding life-pattern changes, clothing and adequate amount of sunscreen is necessary.
> 2. During phototherapy treatment normally photo-exposed sites should only be treated.
> 3. To reduce the incidence of disease flare after phototherapy potent topical corticosteroid is to be applied immediately after each session over the treated area.
> 4. Phototherapy is not curative; symptoms recur after discontinuation of treatment

ACTINOMYCOSIS

1. Penicillin: Parenteral penicillin G 10–20 million U/day intravenously divided every 6 hourly, depending on the severity, for 4 to 6 weeks. Follow-up therapy to be continued with penicillin V 250 to 500 mg, 4 to 6 times daily for 12 to 18 months. Penicillin K (phenoxymethyl penicillin) can also be given.
2. For patients who cannot take penicillin ceftriaxone is an alternative.
3. Amoxycillin 500 mg 4 times daily may be tried in severe cases.
4. *In patients allergic to penicillin/amoxycillin/ceftriaxone*: Doxycycline 100 mg twice daily for 8 weeks
5. Imipenem for 4 weeks in relapsed cases may be successful.
6. *Duration of treatment*: Parenteral therapy for 4–6 weeks followed by oral therapy. Total duration: 2–6 months for mild disease/6–12 months for severe disease.
7. Surgical treatment: More complicated/refractory cases.

> **PRACTICAL HINTS**
> 1. Actinomycosis therapy usually requires long-term antibiotics. However, if detected in early stage, therapy may be successful after short course of antibiotics.
> 2. Polymicrobial infection (found in 75–95% cultures) does not always need other antimicrobial therapy. However, if typical pathogens found in the culture combination of a beta-lactam and a beta-lactamase inhibitor (piperacillin-tazobactam, amoxycillin-clavulanate) may combat penicillin-resistant aerobic and anaerobic pathogens.

3. Mild infection can be eradicated completely by antibiotics while extensive cases may demand combined approach of antibiotics along with surgery.

4. After recovery patients should be specifically instructed to avoid the culprit drug and also all chemically related compound.

ACUTE GENERALIZED EXANTHEMATOUS PUSTULOSIS (AEGP)

1. Immediate withdrawal of offending drug
2. Hospitalization (for fluid, electrolyte, and nutritional support)
3. Usually self-limiting: No specific therapy available
4. Supportive therapy
5. Emollients when superficial desquamation supervenes
6. Topical corticosteroids (medium potency topical corticosteroid/group 4): Twice daily × 1 week
7. For atypical, severe cases: Short course of systemic corticosteroids (methylprednisolone/prednisolone 1 mg/kg for 7–14 days with variable taper)
8. For severe cases low-dose oral cyclosporin (3–5 mg/kg) tapered over 2 weeks

Practical Hints

1. In case of severe involvement management in specialized intensive care unit.
2. Supportive interventions include maintenance of warm temperature, electrolyte balance, nutritional especially high caloric supplementation and prevention of sepsis.
3. Evidence supporting use of systemic corticosteroids/other immunosuppressives for severe AGEP is limited to case reports and small case series. Systemic corticosteroids did not shorten the disease course as per these studies.

ALLERGIC/IRRITANT CONTACT DERMATITIS

1. Acute phase: Topical sterile normal saline soaking, topical corticosteroid solution
2. Subacute phase: Topical corticosteroid cream or pimecrolimus 1% cream
3. Chronic phase: Topical corticosteroid ointment or tacrolimus ointment 0.1%
4. Systemic antibiotics, when signs of secondary infection or associated lymphangitis or cellulitis seen
5. Oral antihistamines to alleviate itching, irritation, if associated
6. Short course of oral corticosteroids in case of severe contact dermatitis
7. Refractory cases: UVB NB, PUVA, azathioprine 100–150 mg/day for 6 months (reported in airborne parthenium contact dermatitis) or cyclosporine 5 mg/kg/day or mycophenolate mofetil 500 mg bid.

Practical Hints

1. Long-term potent topical corticosteroids used for chronic or recurrent contact dermatitis can lead to skin atrophy and even more barrier function defect. This in turn causes more penetration of allergens into the epidermis making the contact dermatitis more refractory. Hence, after getting primary control over the inflammation therapy to be better continued with mid-to-low potent corticosteroids or topical calcineurin inhibitors.
2. Emollients to be used liberally to prevent dryness of skin. This may also help in restoration of barrier

function of the skin. Emollients should preferably be paraben-free, lanolin-free and fragrance-free.
3. Use of soap substitute helps to prevent further damage of epidermal barrier function.
4. Liberal use of barrier creams will aid in protection from contact of offending substances to some extent
5. Gloves should be used by the sufferers, when required. In case of rubber allergy, one may use cotton or polythene gloves underneath the rubber gloves. However, in hot and humid weather prolonged use of occlusive gloves may precipitate maceration, secondary bacterial or fungal infection. Hence, brief and intermittent use of gloves only when required and proper drying of skin in between wearing gloves is mandatory for real benefit.

ALOPECIA AREATA

1. Intralesional corticosteroids (triamcinolone acetonide) in limited patchy cases
2. Potent topical corticosteroids for minimum 3 months especially in children (3 to 10 years)
3. Topical immunotherapy with diphenylcyclopropenone (diphencyprone or DPCP): Initially 2% lotion is applied to a small area (2 to 4 cm^2) of scalp for sensitization. Then lower concentration (0.001 to 0.1%) is weekly applied over a larger area.
4. Topical PUVA/Turban PUVA can be attempted in children
5. Topical minoxidil, topical anthralin, topical retinoic acid or PUVA: Insufficient evidence.
6. Alopecia totalis/universalis: Short course systemic corticosteroids with a tapering schedule can be used.
7. In extensive and refractory cases oral baricitinib (2–4 mg daily) or oral ritlecitinib (50 mg once daily)
8. In rapidly progressive, extensive hair loss an initial, short course of systemic course of systemic glucocorticoids may be beneficial for arresting the progression. These patients may be subsequently switched over to oral baricitinib or ritlecitinib.
9. Psychosocial support and cosmetic interventions may be needed.

Practical Hints

1. The natural evolution of alopecia areata can not be altered by any drug.
2. The extent of the disease reflects the prognostic factor for regrowth especially in alopecia totalis/universalis. Early age of onset also stands as a poor prognostic factor.
3. Topical corticosteroids are more effective in children than in adults. However, alopecia areata in beard or similar thinner skin may show much better benefit even in adults as compared to scalp.
4. Intralesional corticosteroids are not suitable for children.
5. Topical immunotherapy with diphencyprone (DPCP) remains one of the best documented therapies for alopecia areata and also most likely effective therapy in extensive and long-standing cases.
6. DPCP therapy hardly shows adverse effects except local sensitization reaction.

ANDROGENETIC ALOPECIA (AGA)

Men

- Topical minoxidil 5% solution or foam 1 mL twice daily
- Finasteride 1 mg per day.
- Low-dose oral minoxidil (2.5–5 mg daily) [IDOJ 2022]
- Oral dutasteride (0.5 mg/day) (if finasteride is noneffective) [Annals of Dermatology 2022]
- Hair transplantation (for refractory cases)

Women

- Topical minoxidil 2% 1 mL twice daily
- Oral spironolactone 100–200 mg daily [Cureus 2023]
- Systemic antiandrogen cyproterone acetate 52 mg daily on days 1–20 of the cycle.
- Low-dose oral minoxidil (0.25–1.25 mg daily) [IDOJ 2022]
- Low-level laser therapy (LLLT)
- Platelet-rich plasma (PRP) injections

> **PRACTICAL HINTS**
> 1. Patients' counseling should be done before prescribing minoxidil and finasteride stressing the fact that after stopping the products hair loss will resume.
> 2. In male pattern hair loss combination therapy of oral 5-alpha reductase inhibitors (finasteride) with the topical minoxidil may be more effective than treatment with either agent alone.
> 3. In female pattern hair loss a minority of patients might have underlying hyperandrogenism, which should be identified and treated.
> 4. Randomized controlled trial has shown that systemic antiandrogen cyproterone acetate is less effective than topical minoxidil 2% lotion in management of AGA in women.
> 5. Systemic antiandrogen if prescribed in women with AGA increases the risk of deep venous thrombosis and fatal embolism.
> 6. Efficacy data for oral minoxidil are very limited

ANGULAR CHEILITIS

1. *Topical antifungals:* Clotrimazole, miconazole
2. *Topical antibacterials:* Mupirocin, fusidic acid
3. *Systemic antifungals:* Fluconazole

> **PRACTICAL HINTS**
> 1. Proper dentures should be used. Dentures are to be removed at night and adequately cleansed before reintroducing.
> 2. Maintaining optimal oral hygiene is very important.
> 3. Nutritional factors like iron, folate or vit B12 deficiency if present would be corrected.
> 4. Chronic trauma and maceration from habitual lip licking, dental flossing or excessive salivation are to be prevented.
> 5. Treating sicca symptoms (dry mouth) may be necessary if present in association.
> 6. Use of barrier cream (e.g., zinc oxide paste) or petrolatum
> 7. Microlipoinjection of autologous collagen for correction of the deep furrows at the oral commissures may be rewarding for the patients having such ailment provoking angular cheilitis repeatedly.

RECURRENT APHTHOUS STOMATITIS

1. Antiseptic mouth rinse (chlorhexidine gluconate) thrice daily for 6 weeks
2. Sucralfate suspension 4 times daily even up to 2 years
3. Topical corticosteroids (triamcinolone 0.1% in orabase or clobetasol 0.05% gel or ointment): To apply 2–3 times a day
4. Amlexanox (5% oral paste) to apply 4 times daily
5. Tetracycline 250 mg/5 mL to be taken 4 times daily (to be held in the mouth for 2 minutes then swallowed)

For refractory aphthosis:
1. Oral colchicine 0.5 mg once daily, then gradually be increased to twice daily for 4 months
2. Dapsone at starting dose of 25–50 mg daily may be given alone or with colchicine for patients who can tolerate only a low dose of colchicine.
3. *Oral corticosteroids:* Prednisolone 40 mg daily once daily for 5 days, then 20 mg on alternate days for a week. Topical corticosteroids can be added along with.

> **PRACTICAL HINTS**
> 1. The target of the therapy should be prevention of relapse, help in healing, control of pain and maintaining nutrition.
> 2. Topical corticosteroids should be used only for brief span time. Otherwise opportunistic candidial infection may supervene.
> 3. When topical and systemic corticosteroids are inevitable clotrimazole mouth paint or troche is to be prescribed as a preventive measure against candidiasis.

ATOPIC DERMATITIS

1. Topical corticosteroids
2. Topical immunomodulators
3. Emollients
4. Wet-wrap therapy
5. Oral antihistamines
6. UVB NB
7. Antibiotics
8. Systemic corticosteroids
9. Elimination diets
10. Dust mite reduction

In refractory cases:
1. Cyclosporine: 3–5 mg/kg in two divided dose daily × 6 to 26 weeks
2. Methotrexate
3. Injection dupilumab or injection tralokinumab
4. JAK inhibitors: Abrocitinib, upadacitinib

> **PRACTICAL HINTS**
> 1. Frequent use of emollients especially ointment or water-in-oil cream should be encouraged. Such application immediately after bath improves skin hydration and barrier function. Emollients may be used as maintenance therapy and also to prevent relapse.
> 2. Mild nonalkaline cleansers like syndet bar are better choice for atopic patients.
> 3. Application of twice weekly potent cortico-steroids to stable eczema may reduce flares in children and adults but the long-term safety profile this regimen has yet not settled.
> 4. In sensitive skin like face, intertriginous area topical tacrolimus or pimecrolimus may be used instead of topical corticosteroids.

5. Topical corticosteroids are more beneficial during flare but may cause cutaneous atrophy through continuous use. As topical calcineurin inhibitors are not atrophogenic they can be used strategically in rotation with topical corticosteroids according to the stage of the disease for optimal results having minimal side effects.
6. Sedating antihistamines given at night are mostly effective by breaking the 'itch-scratch cycle'. Nonsedating antihistamines are sometimes helpful but usually at higher doses.
7. Due to significant side effects systemic immunosuppressants like corticosteroids are only to be used during acute diseases flares for short-term to medium term periods. Once control is achieved it is better to switch on to standard topical treatment.
8. For children ≥ 6 months and adolescents who are refractory to topical therapy or refuse wet wraps, dupilumab is preferable for favorable safety profile even on long-term use. For children (6 months to 6 years) when dupilumab is undesirable, not accessible or not effective systemic immunosuppressive (cyclosporin or methotrexate) may be given. For children > 6 years in same situation NBUVB is more justified rather than conventional immunosuppressives. In children > 12 years where dupilumab is undesirable, not accessible or not effective tralokinumab, upadacitinib or abrocitinib may be alternative therapy.
9. For refractory adult patients dupilumab can be given as first-line therapy for better long-term safety profile rather than other systemic agents. Injection tralokinumab may be an alternative. If the patient unable or unwilling to take biologics and in whom risks of adverse effect of JAK inhibitors are small, oral abrocitinib or upadacitinib can be advised. Methotrexate can be prescribed for those who cannot afford biologics or JAK inhibitors.
10. In Indian subcontinent especially in hot places with high humidity patients of atopic dermatitis often cannot tolerate well the NBUVB except in the winter months.

NON-TUBERCULOUS MYCOBACTERIAL/ATYPICAL MYCOBACTERIAL SKIN INFECTION

1. In treatment of *Mycobacterium marinum* infection:
   i. There is no consensus regarding treatment regimen and duration of therapy.
   ii. Available effective drugs include doxycycline, azithromycin, ethambutol, minocycline, rifampicin, cotrimoxazole, clarithromycin either used alone or in combination.
   iii. Excision of lesion is controversial. They should better be left for infection involving deeper structure. Chemotherapy should continue.
   iv. The role of wearing gloves during handling of fish should be propagated by public awareness program.
2. In treatment of *Mycobacterium chelonae* infection:
   i. No consensus treatment protocol exists.
   ii. Treatment is dictated by clinical involvement. In minor localized disease single drug therapy is sufficient. Multiple drug is required for disseminated or systemic disease.

iii. Effective drugs include clarithromycin, cefoxitin, fluoroquinolones, tobramycin used either alone or in combination.
iv. Duration of therapy is empirical.
v. Surgical debridement may be adjunctive to medication.
3. In treatment of *Mycobacterium fortuitum* infection:
   i. No consensus treatment protocol exists.
   ii. These group is less drug-resistant compared to *Mycobacterium chelonae* infection.
   iii. Effective drugs include amikacin, cefoxitin, ciprofloxacin, doxycycline, linezolid, minocycline, imipenem, tobramycin, sulfonamides, etc.
   iv. Tetracycline as a group is ineffective.
   v. Surgical debridement may be adjunctive.

> **PRACTICAL HINTS**
> 1. Typically, a treatment duration of 2–4 months is recommended for skin and soft-tissue NTM (non-tuberculous mycobacterial) infection (Wang X, Front Pharmacol 2023)
> 2. Monotherapy or combined therapy depends on the specific situation (NTM species, infection site, and disease severities).
> 3. The surgery operations include excision, debridement, drainage, and amputation, etc.

BASAL CELL CARCINOMA (BCC)

1. Excisional surgery
2. Curettage and electrodessication (C and D)
3. Cryotherapy
4. 5-fluorouracil (5 FU)
5. Topical imiquimod
6. Photodynamic therapy
7. Mohs micrographic surgery
8. Radiotherapy

> **PRACTICAL HINTS**
> 1. For primary, nodular or superficial low-risk BCCs surgical excision (standard excision with 4–5 mm margins and postoperative margin assessment) is preferable. Curettage and electrodessication (C and E) is an alternative, first-line therapy for low-risk BCC.
> 2. For patients with low-risk BCC, who are non-surgical candidates or who prefer to avoid surgery, options may be C and E, topical imiquimod, topical fluorouracil and photodynamic therapy (PDT)
> 3. For high-risk BCCs Mohs micrographic surgery (MMS) is more preferable rather than standard surgical procedure
> 4. Surgery and radiotherapy have been proved to best effective treatment. Maximum cosmetic acceptability is with surgery.
> 5. Cryotherapy has shown reduced cure rate and poorer cosmetic match as compared with surgery. Two free-thaw freeze-thaw cycles has been advocated for nodular and superficial facial lesions for better outcome.
> 6. Imiquimod is highly effective in superficial BCC (once a day for 6 weeks) and moderately effective in nodular BCC (once a day for 12 weeks).

BEHÇET'S DISEASE

1. Sucralfate
2. Topical or intralesional corticosteroids

3. Topical anesthetics
4. Topical tacrolimus
5. Chlorhexidine gluconate
6. Tetracycline suspension
7. Amlexanox 5% paste
8. Colchicine 0.6 mg thrice daily
9. Apremilast uptitrated from 10 mg daily to maximum 30 mg twice daily
10. Dapsone 100 to 200 mg daily
11. Thalidomide 100 to 300 mg daily
12. Systemic corticosteroids
13. Clofazimine 100 to 400 mg daily.

PRACTICAL HINTS

1. The therapeutic aim would mainly be symptomatic relief. However, assessment and management of mucocutaneous and visceral involvement is utmost important.
2. Active aggressive therapy may be warranted in the early phase to prevent recurrence and involvement and damage of vital organs like eye, etc.
3. A coordinated multidisciplinary approach is necessary for optimal care.
4. Treatment should be based on the type of organ system involved and on the severity of disease within that organ system.
5. Oral and genital ulcers, initial treatment with topical corticosteroids may be given. Topical anesthetics can be added to provide temporary relief.
6. Oral colchicine 1–2 mg/day in two to three divided dose can be given rather than oral corticosteroids.
7. Apremilast is a reasonable alternative to colchicine as a glucocorticoid-sparing agent.
8. Cases involving vascular system especially of larger vessels and central nervous system are refractory to therapy.

BULLOUS PEMPHIGOID

1. Potent topical corticosteroids (clobetasol 0.05% cream)
2. *Systemic corticosteroids:* Oral prednisolone 0.5 mg/kg for moderate disease and 1 m/kg for severe disease
3. Tetracycline 500 mg twice to four times daily
4. Tetracycline 500 mg twice to four times daily along with nicotinomide 500 mg thrice daily
5. Doxycycline 100 mg twice daily
6. Dapsone 50 to 100 g daily
7. Azathioprin 2.5 mg/kg daily
8. Mycophenolate mofetil.
9. Rituximab (dose range from 375 mg/m^2 every one to four weeks to 500 mg weekly for 2 weeks)

PRACTICAL HINTS

1. Potent topical corticosteroid in localized disease and low doses systemic corticosteroids in generalized disease: This less aggressive approach may be enough to control the disease and yields less morbidity and mortality.
2. For less extensive disease oral doxycycline may be given instead of systemic steroids alongwith potent topical steroids.
3. Dapsone is specifically indicated when histopathological features predominantly show neutrophils as cellular infiltration.
4. Azathioprine or mycophenolate mofetil can be used as monotherapy or in combination with systemic corticosteroids. Mycophenolate mofetil is much less hepatotoxic than azathioprine.
5. Rituximab may be effective in patients refractory to conventional therapies.

CANDIDIASIS

1. *Topical antifungals:* Topical polyenes or azole antifungals
2. *Systemic antifungals:* Fluconazole or itraconazole
3. Topical antifungals and topical low potent corticosteroids.

> **PRACTICAL HINTS**
> 1. Searching and withdrawal of precipitating factors are very important step along with pharmacological therapy. Relapses and recurrences are almost a rule unless underlying factors are being taken care.
> 2. Topical corticosteroids if used for reducing inflammatory signs and prompt relief should be of lower potency and short term. Patient's counseling is a must before prescribing such combination to prevent overuse or misuse of these products.
> 3. Oral clotrimazole troche can be used for management of oral candidiasis instead of clotrimazole mouth paint where it produces local irritation.
> 4. Assessment of humoral and cell-mediated immune status as well as endocrinal abnormality should be carried out in each case of chronic mucocutaneous candidiasis.
> 5. In chronic mucocutaneous candidiasis if fluconazole or itraconazole is not effective voriconazole or posaconazole may be given.

CELLULITIS/ERYSIPELAS

1. Flucloxacillin
2. Cephalosporins: Cefazolin, ceftriaxone
3. Amoxicillin with clavulanic acid
4. Linezolid
5. Doxycycline
6. Vancomycin
7. Cefepime

> **PRACTICAL HINTS**
> 1. Patients having signs of systemic toxicity, other debilitating diseases like diabetes mellitus or immunocompromised patients should always be treated at indoor with intravenous antibiotics with or without surgery
> 2. Source of infection is to be traced. For example, if this is interdigital tinea at feet, which remains one of the commonest causes of lower leg cellulitis or erysipelas, associated antifungal treatment is mandatory to prevent relapse.
> 3. Patients with chronic eczema, footwear dermatitis, psoriasis or fungal infection of feet should be properly counseled to have adequate control of their disease to prevent cellulitis or erysipelas. They should take special care to avoid immersion of their feet in rain-water and water-logged area. This is especially important when the abovementioned conditions are being treated with topical or systemic corticosteroids or other immunosuppressant agents.
> 4. Red-flag conditions are toxic shock syndrome, necrotizing fasciitis including Fournier's gangrene, clostridial myonecrosis, pyomyositis, deep vein thrombosis and compartment syndrome. These conditions warrant immediate hospitalization and often surgery.
> 5. Specific exposures (from water, soil or recent travel), anatomic sites involvement (periorbital space, neck, over a joint) or pathological sites

(diabetic foot ulcer, pressure ulcer, animal or human bite, puncture wound or surgical wound) needs distinct antibiotic coverage, surgical procedure or specific X-ray or MRI investigations.
6. For regimen covering beta-hemolytic streptococci, methicillin sensitive (MSSA) and resistant (MRSA) in immunocompetent patients oral linezolid, amoxycillin plus doxycycline, or injection vancomycin are more rational. In immunosuppressed conditions initial treatment with injection vancomycin plus cefepime are more justified. For erysipelus oral amoxycillin, cephalexin or parenteral cefazolin can be administered.
7. Duration of antibiotic should be 5 to 6 days rather than longer durations. Extended regimens may be opted for severe or slowly responding cellulitis. Parenteral antibiotics are to be shifted to an oral option once clinical improvement has occurred.
8. Areas of skin breakdown are potential points of entry that should be identified and managed. Common points of entry include intertrigo in the toe webs, tinea pedis, onychomycosis, lower extremity ulcers, atopic dermatitis, and psoriasis.
9. Recurrent infection needs special attention regarding treating points of entry and managing predisposing conditions. Among predisposing conditions patients with lymphedema or venous insufficiency referral to vascular surgeon and compression therapy may be needed.

3. Ciprofloxacin 500 mg twice daily for 3 days
4. Erythromycin 500 mg 3 times daily for 7 days.

Practical Hints
1. Exposed partners must be treated.
2. Single dose treatment is preferable rather than multiple dose regimen.
3. Fluctuant inguinal lymph nodes should be drained, usually by needle aspiration.
4. Associated other STDs especially HIV infection are essential to rule out.
5. If therapy shows no objective improvement after a week few factors may have to be considered: Antibiotic resistance, non-compliance and coinfection with other STDs.
6. In any chancroid case baseline test for syphilis and HIV has been advocated. If these are negative after 3 months the tests should be repeated.
7. In HIV-positive patients, chancroid may present with atypical manifestation or need longer course of treatment. Single dose azithromycin or ceftriaxone are to be given in patients in whom close monitoring would be possible. Some authors have preferred to prescribe 7-day course of erythromycin in HIV patients.
8. The duration of infectivity after initiation of treatment remains uncertain. Chancroid patients should refrain from sex until the ulcer healed completely and must use condom after that. Sex partners of chancroid patients should be treated if they had sexual contact with the patient within 10 days of symptom presentation.

CHANCROID

1. Azithromycin 1 g orally single dose
2. Ceftriaxone 250 mg intramuscularly single dose

CHILBLAINS

1. Nifedipine 20 mg thrice daily for 6 weeks
2. Diltiazem 60 mg thrice daily

3. Pentoxifylline 400 mg thrice daily
4. Topical corticosteroids under occlusions
5. Topical tacrolimus
6. Minoxidil 5% lotion thrice daily application.

> **PRACTICAL HINTS**
> 1. Avoiding cold exposure especially at night and morning and using protective gloves and socks are to be followed by the patients strictly in cold weather.
> 2. Topical minoxidil may help those patients who are intolerant to systemic medicines.
> 3. Usually the ailment persists only during the coldest days.
> 4. Chilblains may mimic chilblain lupus or other peripheral vascular diseases.

CHRONIC ACTINIC DERMATITIS (CAD)

1. Topical corticosteroids
2. Topical tacrolimus
3. Topical pimecrolimus
4. Hydroxychloroquine 200 mg once to twice daily
5. Azathioprine 50 mg thrice daily for 6 to 8 weeks.
6. Oral tofacitinib
7. NB-UVB
8. PUVA

> **PRACTICAL HINTS**
> 1. Proper protective cloths, hat and umbrella as well as frequent sunscreen are must for successful management along with medications.
> 2. To identify photoallergens by photopatch testing may aid much in control of the disease. Common photoallergens are parthenium, para-phenylenediamine, sunscreen (containing oxybenzone), fragrance mix, colophony, etc.
> 3. NB-UVB or PUVA can be given in low dose, initially with oral glucocorticoids to decrease treatment-induced flare.

CONDYLOMA ACUMINATA

1. Initial evaluation for other sexually transmitted infections
2. Patient self-administered podophyllatoxin (0.5%) twice daily for 3 days per week for 4 weeks.
3. Weekly painting of lesions with 25% of podophyllum resin by dermatologist and washing off after 1 hour.
4. Topical imiquimod (5%) applied on and around lesion thrice weekly for a maximum of 16 weeks.
5. Application of trichloroacetic acid by dermatologist especially in cases of pregnant ladies.
6. Topical sinecatechins can be applied by patients thrice daily to external genital and perianal warts until all warts have been cleared (maximum duration = 16 weeks)
7. Liquid nitrogen cryosurgery every 1 to 3 weeks till the lesion clears.
8. Electrosurgery, curettage or carbon dioxide LASER can be used in larger or resistant lesions.
9. Women with genital wart require to undergo periodic papsmear routinely and colposcopy when indicated.
10. Presence of genital ulcer does not mandate cesarean delivery.
11. *HPV vaccine:* A quadrivalent (types 6, 11, 16, 18) and a bivalent (types 16, 18) recombinant vaccine can reduce the incidence of genital wart and cervical cancer significantly if used in time. 9-valent vaccine (types 6, 11, 16, 18, 31, 33, 45, 52, and 58) has also been available.

> **PRACTICAL HINTS**
> 1. A thin petrolatum cover should be applied around wart before podophyllum application. After drying the area should be liberally powdered.
> 2. Podophyllum resin and podophyllotoxin are contraindicated in pregnancy.
> 3. In pregnant patients trichloroacetic acid cautery and cryoablation are only option.
> 4. In immunocompromised persons self treatment with imiquimod is the first line option in localized and small lesions.
> 5. The risk of genital ulcer increases with any amount of smoking. Patients should be counseled that cessation of smoking may impact the resolution of lesion.

CUTANEOUS AMYLOIDOSIS

Macular Amyloidosis

1. Potent topical corticosteroids with or without occlusion
2. UVB NB.

Lichenoid Amyloidosis

1. Potent topical corticosteroids with or without occlusion
2. Topical tacrolimus 0.1% ointment
3. Topical keratolytic agents like salicylic acid or urea
4. Dermabrasion
5. Oral retinoids (acitretin 25 mg daily for 6 months)
6. UVB or PUVA.

Nodular Amyloidosis

1. Intralesional corticosteroids
2. Excision
3. Dermabrasion
4. Laser (CO_2, Nd:YAG, pulsed dye).

> **PRACTICAL HINTS**
> 1. The basic aim of the treatment is to break off the itch-scratch cycle.
> 2. Patients' counseling to be done to avoid precipitating factors like friction, scratching, rubbing, etc.
> 3. Any of the treatment modalities available is neither curative nor uniformly effective.

CUTANEOUS LARVA MIGRANS (CREEPING ERUPTION)

- Oral albendazole 400 mg single dose or daily for 3 to 7 days
- Oral ivermectin 12 mg (200 mcg/kg) single dose.
- Topical thiabendazole 15% in lipophilic vehicle twice daily for 5 days.
- Topical albendazole 10% ointment, prepared by crushing three 400 mg tablets of albendazole in 12 g of petroleum jelly to be applied thrice daily for 10 days
- Antihistamines for control of itching
- Topical corticosteroids for symptomatic relief

> **PRACTICAL HINTS**
> 1. Usually the lesions are self-limited. How- ever, symptoms especially severe pruritus may demand treatment.
> 2. A clinical trial has shown that single dose of ivermectin may be more effective than single dose of albendazole.

3. Albendazole can be safely administered in children.

CUTANEOUS LEISHMANIASIS

First Line Therapies

Oral miltefosine: 2.5 mg/kg (maximum 150 mg) orally in three divided doses for 28 days (for weight 30–40 kg: 50 mg orally twice daily)

Pentavalent Antimonials

- *Meglumine antimoniate:* Intralesionally with local anesthetic or systemically 10 mg/kg daily for 2 weeks
- *Sodium stibogluconate:* Intralesionally 1 to 2 mL weekly or 10 mg/kg IM/IV daily for 2 weeks.

Second Line Therapies

- Liposomal amphotericin B
- Allopurinol plus low dose meglumine antimoniate
- Azoles (itraconazole, ketoconazole, fluconazole)
- Topical paromomycin cream
- Cryotherapy.

> **PRACTICAL HINTS**
> 1. Oral miltefosine has reasonable efficacy against many New World cutaneous leishmaniasis (CL) species. Regarding use of miltefosine for Old World CL data are limited but it appears to have some efficacy.
> 2. Toxicity of sodium stibogluconate is common and dose-related.
> 3. *Leishmania recidivans* needs higher doses of antimonials for longer period.
> 4. Cutaneous leishmaniasis may heal spontaneously sometimes but may leave scar. To minimize scar therapy should be offered.

DARIER'S DISEASE

1. Keratolytic emollients
2. Antiseptic cleansers
3. Sunscreen
4. Thin clothes
5. Intermittent antibiotics and antifungals
6. Mid-potent topical corticosteroids
7. Topical calcineurin inhibitors
8. Topical retinoids
9. *Oral retinoids:* Isotretinoin or acitretin (0.5 mg/kg/day as starting dose), alitretinoin (10–30 mg/daily).
10. Surgery.

> **PRACTICAL HINTS**
> 1. In acute flare topical corticosteroids are preferable rather than topical calcineurin inhibitors
> 2. Irritation due to topical retinoids can be minimized by frequent use of emollients, short duration of use of topical retinoids and combination of topical corticosteroids with retinoids.
> 3. Systemic retinoids are to be considered only in refractory cases not responding to topical therapy due to their adverse effects and relapse after their withdrawal.
> 4. Systemic retinoids are contraindicated in patients with major features of bullous lesions or intertriginous involvement where these can cause flare up. Maintenance dose of systemic retinoids may be alternate day or even alternate week.

DECUBITUS ULCER

1. Removal of pressure
2. Frequent change of position
3. Air-fluidized or liquid-filled bed
4. Wound dressings without trauma
5. Debridement of necrotic debris

6. Wound swab for bacterial culture and sensitivity
7. Moist dressing
8. Nutritional assessment and care
9. Topical antibacterials
10. Hydrocolloid dressing
11. *Stage IV ulcer:* Surgical intervention.

> **PRACTICAL HINTS**
> 1. Wound cleaning should preferably be done with sterile normal saline rather than corrosive agents like hydrogen peroxide or povidone-iodine.
> 2. Skin surrounding the ulcer would not be dried to prevent maceration.
> 3. Dermatitis around the decubitus ulcer may be treated with moisturizer preferably without fragrances, paraben and lanolin.

DERMATITIS HERPETIFORMIS

- Gluten-free diet
- Dapsone
- Tetracycline and nicotinamide
- Colchicine
- Sulfapyridine (0.5 g/thrice daily per day at onset/may be increased upto 6 g/day)
- Sulfasalazine (1–2 g/day)
- Systemic corticosteroids
- Topical corticosteroids.

> **PRACTICAL HINTS**
> 1. Maintenance of strict gluten-free diet along with dapsone may help in adequate control over the symptoms. Dose of dapsone may also be minimized by this combination. Patients with granular IgA deposits may even respond only with gluten-free diet without dapsone.
> 2. Starting dose of dapsone are to be kept between 25 to 50 mg in adults and 0.5 mg/kg in children to reduce the side effects of dapsone. Usual maintenance dose in adult is 100 mg daily. Dose to be monitored in such a way that one or two lesions per week can be accepted. Unnecessary high dose may induce toxicities.
> 3. Colchicine may be tried in patients in whom dapsone causes adverse effects.

DERMATOMYOSITIS (DM)

Cutaneous Involvement

1. Sunscreen (high SPF with UVA protective agents)
2. Topical corticosteroids
3. Topical tacrolimus or pimecrolimus
4. Hydroxychloroquine or chloroquine
5. Methotrexate (low dose: 5–15 mg weekly)
6. Mycophenolate mofetil (1 g twice daily).

Systemic Involvement

1. Systemic corticosteroids (1 mg/kg gradually tapered to half dose over 6 months and very slowly reduced to stop totally after 2 to 3 years; may be given on alternate days or as pulse)
2. Methotrexate (15 mg/m² weekly)
3. Azathioprine (2–3 mg/kg/day)
4. Mycophenolate mofetil (1 g twice daily)
5. Intravenous immune globulin (2 g/kg body weight monthly infusion for 3 months with systemic steroids)

> **PRACTICAL HINTS**
> 1. Cutaneous DM may improve during treatment of other manifestations of DM, e.g., myositis. Systemic treatment particularly for cutaneous ailment are required when active skin lesions persist inspite of control of other manifestations.

2. In mild cutaneous DM (< 10% body surface area involvement, tolerable pruritus, and nondisabling) hydroxychloroquine rather than methotrexate would be preferred as initial therapy.
3. In severe cutaneous DM (> 10% body surface area involvement, intolerable pruritus, and otherwise disabling) methotrexate rather than hydroxychloroquine would be preferred as initial therapy. Methotrexate and hydroxychloroquine may be started simultaneously or hydroxychloroquine may subsequently be added later on if there is inadequate response to methotrexate.

DIAPER DERMATITIS

1. Frequent change of diaper
2. Air exposure for a few hours per day
3. Disposable absorbent diapers
4. Barrier creams (e.g., petrolatum jelly, zinc oxide creams)
5. Topical antifungal (azole) for *Candida* superinfection
6. Topical hydrocortisone 1%.

> **PRACTICAL HINTS**
> 1. Cleansing of the skin should be done very gently with water or soap-free cleansers preferably alcohol-free and fragrance-free. Soap may damage barrier layer of the skin.
> 2. Any topical preparations containing fragnance, preservatives (paraben) and lanolin should be avoided.
> 3. Products containing boric acid, camphor, phenol, benzocaine and salicylates should be avoided for risk of systemic toxicity.
> 4. Topical steroids if used should be confined only to refractory cases not responding to conventional treatment. This should be of lowest potency and of very short-term.
> 5. Occlusive plastic pants and topical corticosteroids may induce granuloma gluteale infantum as a complication of diaper dermatitis.

DISCOID ECZEMA (NUMMULAR ECZEMA)

1. Decrease exposure to irritants like soap, over the counter moisturizer, etc. Infrequent washing by mild bar type soap or soap-free cleanser is recommended.
2. Dryness must be controlled by proper bath and moisturizer application.
3. Acute lesions are treated by wet dressing till dryness. Then discontinue to avoid excessive dryness.
4. Topical application of class 2 to 4 corticosteroid is mainstay of therapy.
5. Tar preparations may be used alone or in combination with topical steroid.
6. Calcineurin inhibitors (tacrolimus and pimecrolimus) are also useful.
7. Secondary infection should be treated with systemic anti-staphylococcal antibiotics.
8. Sedative oral antihistaminic reduces itch.
9. In widespread disease, systemic corticosteroids may be considered for a short period. Flare after drug withdrawal is expected.
10. UVB (both broadband and narrowband) is useful in extensive disease. In resistant cases PUVA can be given.

> **PRACTICAL HINTS**
> 1. Patch testing should be considered in refractory cases to exclude allergic contact dermatitis and systemic contact dermatitis.
> 2. Active tinea pedis lesion should be searched to exclude id reaction.

DISCOID LUPUS ERYTHEMATOSUS (DLE)

1. Broad spectrum sunscreen
2. Topical or intralesional corticosteroids
3. Topical tacrolimus or pimecrolimus
4. Chloroquine or hydroxychloroquine
5. Methotrexate
6. Systemic retinoids
7. Mycophenolate mofetil
8. Clofazimine (100 mg thrice in a week to daily)
9. Dapsone (25 to 150 mg daily).
10. Thalidomide

> **PRACTICAL HINTS**
>
> 1. No difference has been evidenced in efficacy as well as toxicity between chloroquine and hydroxychloroquine.
> 2. Patients not responding to hydroxy-chloroquine may be tried with methotrexate.
> 3. Systemic retinoids like isotretinoin or acitretin may also be useful in patients with intolerance to antimalarials. These retinoids are especially effective in hyper- trophic variety of DLE.
> 4. Dapsone may have a specific role in bullous lupus erythematosus.

DRUG ERUPTION

1. The first step in any cutaneous adverse drug reaction is to confirm the diagnosis and identify the implicated agent. These may not be possible in many cases because coexistence of viral exanthem, course of multiple drugs and in Indian perspective random availability of non-prescription medicine.
2. The second step is assessment of severity. The presence of following indicate severe drug reaction:
   - Fever, malaise, cough, arthralgia.
   - Erythroderma, facial edema, purpura, skin tenderness and mucosal involvement and lymphadenopathy.
3. The third step is to take decision whether to withdraw or continue with the drug. This is done on a case-to-case basis depending upon the severity of reaction, importance of the implicated medication and presence of alternative.
4. The fourth step is general care of the patient which is according to the clinical presentation.
5. The fifth step is symptomatic management. This is done with systemic antihistamines, topical corticosteroid, topical calamine and/or moisturizer. Exception is acneiform drug eruption where topical tretinoin is used.
6. Systemic steroid is used in severe drug eruption except in SJS-TEN (see below). The initial dose is 0.5–2 mg/kg prednisolone per day. The duration is dependent upon the reaction pattern and is usually longer in drug hypersensitivity syndrome.
7. The next step is prevention of future reaction. Counseling the patient and providing with a probable drug list is essential. As SJS-TEN or drug hypersensitivity syndrome may run in families, a prior personal and family history is essential to reduce incidence of drug reaction.
8. The final step is reporting the reaction to authority.

> **PRACTICAL HINTS**
>
> 1. Even drug taken before many times may produce allergy suddenly. We have to consider drug and viral interaction in such cases where a drug normally not inducing allergy in a subject may create allergy in prodormal or active phase of a viral infection. Classical

example is ampicillin producing eruption in infectious mononucleosis patients.
2. A maculopapular drug eruption can later be turning into a full-blown SJS/TEN or drug hypersensitivity syndrome in certain cases. Cutaneous features like skin tenderness, positive Nikolsky's sign or systemic signs like fever, arthralgia, blood eosinophilia may give some clue.

ERYTHEMA MULTIFORME (EM)

1. Acyclovir 400 mg twice daily before food for 6 months to 2 years in recurrent EM.
2. Oral valacyclovir 500 mg daily or famciclovir 250 mg twice daily (where inadequate response to oral acyclovir)
3. Topical corticosteroids in adhesive base for oral EM
4. Clotrimazole troche or mouth paint and if required oral fluconazole in oral EM to combat secondary candidiasis.
5. For patients with severe, recurrent HSV-associated or idiopathic EM who are refractory to continuous systemic antiviral therapy and where other causes have been ruled out, mycophenolate mofetil, dapsone or azathioprine have been advocated.

Practical Hints

1. Oral acyclovir is not only effective in preventing recurrent herpes-associated EM but also in EM where erythema multiforme not directly provoked by herpes.
2. Systemic corticosteroids has only very limited role in acute attacks of EM where these can shorten the fever duration. This regimen, however, can induce side effects and remains controversial.

ERYTHEMA NODOSUM

1. Bed rest with leg elevation
2. To treat underlying diseases (especially infectious ones)
3. To withdraw provoking drugs, if any
4. NSAIDs (indomethacin 25 mg thrice daily or naproxen 250 mg twice daily for 1 month)
5. Potassium iodide (Saturated solution of potassium iodide or SSKI)
6. Colchicine (2 mg daily for 3 days, then 1 mg daily for 2 to 4 weeks)
7. Hydroxychloroquine (200 mg twice daily for 3 months).
8. Dapsone (50 to 100 mg daily)
9. Short course of systemic steroids

Practical Hints

1. NSAIDs can be used as first-line therapy. Potassium iodide may be reserved for patients requiring rapid resolution.
2. SSKI may be started as 5 drops thrice daily in orange juice to make it more palatable. This dose may be increased by one drop per dose per day until clinical remission is obtained. Side effects from SSKI should be monitored.
3. Patients are to be properly counseled for not to be satisfied only with symptomatic relief. They should fully cooperate with the doctors to search and remove the cause if playing any underlying role.
4. For patients who fail to respond to NSAIDs and SSKI or who have severe debilitating symptoms a short course of systemic glucocorticoids can be attempted.
5. Colchicine may be effective in erythema nodosum associated with Behçet's disease.

6. For recalcitrant, chronic, or recurring erythema nodosum colchicine, hydroxychloroquine or dapsone can be prescribed.

ERYTHRASMA

1. Topical benzoyl peroxide 2.5% gel daily after shower for 7 days
2. Topical erythromycin or clindamycin twice daily for 7 days
3. Sodium fusidic acid 2% twice daily for 2 weeks
4. Erythromycin 250 mg 4 times daily for 7 days (in extensive/refractory case).
5. Clarithromycin 500 mg twice daily for 7 days (in extensive/refractory case).

> **PRACTICAL HINT**
> Prevention of erythrasma may be done with regular use of benzoyl peroxide wash. Medicated powder containing clotrimazole or miconazole may also be used.

ERYTHRODERMA (EXFOLIATIVE DERMATITIS SYNDROME)

General Measures

1. Hospitalization
2. Single room for the patient
3. Control of room temperature (usually warm humid room with many blanket)
4. Monitoring body temperature
5. Monitoring of fluid intake and output and renal function
6. Electrolyte balance
7. To assess and manage of oral mucosa, eyes and genitourinary tract
8. To watch for signs of cardiac failure
9. Protein-fortified diet (approx 130% of normal balanced diet protein)
10. Folate supplementation
11. Bland emollients
12. To avoid irritating topical agents like tar, anthralin, etc.
13. To avoid salicylic acid to avoid salicylism through increased absorption.
14. Systemic antibiotics (to treat cutaneous superinfection)
15. Oral antihistamines.

Specific Measures

1. Work-up to search underlying diseases or precipitating drugs
2. Topical corticosteroids
3. Systemic corticosteroids (only in idiopathic and drug-induced variant. Starting dose prednisolone 0.5 to 1 mg/kg/day for 7 to 10 days)
4. Cyclosporine (in refractory psoriasis and atopic dermatitis)
5. UVA1 phototherapy.

> **PRACTICAL HINTS**
> 1. In erythroderma systemic absorption may be increased up to 20 percent of the topical agents. Hence choice of topical cortico- steroids would be of mild-to-moderate potency.
> 2. Clinicians can consider systemic antibiotics in all cases as staphylococcal colonization may aggravate erythroderma and patients are sometimes at the risk of fatal staphylococcal septicemia.
> 3. In neonates and children having erythroderma monitoring fluid and electrolyte balance is of prime importance to avoid hypernatremic dehydration.
> 4. For idiopathic erythroderma not responding to topical therapy systemic corticosteroids rather than other immunosuppressant would be better

choice. After 7–10 days prednisolone to be slowly tapered over several weeks to avoid rebound while introducing other immunosuppressive therapy like cyclosporin or methotreaxate.
5. Cyclosporine may be the initial choice in refractory cases if systemic corticosteroids are otherwise contraindicated.

FURUNCULOSIS

1. *Topical antibiotics:* Mupirocin, fusidic acid, ozenoxacin, retapamulin
2. *Systemic antibiotics:* Flucloxacillin, clindamycin (low dose: 150 mg 4 times daily or 300 mg twice daily for 7 to 14 days), fluoroquinolones, linezolid
3. Parenteral antibiotics: In cases with signs of systemic toxicity, rapidly progressive or extensive erythema or inability to absorb oral therapy and in immunosuppressed patients
4. *Surgery:* Incision and drainage.

Recurrent Furunculosis

1. Bacterial culture and sensitivity from the fresh lesion.
2. Rifampicin 600 mg daily for 7 to 10 days along with semisynthetic penicillin, cephalosporin, minocycline, or ciprofloxacin
3. Mupirocin cream or ointment to apply twice daily to the anterior nares for a week. This procedure can be repeated every month at a fixed week for 3 months
4. Antiseptic soaps.

> **PRACTICAL HINTS**
> 1. Recurrent furunculosis throws special challenge. Treatment of family members may be required.

2. Chronic folliculitis of moist area especially of the buttocks may be treated with 6.25% aluminium chloride hexahydrate in absolute ethyl alcohol once daily at bedtime for direct antibacterial as well as antiperspirant effect.

GONORRHEA

Uncomplicated Infection (Urethral, Cervical, Rectal)

1. Ceftriaxone 500 mg IM single dose

Alternative Regimens

2. Cefpodoxime 400 mg orally single dose
3. Ciprofloxacin 500 mg orally single dose
4. Cefixime 400 mg orally single dose.

Pregnant Women

1. Ceftriaxone 125 mg IM single dose
2. Spectinomycin 2.0 g IM single dose (if cannot receive ceftriaxone).

Cotreatment for *Chlamydia*

1. Doxycycline 100 mg twice daily for 7 days
2. Azithromycin 1 g orally single dose
3. Erythromycin 500 mg 4 times daily for 7 days

> **PRACTICAL HINTS**
> 1. Higher dose doses of ceftriaxone are to be used because of decreased susceptibility.
> 2. Alternative regimen have very limited role except in the cases of ceftriaxone allergy or unavailability.
> 3. All patients with gonorrhea should be monitored 3 to 4 months after the treatment to exclude repeat infection.

> 4. Cotreatment for *Chlamydia* is a must in each case of gonorrhea unless *C. trachomatis* infection has been excluded otherwise.
> 5. Treatment of sex partners is essential for preventing reinfection and controlling the spread of infection.

GRANULOMA INGUINALE

1. Azithromycin 500 mg orally daily for 7 days or 1 g orally weekly for 4 weeks
2. Erythromycin 500 mg orally 4 times daily for minimum 3 weeks
3. Trimethoprim-sulfamethoxazole double strength 1 tab twice daily for minimum 3 weeks
4. Doxycycline 100 mg orally twice daily for minimum 3 weeks
5. Ciprofloxacin 750 mg orally twice daily for minimum 3 weeks.

> **PRACTICAL HINTS**
> 1. The therapy should be continued until all the lesions healed completely. However, azithromycin should not be continued beyond 4 weeks.
> 2. Surgical intervention may be required in refractory and extensive cases where medical management has failed.
> 3. In spite of adequate treatment relapse can take place after 6 to 18 months.

HERPES SIMPLEX (INCLUDING HERPES GENITALIS)

1. Oral acyclovir
2. Oral valacyclovir
3. Oral famciclovir
4. Foscarnet (40 mg/kg once to thrice daily for acyclovir-resistant HSV usually in AIDS)
5. Cidofovir (topical 0.3 or 1% gel for acyclovir-resistant HSV usually in AIDS)

> **PRACTICAL HINTS**
> 1. *Dose:* Primary and recurrent cutaneous or genital infection: Acyclovir 200 mg 5 times daily for 5 days; Valacyclovir 500 mg twice daily for 5 days; Famciclovir 250 mg twice daily for 5 days.
> 2. Suppressive therapy for recurrent herpes (more than 6 to 10 episodes per year): Acyclovir 400 mg twice daily, valacyclovir 1 g daily, famciclovir 250 mg twice daily for up to 1 year.
> 3. Oral valacyclovir are preferable as dose frequency is less and all three drugs are almost similar in efficacy and safety profile.
> 4. There is no role for topical antiviral therapy and there does not appear to be any advantage of adding topical therapy to oral agent.

HERPES ZOSTER

1. Acyclovir 800 mg 5 times daily for 7 to 10 days
2. Famciclovir 500 mg thrice daily for 7 days
3. Valacyclovir 1 g thrice daily for 7 days
4. IV acyclovir (10 mg/kg every eight hourly) in immunocompromised patients.
5. Foscarnet 40 mg/kg every 8 to 12 hourly for 7 to 10 days in patients with suspected acyclovir-resistant herpes zoster
6. Amitriptyline 75 to 100 mg daily for postherpetic neuralgia
7. Nortriptyline 50 to 100 mg daily for postherpetic neuralgia (to start with 10 to 20 mg daily)
8. Gabapentin for postherpetic neuralgia (300 mg daily as starting dose; may be increased over 4 weeks up to 3,600 mg/day in divided dose until therapeutic result is obtained or intolerable adverse effects set in).

9. Herpes zoster vaccine: For all above 50 years old—recombinant (glycoprotein E) zoster vaccine intramuscularly one dose followed by second dose after 2 to 6 months.

> **PRACTICAL HINTS**
> 1. As varicella zoster virus shows less therapeutic response to antivirals their dose should be much higher as compared to herpes simplex virus. Clinicians should counsel the patients to take adequate dose of the drugs for proper benefit.
> 2. Systemic corticosteroids with acyclovir compared with acyclovir alone in a randomized placebo-controlled study did not show any superiority of steroids combination in reduction of postherpetic neuralgia.
> 3. Low dose of amitriptyline or nortriptyline (10 to 20 mg at night) started at the time of diagnosis of herpes zoster as preventing measure along with antivirals may be helpful in reducing postherpetic neuralgia in the high-risk group (over the age of 60 years).
> 4. For pregnant patients oral acyclovir is preferable as there is most experience with this medication in pregnancy with extensive safety reports.

HIDRADENITIS SUPPURATIVA

1. Topical clindamycin for 3 months
2. Systemic tetracycline 250 to 500 mg 4 times daily until lesions resolve
3. Erythromycin 250 to 500 mg 4 times daily until lesions resolve
4. Doxycycline 100 mg twice daily until lesions resolve
5. Minocycline 100 mg twice daily until lesions resolve
6. Intralesional triamcinolone 3 to 5 mg/mL into the painful nodules
7. Prednisolone 60 to 80 mg/day for 2 to 3 days tapered over 14 days may improve severe pain and inflammation dramatically. After stopping usually there occurs flare
8. Oral isotretinoin not effective in established severe disease. In early disease, this may help to prevent follicular occlusion
9. Cyproterone acetate may be effective only in high doses, which may yield adverse effects. Combination of cyproterone acetate plus ethinyl estradiol (30 µg/day for 21 days) may be more useful than any of these two single drugs
10. Spironolactone
11. Metformin
12. Adalimumab: Where atleast one oral antibiotic fails
13. Secukinumab and infliximab: Alternatives to adalimumab
14. *Surgery:* In acute abscess, recurrent painful nodules and sinus tract, extensive involvement.

> **PRACTICAL HINTS**
> 1. Weight reduction, wearing loose clothes, avoiding friction and moisture accumulation on the skin, use of antibacterial soaps and topical aluminium chloride may be useful adjuvant methods which can be added with the medical therapy.
> 2. Monthly 5-day course of intranasal mupirocin may be used to eradicate nasal carrier of *S. aureus*.

HIRSUTISM

1. Initial assessment must include a scoring in modified Ferriman and Gallwey scale. Associated feature of androgen excess like thinning of hair or pustular acne should be looked for.
2. Evaluation for presence of hyperandrogenism should follow. If present source of the excess androgen is sought.

3. The treatment modality has three parts:
   i. Physical/chemical
   ii. Pharmacological.
   iii. Bleaching
4. The physical/chemical part is essential for all. It targets the present terminal hair. It should be used alone or in combination with pharmacological therapy. Modalities of physical/chemical therapy includes:
   i. *Depilatory process:* Hair is removed at skin surface. Follicle remains intact. Popular methods are:
      - *Shaving*: Cheap and safe. Does not change rate and density of hair growth. Socially unacceptable.
      - *Depilatory creams (hair removing cream)*: Malodorous and potentially irritant. Less chance of both with thioglycollate containing creams, but they are more time consuming.
   ii. *Epilatory process:* Hair is removed at follicle level. Procedures include:
      - *Plucking:* Painful. May give rise to folliculitis and postinflammatory hyperpigmentation in Indian skin.
      - *Waxing:* It is a widespread plucking with all its disadvantages.
      - *Electrolysis and electrothermolysis (using radiofrequency):* Done under topical anesthesia (EMLA). Skin type and hair color are not a concern. Successful for white hair as well. Scarring may occur. Pretreatment with tretinoin cream reduce healing time.
      - *Laser:* Different lasers are efficient in removing pigmented hair only. White hairs are resistant. In Indian skin longer wavelength lasers like Nd:YAG laser is safe. Safety of other laser or IPL is less in type V and VI skin. Side effects include thermal burn, postinflammatory hyper-pigmentation and scarring. Single session reduces 10–20% of existing hair making multiple sessions necessary.
5. *Pharmacological therapy*: Essential in hirsutism with androgen excess but also effective in idiopathic hirsutism with normal androgen level. Usually ineffective on existing hair. Visible effect is seen in 6–12 months. Available agents marginally differ in efficacy. Choice of agent depends on patient profile, associated disease or need of patient and experience of clinician with that particular agent. Available therapies are:
   - *Oral contraceptive pill:* The selection of the progestin component is important. Drospirenone is the preferred agent. Initial evaluation should concentrate on OCP side effect like DVT.
   - *Cyproterone acetate:* Available in combination with ethinyl estradiol in India. High estrogen content increases the chance for DVT and weight gain.
   - *Spironolactone*: Used in 100–200 mg/day, it is effective but associated with menstrual irregularity. Combined use with OCP offers good menstrual control and offers protection from pregnancy (spironolactone in pregnancy cause feminization of male fetus).
   - *Finasteride*: Used in 2.5–5 mg daily dose (with OCP in female of child-bearing age group to prevent feminization of male fetus).
   - *Metformin*: Particularly useful in PCOS and other form of insulin resistance.
   - *Bromocriptine:* Useful in hyperpro-lactinemia.
   - *Systemic corticosteroid*: Prednisolone (5–10 mg) or dexamethasone (0.2–0.5 mg) taken at bedtime is useful in hirsutism with congenital adrenal hyperplasia.

- Eflornithine hydrochloride 13.9% cream applied twice daily is effective in 8 weeks. They act by blocking ornithine decarboxylase. Result is temporary. Regrowth seen within 8 weeks of drug withdrawal. Should be combined with other mode. May cause irritation.
6. Bleaching: 6% hydrogen peroxide bleach makes hair less visible.
7. Weight reduction is an essential component to reduce circulatory androgen level.

> **PRACTICAL HINTS**
> 1. Drug history to be taken to rule out drug-induced hirsutism.
> 2. Cut off value of modified Ferriman and Gallwey scale in Indian skin is not delineated.

HYPERHIDROSIS

1. Treatment modality is to be decided on severity of disease and occupation of the patient.
2. General measures like frequent wash with deodorant soap, changing socks daily, wearing cotton socks and leather shoes without rubber or leather soles should be stressed.
3. Palmoplantar and axillary hyperhidrosis is treated with 20% aluminium chloride hexahydrate in absolute alcohol. Initially applied high time with or without occlusion every night till desired reduction in sweating achieved. Then once weekly maintenance regimen is followed. Local irritation is important adverse effect.
4. Tap water iontophoresis for 15–30 minutes daily and then 2–3 times weekly is effective. Direct current is more effective though less tolerated. Addition of glycopyrrolate solution potentiates effect but may be associated with systemic absorption.
5. Local injection of botulinum toxin A placed 1–2 cm apart in a checkerboard pattern to deliver the drug in superficial dermis is the most effective treatment. A single session effect lasts for 6–9 months.
6. Sympathectomy and sympathotomy may offer benefit in severe and recalcitrant cases. Nowadays endoscopic method is preferred.
7. Topical glycopyrronium: Alternative initial treatment of axillary hyperhidrosis.
8. Liposuction and curettage of sweat gland can be done in axillary hyperhidrosis.
9. Systemic anticholinergic drugs are effective but seldom tolerated.
10. Sedatives are sometime helpful.
11. Relaxation techniques like biofeedback training may reduce sweating.

> **PRACTICAL HINTS**
> 1. Secondary causes of hyperhidrosis are to be ruled out before initiating therapy.
> 2. Aluminium chloride hexahydrate should be applied on dry skin to reduce irritation. Morning application of 1% hydrocortisone cream may be considered.

ICHTHYOSIS

1. Skin hydration is maintained with adequate bath or soak and immediate application of moisturizer. Drying agents are discouraged.
2. Mild keratolytics like α-hydroxy acids (lactic acid, glycolic acid), β-hydroxy acid (salicylic acid) and urea help in scale removal.
3. Propylene glycol (40–60% in water) with or without occlusion helps in scale removal.
4. Topical retinoids or vitamin D3 analogues though effective is poorly tolerated. Tazarotene, the most potent topical retinoids may be used very judiciously.
5. Systemic retinoids like acitretin or isotretinoin are indicated in severely

affected patients like lamellar ichthyosis, congenital ichthyosiform erythroderma.
6. In epidermolytic hyperkeratosis anti-staphylococcal agents (topical or systemic) are required to reduce bacterial infection.
7. Nutritional supplementation is required in severe variety of congenital ichthyosis to prevent growth failure.
8. Proper eye and lip care should be undertaken. Opinion from ophthalmologist is essential in ectropion seen in lamellar ichthyosis.

> **PRACTICAL HINTS**
> 1. Acquired ichthyosis should be thoroughly evaluated to find out the cause.
> 2. Due to lack of barrier function drug absorption from skin surface is enhanced increasing toxicity of topically applied salicylic acid, corticosteroid, calcineurin inhibitors, etc. Children are more vulnerable.
> 3. Systemic retinoids can increase blistering in epidermolytic hyperkeratosis. Starting dose should be low.
> 4. Fungal infection is common in ichthyotic disease. Localized itching or change of scale pattern is suggestive.

IMPETIGO

1. Wet-dressing with burrow's solution or potassium permanganate can reduce oozing and removes crust.
2. In limited disease, topical antibiotic like mupirocin or fusudic acid is sufficient.
3. More extensive lesion requires systemic antibiotic therapy.
4. Antibiotic is chosen with compatibility to age, sex and the demographic sensitivity profile.
5. Most clinicians prefer dicloxacillin or 1st generation cephalosporins.
6. In penicillin sensitive patients macrolides may be used though emerging resistance pattern restrict their use.
7. Clindamycin is a suitable alternative.
8. In recurrent diseases colonization (particularly nasal) should be eliminated by application of 2% mupirocin ointment.
9. Weight reduction, frequent bath with antibacterial soaps, change of clothing and maintenance of personal hygiene is recommended.
10. In resistant cases, oral rifampicin can be used.
11. Predisposing factors like diabetes mellitus and HIV in suspected cases should be investigated.

> **PRACTICAL HINT**
> Recurrent impetigo may be a manifestation of undiagnosed scabies or insect bite hypersensitivity. Treat the primary cause.

INFANTILE HEMANGIOMAS (IH)

1. Topical beta blockers (topical propanolone, topical timolol, topical carteolol)
2. Oral propanolone (1 mg/kg/day; may be increased to target dose of 2–3 mg/kg/day)
3. Systemic corticosteroids (3 to 5 mg/kg daily for 6 to 12 weeks): Alternative agents for patients with contraindications for betablocker.
4. Sirolimus
5. Laser (continuous wave or pulsed dye)
6. Surgical excision.

> **PRACTICAL HINTS**
> 1. Each case should be assessed individually.
> 2. Decision should be taken considering all factors: To treat or not to treat
> 3. For majority lesions active nonintervention may be the rational approach

as spontaneous resolved hemangioma may yield best cosmetic result.
4. Active intervention may be required in:
   (a) ulcerated IH (b) IH obstructing vital structures like eyes, ears, larynx, etc., and (c) life-threatening IH.

INSECT BITE HYPERSENSITIVITY

1. Avoidance of insect contact is essential.
2. Use of dress cover, mosquito net and insect repellants should be advised according to patient profile.
3. Existing lesion can be treated with class 3 or 4 topical corticosteroid.
4. Secondary pyodermas are treated with topical or systemic antibiotic.
5. In pediatric patient, parent counseling about the self-resolving nature of the disease is important to alleviate anxiety.

Practical Hints
1. Atopic persons may have this disease for indefinite duration.
2. Change of place may bring out fresh lesion in predisposed individual.
3. Cancer patient under chemo/radiotherapy may develop insect bite hypersensitivity without change of place.

KELOID

1. Treatment modality is decided according to:
   i. Location and size of lesion.
   ii. Experience of the clinician with particular therapeutic option.
   iii. Patient profile.
   iv. Cost of therapy.
2. Intralesional triamcinolone remains the primary mode with dermatologists because most patients have smaller lesion without functional impairment.
3. Cryotherapy immediate prior intralesional injection reduces toughness of keloid and makes injection easier.
4. Mixing triamcinolone with lignocaine reduces pain.
5. Initial concentration of triamcinolone is kept high (40 mg/mL). Later lower concentration (2–5 mg/mL) is chosen to avoid unnecessary atrophy.
6. Role of silicone gel is controversial. It can be chosen as a modality after consulting the patient.
7. Cryotherapy alone is effective in smaller and newer lesion. Associated depigmentation restricts use in Indian skin. Combination with intralesional triamcinolone is helpful (see 3).
8. Surgical excision is helpful in removing larger and functionally impairing keloid.
9. To prevent recurrence excision is combined with skin grafting and pressure dressing of donor and recipient site along with any one of the following
   i. Radiotherapy.
   ii. Intralesional corticosteroid or interferon-α
   iii. Topical imiquimod.
10. Laser (carbon-dioxide, Nd:YAG) therapy in keloid is associated with high recurrence rate and not recommended routinely. Pulse dye Laser is claimed to be successful in trials; clinical application is not delineated.
11. In predisposed patients keloid formation can be reduced by:
    i. Avoid unnecessary surgery.
    ii. When essential prior radiotherapy of the proposed surgical site may be considered.

iii. Clean cut scalpel surgery is preferred over electrosurgery.
iv. Wound closure should take place without tension.
v. Infection rate to be kept at minimum.
vi. Pressure dressing is mandatory.

> **PRACTICAL HINTS**
> 1. Patient expectation should be addressed before initiating therapy.
> 2. Photographic documentation is mandatory.
> 3. Use of intralesional 5-FU, bleomycin, etc., is better left for person conversant with individual agent.
> 4. Topical retinoic acid and UVA1 may be used in selected cases.

KERATOSIS PILARIS (KP)

1. Keratosis pilaris is mostly a cosmetic concern.
2. Comorbidity like atopic dermatitis, ichthyosis vulgaris or nutritional deficiencies should be sought and treated.
3. Majority improves by adulthood.
4. Aggravating factors like tight fitting clothes, abrasive scrubs are to be avoided.
5. Use of moisturizer on regular basis reduces the dryness and inflammation.
6. Topical tretinoin or adapalene imparts temporary and partial improvement. Irritation may be a limiting factor.
7. Application of 12% ammonium lactate cream/lotion twice daily improves roughness.
8. Low potent topical steroid may be used to reduce associated inflammation. Long-term use is not recommended.

> **PRACTICAL HINT**
> Inflammatory KP may be confused with acne vulgaris. Absence of comedone and associated xerosis clinches diagnosis.

LEG ULCERS

Venous Ulcer

1. Leg elevation
2. Compression stockings
3. Local wound care
4. Dressings
5. Debridement (autolytic, chemical and/or mechanical)
6. Wound swab for culture and sensitivity
7. Antimicrobial treatment (topical and/or systemic)
8. Management of surrounding stasis dermatitis, if any
9. Referral to vascular surgeon
10. Surgery.

Arterial Ulcer

1. To stop smoking, if present
2. Low cholesterol diet
3. To control hypertension, DM, hyperlipidemia
4. Lipid-lowering agents
5. Anti-platelet agents (aspirin or clopidogrel)
6. Cilostazol, an inhibitor of phosphodiesterase III
7. Exercise to develop collateral circulation
8. Elevation of head of the bed by 4 to 6 inches
9. Local wound management
10. To keep the legs warm
11. Hyperbaric oxygen.

> **PRACTICAL HINTS**
> 1. Compression for venous ulcer to be done only in the absence of associated arterial diseases.
> 2. Clopidogrel has been approved by FDA for arterial leg ulcer and is more effective than aspirin
> 3. Topical preparations are to be used with utmost care in and around any leg ulcer as there is high chance of contact sensitization at this place.

LEPROSY AND ITS REACTION

Paucibacillary

1. Dapsone 100 mg daily
2. Rifampicin 600 mg monthly once (supervised).
3. For 6 months

Multibacillary

1. Dapsone 100 mg daily
2. Clofazimine 50 mg daily
3. Rifampicin 600 mg and clofazimine 300 mg one monthly (supervised).
4. For 12 months

Second Line of Drugs

1. Minocycline 100 mg daily
2. Ofloxacin 400 mg daily
3. Levofloxacin 500 mg daily once or twice
4. Clarithromycin 500 mg twice daily.

Reactions

Mild Type 1 Reversal Reaction (RR) or ENL
NSAIDs (ibuprofen or aspirin)

Severe RR

Prednisone 0.5 to 1.0 mg/kg once to twice daily to start immediately and to continue for 3 to 6 months, then to be slowly tapered.

Severe RR or ENL

Clofazimine 100 mg thrice daily for 6 weeks and then reduced to 100 mg daily for several months.

Severe ENL

- Thalidomide 100 mg at night; may be increased up to 400 mg daily
- Prednisolone 0.5 to 1.0 mg/kg daily

> **PRACTICAL HINTS**
> 1. Close follow-up of the patients are to be done who have completed antileprosy treatment.
> 2. Downgrading reactions are to be treated with antileprosy drugs only.

LUPUS ERYTHEMATOSUS (LE): SPECIFIC SKIN LESION

Management of LE specific skin lesion is primarily a dermatologist's job. Systemic involvement is managed by an internist/rheumatologist.

Following measures are to be taken in a step-ladder pattern:

1. *Photoprotection:*
   a. *Physical photoprotective measures:*
      i. Outdoor activities to be restricted before 10 AM and after 4 PM even on cloudy days (more than 80% of sunray penetrate cloud cover).
      ii. UV rays are reflected from water, concrete, sand, snow, tile, and reflective window glass in buildings. The window glass blocks some UV rays, especially UVB, but significant UVA pass through. Plastic adherent films that block all UVB and UVA rays should be applied to home and car windows.
      iii. Clothing can provide sun protection. Dark colored tightly woven fabric gives best protection. Umbrella or 4 inch wide brimmed hats should be used while outdoor.
   b. *Sunscreens:* Sunscreens should be applied liberally to all exposed parts 15 to 30 minutes before sun exposure with particular attention to the posterior neck, the ears, and the areas of the

scalp covered with thin hair. Choose a sunscreen with at least 30 SPF with additional UVA—blocking property. Adults using sunscreen regularly should take daily oral supplementation (400 to 800 units) of vitamin D.
2. Topical corticosteroids (class 1–2), tacrolimus and/or pimecrolimus (on face mainly), intralesional triamcinolone in isolated lesion.
3. If no response
   a. Start hydroxychloroquine at 6.5 mg/kg/day
   b. Measures for smoking cessation in smokers.
   c. If no response seen by eight weeks quinacrine 100 mg/day should be added.
   d. If no improvement felt in next 4 weeks replace hydroxychloroquine with chloroquine 250 mg/day and continuing quinacrine.
4. If no response after several weeks, dapsone, a systemic retinoid, clofazimine or gold remain therapeutic options.
5. If the above treatments fail, or cannot be tolerated, thalidomide or immunosuppressive agents like short-term systemic steroids, methotrexate, azathioprine, mycophenolate mofetil or cyclosporine should be considered.
6. Patients with severe disease may be treated with immunosuppressive agents, in combination with the antimalarials in the initial phase.
7. *Biologics:* Efalizumab, rituximab, abatacept have been shown to be effective in recalcitrant disease. They themselves may induce DLE. More experience required regarding their use in LE.

> **PRACTICAL HINTS**
> 1. Dapsone would be tried before antimalarials in bullous LE.
> 2. No evidence of any difference in ocular toxicity has been found between chloroquine and hydroxychloroquine.

LICHEN NITIDUS

1. Mostly asymptomatic and self-limiting. So, no intervention is required.
2. Treatment is given either in symptomatic ground (severe itching) or cosmetological concern.
3. Topical glucocorticoid induce remission. Short course of oral glucocorticoid may be helpful in extensive or symptomatic disease.
4. Topical tacrolimus or pimecrolimus can be tried.
5. Phototherapy, both narrow and broad band UVB and systemic PUVA are also helpful.

> **PRACTICAL HINT**
> Assurance to parents is needed to explain the benign nature of the disease.

LICHEN PLANUS

1. Topical or intralesional corticosteroids is the mainstay of therapy.
2. Systemic steroid (short course) is indicated in eruptive lichen planus, erosive mucosal lichen planus.
3. Topical calcineurin inhibitors show variable response.
4. Systemic retinoids, like acitretin (30 mg/day) or isotretinoin (20–40 mg/day) shows marked improvement in cutaneous, oral and nail lesion with a mean treatment duration of 4 months.
5. Cyclosporine mouthwash is useful in unresponsive, erosive oral lichen planus.
6. Systemic cyclosporine with a low dose range of 3–10 mg/kg/day is used in recalcitrant lichen planus. Azathioprine and

mycophenolate mofetil may also be used in recalcitrant generalized lichen planus.
7. Use of dapsone, hydroxychloroquine or thalidomide can be considered in a case-to-case basis.
8. PUVA therapy is useful in generalized cutaneous disease. Success is also reported with narrow band UVB and UVA1 phototherapy.
9. Symptomatic therapy includes lignocaine and diphenhydramine in painful, erosive mucosal lichen planus and sedative antihistamine in cutaneous disease.
10. Lichen planopilaris is best-treated with potent topical glucocorticoid along with systemic glucocorticoid. Concomitant use of topical glucocorticoid with systemic glucocorticoid arrests progression.
11. Lichen planus hypertrophicus is treated with potent corticosteroid under occlusion or intralesional corticosteroid.

> **PRACTICAL HINTS**
> 1. Drug and contact history should be evaluated in all patients to rule out lichenoid drug eruption and lichenoid contact dermatitis.
> 2. Histology should be considered in all atypical and unresponsive case.
> 3. Erosive mucosal lichen planus and lichen planus hypertrophicus have malignant potential.
> 4. Evaluation and counseling is required.

LICHEN SCLEROSUS (LS)

1. Treatment of mucous membrane lichen sclerosus is started with class 1 topical corticosteroid like clobetasol.
2. The duration is kept below 4 weeks to reduce atrophy.
3. The continuation phase treatment includes either less potent corticosteroid or calcineurin inhibitors like tacrolimus.
4. Intralesional corticosteroid like triamcinolone acetonide are useful for isolated unresponsive plaque.
5. Acitretin (20–0 mg/day) is useful in severe recalcitrant disease. Isotretinoin may also be used.
6. Oral methotrexate also may be given in refractory cases.
7. Cryotherapy and laser (both ablative and non-ablative) are useful in selected cases.
8. Vulvectomy is necessary in secondary squamous cell carcinoma.
9. Circumcision resolves penile LS and associated phimosis.
10. Asymptomatic extragenital LS seldom require any treatment.

> **PRACTICAL HINTS**
> 1. Female LS patients should be closely monitored for secondary genital malignancies.
> 2. The efficacy of testosterone propionate ointment in LS is questioned.

LICHEN SIMPLEX CHRONICUS

1. Potent topical steroid of class 1 to 3 with or without occlusion is the mainstay of therapy.
2. Nonsteroidal topical anti-inflammatory agents like menthol or pramoxine can also reduce itch.
3. Adequate moisturization increases therapeutic efficacy of the above agents.
4. The role of scratching in the disease process needs to be explained to the patient. Cutting of nails and occluding the lesion with plastic films or steroid impregnated tape is essential.
5. Stress plays a role in aggravation. Stress reduction should be attempted.
6. Night-time itch should be controlled by sedative antihistamines or tricyclic antidepressants.

7. Selective serotonin reuptake inhibitors are helpful in daytime pruritus or in obsessive-compulsive disorder.

> **PRACTICAL HINTS**
> 1. Patch test is to be considered in lichen simplex chronicus involving periorbital area, dorsal hand and feet and anogenital area
> 2. Systemic causes of pruritus should be investigated in unresponsive cases.

LYMPHOGRANULOMA VENEREUM (LGV)

1. Oral doxycycline 100 mg twice daily for 21 days is the treatment of choice.
2. If doxycycline is contraindicated erythromycin base at a dose of 500 mg four times a day is given orally for 21 days.
3. Oral azithromycin 1 g weekly for 3 weeks is curative but safety in pregnancy is not established.
4. Sexual partner within prior 30 days should also be treated.
5. Therapy may be prolonged in HIV-positive patients. Treatment should continue till complete resolution of all signs and symptoms take place.
6. Aspiration of buboes is required if they do not respond to medical therapy.
7. Aspiration is done by a lateral approach through healthy skin to avoid fistula formation.
8. In late complication surgery is required to reduce morbidity. It includes rectal stricture dilatation, rectovaginal fistula repair, genital reconstruction, etc.

> **PRACTICAL HINT**
> Test for other STIs including HIV/AIDS should be done.

MELASMA

1. Initial evaluation should be based on clinical parameter instead of Wood's lamp finding because in Indian skin that is seldom yielding.
2. Melasma should be differentiated from pigmented contact dermatitis by allergic patch test whenever needed.
3. Patient should be counseled about the slow response to treatment, persistence of dermal pigmentation, importance of sun avoidance and effect of drugs particularly hormonal contraceptives on therapeutic outcome.
4. Art of sun-protection by physical method should be explained. These will be supplemented by a SPF50 sunscreen with avobenzone as a component for UVAI protection. Sunscreens containing iron oxide provide additional protection from visible light and can be used for cosmetic camouflage.
5. Classical depigmentary agents like hydroquinone (2–4%), azelaic acid (15–20%), kojic acid or arbutin are the mainstay of therapy.
6. Tretinoin (0.025–0.1%) is also helpful alone or in combination.
7. Class 4 to 6 corticosteroids are useful but side effect like atrophy and telangiectasis restrict their use.
8. Modified Kligman formula incorporates the above three drugs to increase efficacy and reduce toxicity.
9. Non-hydroquinone products (azelaic acid, kojic acid, niacinamide) can be used for longer duration.
10. Chemical peel by α-hydroxy acids are effective in unresponsive cases.
11. Efficacy of laser is not well established. They should used with cautions in darkly pigmented skin.

> **PRACTICAL HINTS**
> 1. Hydroquinone should not be used more than 6 months because of chances of development of exogenous ochronosis.
> 2. Pure dermal pigmentation responds poorly to treatment. Cosmetic camouflage is recommended.
> 3. All topical therapies except steroids are potential irritant. They may induce an irritant contact dermatitis with resultant hyperpigmentation.

MILIARIA

1. Heat exposure must be terminated to alleviate symptom.
2. Air conditioning or frequent cold bath is recommended.
3. Topical coolant like calaminol may be appreciated by the patient.
4. Eczematous change is treated with topical corticosteroid.
5. As miliaria causes destruction to sweat duct an attack is followed by reduction in sweat volume and resultant xerosis for a few days. Advice emollients.

> **PRACTICAL HINTS**
> 1. Clothing should be loose and breathing (cotton clothes). Workplace should be aerated.
> 2. Systemic antibiotic may be necessary in secondary infected cases.

MOLLUSCUM CONTAGIOSUM

1. Majority molluscum contagiosum lesions are self-limiting. So watchful expectancy is the primary mode of management.
2. Curettage to remove the infectious core is rapid and painless though in children topical EMLA cream should be considered.
3. Liquid nitrogen cryotherapy is also rapid but painful particularly in genital lesion. Topical anesthesia is mandatory.
4. Cantharidin (0.7 or 0.9%) is applied with a wooden stick on lesion. It is left for 4 hours. A blister develops in 24 hours that resolves along with the lesion.
5. Topical application of podophyllin in 10 to 25% suspension in physician's office is useful. It is washed after 1 to 4 hours. Podophyllotoxin is equally effective with less adverse effect and can be home applied.
6. 5% imiquimod cream applied alternate day cures 80% of molluscum.
7. Topical cidofovir (1%, 3% cream or gel) is effective but costly.
8. Topical retinoids, salicylic acid, 5-fluorouracil, silver nitrate paste, 10% KOH and trichloroacetic acid (25–50%) are alternative mode of therapy.
9. Oral cidofovir and subcutaneous interferon-α are indicated in resistant lesions in immunocompromised patients.
10. Oral cimetidine (40 mg/kg/day) is used in extensive lesions.
11. Anti-retroviral therapy is effective in molluscum contagiosum in HIV/AIDS.

> **PRACTICAL HINTS**
> 1. As the disease is self-limiting in immunocompetent person therapy with scarring potential should be avoided.
> 2. Molluscum is a sexually transmittable disease. Investigation for HIV and other STIs should be considered in pertinent cases.
> 3. In children, lesion should be kept covered. Pricking is discouraged.
> 4. Adults should be warned against beauty parlor derived infection.
> 5. Children with molluscum contagiosum should not be excluded from daycare

> or school. Lesions should be covered with clothing or a bandage to reduce the risk of transmission.

MORPHEA

1. Intervention is necessary in more severe disease which can cause irreversible fibrosis and damage.
2. Topical or intralesional steroids are mainstay of therapy. Systemic steroid may be required in more aggressive disease.
3. Topical tacrolimus can be tried
4. Calcipotriol with or without UVAI phototherapy is beneficial in children.
5. Antimalarials may be used as substitute.
6. For rapidly progressive and extensive morphea immunosuppressants like cyclosporine, methotrexate, mycophenolate mofetil, cyclophosphamide, azathioprine, etc., have been reported to be successful.
7. Penicillin and depenicillamine are effective.
8. PUVA, broadband UVA and UVAI phototherapy alone or in combination is efficacious.
9. Tofacitinib, ruxolitinib, and abatacept are potentially beneficial in extensive and refractory morphea.
10. Physical therapy in the early stage maintains joint mobility and reduces morbidity.

> **PRACTICAL HINTS**
> 1. Spontaneous resolution may take place without intervention.
> 2. Surgical intervention is required in selected cases.

MYCETOMA

1. In eumycetoma medical therapy is mostly unsuccessful.
2. Ketoconazole, itraconazole, fluconazole, voriconazole, posaconazole and terbinafine have all been used in eumycetoma caused by sensitive organism in different studies. Their role in clinical set-up is not clear.
3. Amputation is the only definitive curative procedure in advanced cases but the value of such procedure in a non life-threatening infection should be weighted in a case-to-case basis.
4. In actinomycetoma caused by nocardial species trimethoprim-sulfamethoxazole is the drug of choice.
5. Amikacin injection can be combined for better result.
6. In nocardia infection third generation cephalosporins (ceftriaxone and cefotaxime) may also be effective.
7. In patients sensitive to sulfaminocycline or amikacin-imipenem combination gives good result.
8. In actinomycetoma caused by actinomycetes a combination of dapsone with streptomycin or trimethoprim-sulfamethoxazole with streptomycin or amikacin is used.
9. Duration of therapy is long and patient specific.
10. Surgical debridement is considered on a case-to-case basis.

> **PRACTICAL HINTS**
> 1. The ideal condition of selecting chemotherapeutic agent from culture-sensitivity is mostly unavailable in clinical practice.
> 2. Amputation in eumycetoma should be considered after assessing the availability of suitable prosthesis.

MYCOSIS FUNGOIDES

Stage IA

1. Emollients
2. Topical corticosteroids
3. Topical mechlorethamine

4. Topical bexarotene
5. Topical imiquimod
6. PUVA or UVB or Excimer Light

Stage IB or IIA

1. Topical corticosteroids
2. Topical mechlorethamine
3. NBUVB
4. Local radiotherapy

Stage IIB (Tumor Stage)

Limited
1. Radiation therapy plus topical therapy

Generalized tumors
1. Brentuximab vedotin
2. Romidepsin

Stage III (Erythrodermic MF)

1. Like Sezary syndrome
2. Extracorporeal photochemotherapy
3. Mogamulizumab

Stage 4

Like Sezary syndrome
1. Brentuximab vedotin
2. Romidepsin
3. Pralatrexate

> **PRACTICAL HINTS**
> 1. Therapy choice, prognosis and mortality depends on stage of the disease.
> 2. Both PUVA and UVB-NB are effective in mycoses fungoides.

PALMOPLANTAR PUSTULOSIS

1. Wet soaks followed by class 1 corticosteroids application is primary mode of therapy. Unresponsive cases may require occlusion.
2. Maintenance is done with anthralin, tazarotene or calcipotriol.
3. In persistent cases, PUVA can be used alone or in combination with acitretin.
4. In disabling disease or disease with frequent recurrence systemic retinoid acitretin can be used. Teratogenicity restricts use in child-bearing age group.
5. Methotrexate or cyclosporine can be used as an alternative.

> **PRACTICAL HINTS**
> 1. Gram-stain and KOH preparation are needed to rule out infection.
> 2. Avoidance of smoking

PARAPSORIASIS

1. In small plaque parapsoriasis (SPP) treatment is not mandatory and patient may opt for no treatment. So counseling is essential before initiating therapy.
2. Treatment is initiated with topical corticosteroid (class 3 to 5) along with emollient.
3. If not responsive to the above regimen. Narrowband UVB or PUVA should be considered.
4. In the initial phase re-evaluation is done 3 monthly to identify any deviation from the stable nature of SPP.
5. In the later phase, yearly evaluation is sufficient.
6. Large plaque parapsoriasis (LPP) is potentially malignant and every effort is spent to arrest progression of the disease and early identification of a lymphomatous change.
7. Initial therapy is started with topical corticosteroid (class 1 to 3) with phototherapy (NBUVB or PUVA).
8. Poikilodermatous type can be treated with topical nitrogen mustard.

9. Patient evaluation is done every 2–3 months to assess progression.
10. If sign of spread detected multiple biopsies should be taken from suspected areas.
11. Cases satisfying clinicopathological criteria of patch stage MF should be treated as cutaneous lymphoma.
12. Stable cases are evaluated yearly.

> **PRACTICAL HINT**
> In large plaque disease use of immunohistochemistry and T-cell receptor gene rearrangement testing should be used if available to rule out lymphoma.

PARONYCHIA

1. Acute paronychia is bacterial in origin.
   - Treated with systemic antibiotic initially. As most cases are staphylococcal or streptococcal a semi-synthetic penicillin (dicloxacillin) or 1st generation cephalosporin (cephalexin) is chosen.
   - In β-lactam sensitive person a macrolide (erythromycin or azithromycin) is used.
   - If no response is seen in 48 hours, incision and drainage should be considered.
   - Further antibiotic selection is dictated by the culture-sensitivity of the drained pus.
2. Chronic paronychia is multifactorial in origin. Treatment centers on:
   - *Hand care:*
     a. Water and irritant contact should be kept to minimum.
     b. Wearing cotton gloves under rubber gloves is mandatory during work.
     c. Frequent application of thick moisturizer like white soft paraffin is helpful.
   - *Treatment of the infection:*
     a. Secondary candidal colonization should be treated by topical or if required systemic antifungal.
     b. Systemic antifungals (fluconazole or itraconazole) are particularly effective when candidal onychomycosis is present.
     c. Topical antibiotic can be used in the initial phase.
     d. Systemic antibiotic is needed when acute paronychia sets in.
   - *Treatment of the inflammation:*
     a. Dry heat application.
     b. Application of topical corticosteroid (class 3)

> **PRACTICAL HINTS**
> In unresponsive cases, despite above measures:
> 1. Peripheral circulation should be assessed.
> 2. Cushing's disease and Raynaud's phenomenon should be ruled out.
> 3. Chronic paronychia may be manifestation of protein contact dermatitis.

PEDICULOSIS

1. Permethrin 1 to 5% is applied on dry scalp for 10 minutes is an effective pediculocide.
2. 0.5% malathion applied for 8–12 hours is also effective but use is limited by adverse effects.
3. Second application for all pediculocide except lindane is recommended due to variable ovicidal activity and lack of patient compliance.
4. Cotrimoxazole is an effective antibacterial agent with an ability to kill adult lice.
5. Topical ivermectin 0.5% lotion to be applied only once on dry hairs.

6. Oral ivermectin at a dose of 250 µg/kg body weight given 7–10 days apart is very effective. Use not recommended for patient below 15 kg.
7. All members of household needs to be examined and affected one has to be treated.
8. Bedding, clothing, comb, floor should be cleaned according to recommendation to prevent recurrence.
9. The treatment modality for pediculosis pubis is same as above. Sexual contacts should be treated along with the affected household members.
10. Petrolatum applied thickly over eyelid twice daily for 2 weeks removes eyelid lice.
11. For pediculosis corporis, bathing, laundering infested clothing in hot water followed by hot ironing (especially the seam of the clothing) and maintenance of personal hygiene is only required.
12. Some prefer to treat with 5% permethrin cream, left for 8–10 hours.
13. Dusting of clothing with malathion or permethrin based tick repellant is recommended to prevent recurrence.

> **PRACTICAL HINTS**
> 1. In pediculosis capitis secondary pyodermas should be treated before application of pediculocide.
> 2. All pediculocide will kill but not remove the organism. Proper combing is essential for that.

PEMPHIGUS VULGARIS AND FOLIACEOUS

1. *Glucocorticosteroids:* 0.5 to 1.5 mg/kg of body weight daily till new bullae formation stops and Nikolsky's sign becomes negative. Then the dose can be rapidly tapered to half of the starting dose when the patient's skin is almost free of blisters. From this point very slow tapering of dose is to be done to attain a minimally effective maintenance dose.
   Mild pemphigus 0.5 mg/kg/day
   Moderate to severe pemphigus 1 mg/kg/day
2. Rituximab: Typical initial dosing: Two 1,000 mg intravenous infusion separated by two weeks. Intravenous methylprednisolone 100 mg should be given 30 minutes prior to each tituximab infusion.
3. *Adjuvant immunosuppressives:*
   a. *Azahiprine:* 1 to 2.5/kg body weight (dose depending on TPMT level) till complete clearing, then tapering to 1 mg/kg
   b. *Cyclophosphamide:* 100 to 200 mg daily; tapering to 50 to 100 mg/day. Or in 'pulse' therapy: 1,000 mg IV once in a week or every 2 weeks in 'staring' dose, then 50 to 100 mg /day as maintenance
   c. *Mycophenolate mofetil:* 1.5 to 2 g daily
3. Fluid and electrolyte balance
4. Antimicrobial therapy, when required
5. Topical or intralesional corticosteroids
6. Wet dressings
7. Cleansing baths

> **PRACTICAL HINTS**
> 1. Strict monitoring is essential for watching therapeutic response and drug-related side effects by clinical assessment and laboratory work-up.
> 2. Mycophenolate mofetil remains a promising adjuvant for this group of immunobullous disease.
> 3. Combined rituximab and prednisolone is an effective initial therapy. For practical reasons for obtaining and administering rituximab, glucocorticoids therapy often begins before rituximab therapy. Initial signs of clinical improvement by systemic glucocorticoids usually appear within 2 to 3 weeks. Effects of rituximab may not appear for 8 to 12 weeks.

PITYRIASIS LICHENOIDES CHRONICA

1. There is no consensus treatment modality. Even no treatment remains an option.
2. Topical corticosteroids are first line therapy.
3. Calcineurin inhibitor tacrolimus can be used, particularly in maintenance.
4. Phototherapy (BBUVB, NBUVB or PUVA) is the most effective mode.
5. Systemic antibiotics like erythromycin (500 mg twice to four times daily), tetracycline (500 mg twice to four times daily) or minocycline (100 mg twice daily) are other options.
6. Systemic corticosteroid, methotrexate, ciclosporin, dapsone or IVIG are very rarely required.

> **PRACTICAL HINTS**
> 1. Incidence of conversion to CTCL is very rare.
> 2. Follow-up is decided on case-to-case basis.

PITYRIASIS LICHENOIDES ET VARIOLIFORMIS ACUTA (PLEVA)

1. Treatment is initiated with topical corticosteroid with phototherapy (NBUVB, PUVA, natural sunlight) in mild-to-moderate disease.
2. Oral antibiotics like erythromycin (500 mg twice to four times daily), tetracycline (500 mg twice to four times daily) or minocycline (100 mg twice daily) are other options.
3. Severe disease is treated with tapering dose of systemic corticosteroid initially.
4. Dapsone can be used as a steroid sparing agent.
5. Steroid unresponsive cases are managed with methotrexate (10–25 mg PO/week), cyclosporine (2.5–4 mg PO divided in 2 doses/day) or acitretin (25–50 mg PO/day)

> **PRACTICAL HINT**
> Lymphomatoid papulosis should be ruled out by immunohistochemistry in suspected cases.

PITYRIASIS ROSEA

1. Most patients do not require treatment. Counseling regarding the self-resolving nature of PR is sufficient.
2. If the pruritus is troublesome topical menthol, pramoxine or topical corticosteroid (class 4–6) can be considered.
3. Night-time sedative antihistamines also reduce itch.
4. Role of oral erythromycin is controversial.
5. Oral acyclovir 800 mg 5 times daily for 7 days has shown to be effective in patients of PR with flu-like symptom or extensive skin lesion.
6. Phototherapy with NBUVB or sunlight is also effective but may result in postinflammatory-hyperpigmentation particularly in Indian skin.
7. Systemic corticosteroid may be required in very few patients with severe disease. Tapering must be slow to avoid resurgence.

> **PRACTICAL HINTS**
> 1. In suspected cases serology is to be done to rule out secondary syphilis.
> 2. Drug history is essential particularly in patients with atypical lesion and severe pruritus.

PITYRIASIS RUBRA PILARIS

1. Therapeutic regimen is chosen according to the clinical severity, patient profile and personal experience of concern physician.

2. For erythrodermic stage acitretin (0.5–0.75 mg/kg body weight) is the drug of choice along with general management for erythroderma. Isotretinoin (0.5–1 mg/kg/day) is preferred in pediatric population.
3. Methotrexate (10–25 mg weekly) remains 2nd option medication. It is used alone when acitretin cannot be started or in combination when acitretin alone is partially effective.
4. Phototherapy (NBUVB, PUVA, UVA1) alone or in combination with acitretin is useful. Due to possibility of photoaggravation phototesting prior starting of therapy is mandatory.
5. IL-17 or IL-23 inhibitors may be administered.
6. Extracorporeal photopheresis is useful in patients with severe symptom when the above regimens fail.
7. The role of other systemic agents like azathioprine, cyclosporine, fumaric acid esters and TNF-α antagonist is yet not clear.
8. Vitamin D3 analogs and topical retinoid tazarotene is also effective.
9. Topical corticosteroid (class 1–3) is considered a 2nd line therapy when step 6 and 7 fails.
10. Phototherapy remains another option in localized disease.
11. For patients of PRP who are suffering from HIV/AIDS, HAART is very effective.

> **PRACTICAL HINTS**
> 1. Systemic steroid has no role.
> 2. Localized disease is treated primarily with moisturizer and topical keratolytics like urea or salicylic acid.

PITYRIASIS VERSICOLOR

1. 2% ketoconazole in a shampoo base applied on affected areas for 5 minutes for 3 consecutive days is curative.
2. 2.5% selenium sulfide shampoo is a cheaper alternative but requires 10 minutes contact for 7–14 days and has got a bleaching effect.
3. Monthly application of both the agents is recommended for prevent recurrence.
4. In resistant cases, oral antifungals like itraconazole (100–200 mg twice daily for 7 days) or fluconazole (400 mg single dose) can be used.
5. Associated hypopigmentation may remain for longer period. Phototherapy can be used in persistent cases.
6. Topical tretinoin is effective in hyperpigmented variety.

> **PRACTICAL HINTS**
> 1. Though effective the use of terbinafine 1% solution should never be the first line of management due to cost and approval issue.
> 2. Systemic allylamines have no place in management of PV.
> 3. For prophylaxis topical rather than oral agents are always preferable.

POLYMORPHOUS LIGHT ERUPTION

1. Avoidance of sun including UVA. It should be explained to the patient that UVA penetrates the glass and so sunray in a room coming through glass window may precipitate PMLE lesion.
2. Proper sunscreen should be chosen. It should have a high SPF with additional UVA blocking property. Application method and the common mistakes in sunscreen application should be emphasized to the patient.
3. Mild variety responds to topical corticosteroid (class 3–5) or calcineurin inhibitors.
4. A small burst of systemic corticosteroid may be helpful.
5. Prophylactic phototherapy in spring can be considered in severely affected

patients. PUVA is most effective followed by NBUVB. Some patient can have a flare with initiation of phototherapy. It should be treated with systemic corticosteroid.
6. Efficacy of hydroxychloroquine is moderate.
7. If the above modes fail, introduce other immunosuppressives like azathioprine or cyclosporine.

> **PRACTICAL HINTS**
> 1. Assessment of antinuclear antibody titer is routine in all patients.
> 2. Rule out use of photosensitizing agents particularly in unresponsive cases before switching to prophylactic phototherapy or immunosuppressants.

POMPHOLYX

1. Wet dressing with Burrow's solution or diluted potassium permanganate (1:8,000) reduces vesiculation.
2. Oral antihistamines can reduce pruritus. Patient should be counseled about stress reduction.
3. Topical corticosteroids (class 1–3) with or without occlusion are mainstay of therapy, ointment preparation is preferred over cream.
4. Topical calcineurin inhibitors (tacrolimus and pimecrolimus) are also effective but lack the potency of corticosteroids. They are used in rotation with corticosteroids to avoid steroid-induced atrophy.
5. Oral alitretinoin (10 to 30 mg) can be administered
6. Short course of systemic corticosteroids (0.5–1 mg/kg/day tapered over 1–2 weeks) is sometimes useful in recurrent pompholyx, if initiated at the beginning of pruritus. Long-term use is prohibited.
7. Phototherapy is effective in recurrent disease. Among phototherapeutic options PUVA and UVAI is more effective than UVB.
8. Grenz-rays can also be beneficial.
9. Patients of pompholyx who also suffer from hyperhidrosis may benefit from iontophoresis, intradermal botulinum toxin or sympathectomy.

> **PRACTICAL HINTS**
> 1. Bullous tinea and dermatophytid should be excluded before initiating therapy.
> 2. In unresponsive cases patch testing should be considered to rule out allergic contact dermatitis and systemic contact dermatitis
> 3. Elimination diet and use of disulfiram can be helpful in patients allergic to nickel.
> 4. The role of methotrexate, cyclosporine and mycophenolate mofetil is not well delineated in pompholyx. They may be tried on a case-to-case basis depending upon the clinician's experience with individual agent.

PREGNANCY DERMATOSES

Polymorphic Eruption of Pregnancy (PUPPP)

1. Important differential diagnosis is from pemphigoid gestationis, which is a rarer and more significant disorder.
2. Treatment is usually with topical corticosteroids and chlorpheniramine; however, corticosteroids may add to the tendency for striae, and sedating antihistamines may be best avoided prior to delivery to avoid fetal sleepiness manifesting as poor fetal movement

Atopic Eruption of Pregnancy

1. Low to mid-potency topical corcisteroids
2. Skin hydration by frequent use of emollients

Pemphigoid Gestationis

1. Treatment of typical cases is with systemic corticosteroids, (dose 0.5 mg/kg) [should not exceed 80 mg/daily] which may need to be continued for several months after completion of the pregnancy. Even when most activity has settled, premenstrual exacerbations may occur.
2. If blisters occur in the baby, these are transient, as they are due to passively transferred immunoglobulin across the placenta.
3. It is important to recognize that milder versions do occur and may be amenable to control with topical corticosteroids alone, although proof of the disorder by biopsy for immunofluorescence is worthwhile in view of the risks of recurrence.
4. *Refractory cases:* Plasmapheresis, IVIG, cyclosporine.
5. *Maternal complications:* Nil/increased risk of Grave's and other autoimmune disease.
6. *Fetal risk:* Small for their gestational age, prematurity.

Impetigo Herpetiformis

1. Treatment is usually limited to systemic steroids (15–20 mg/day) and UV therapy
2. *Other choice:* Cyclosporine (category C drug).

Cholestasis of Pregnancy

1. Weekly fetal monitoring since 34 weeks
2. *Early induction of labor:* 37–38 weeks
3. *Pruritus:* Cholestyramine (may precipitate Vit K trigger coagulopathy), ursodeoxycholic acid (UDCA) 450–1,200 mg daily: Safe, well-tolerated, decreases fetal mortality)

Pruritic Folliculitis of Pregnancy

10% benzoyl peroxide + 1% hydrocortisone

Papular Dermatitis of Spangler

High dose of prednisone (40–200 mg/day)

> **PRACTICAL HINTS**
>
> 1. *Pregnancy dermatoses with fetal risk:* Pemphigoid gestationis, cholestasis of pregnancy, impetigo herpetiformis (Pustular Ps of pregnancy), papular dermatitis of Spangler.
> 2. *Pregnancy dermatoses without fetal risk:* Polymorphic eruption of pregnancy (PUPPP), pruritic folliculitis of pregnancy, prurigo of pregnancy (prurigo gestationis), prurigo gestationis of Besnier (atopic eruption of pregnancy).

PRURIGO NODULARIS

1. Treatment of prurigo nodularis is a clinical challenge.
2. Itching should be alleviated with nighttime use of sedative antihistaminic or tricyclic antidepressant.
3. Selective serotonin reuptake inhibitors can be used to control daytime pruritus.
4. Topical antipruritic agent like menthol, calamine or pramoxine can reduce itch. Emollients are also effective particularly if itch is associated with xerosis.
5. Topical corticosteroids (class 1–2) are mainstay of initial therapy. Occlusion potentiates their efficacy.
6. Intralesional corticosteroids are effective but sometimes the lesions are too many to be injected.
7. Vitamin D3 analogue calcipotriene or calcineurin inhibitor tacrolimus may have steroid sparing effect but lacks potency.
8. Phototherapy particularly PUVA is effective in certain cases.
9. Thalidomide is very effective. Therapy is initiated at 100 mg/day and later titrated

to lower dose to avoid dose-dependent neuropathy (appears at a cumulative dose of 40–50 g).
10. UVB and thalidomide can be sequentially used to reduce toxicity of both.
11. Cyclosporine at a dose of 3–4.5 mg/kg is very effective in resistant cases. Long-term use is restricted due to adverse effect.
12. Methotrexate can be an alternative.
13. Injection dupilumab for refractory cases
14. Cryotherapy can be adjunctive.

> **Practical Hints**
> 1. Patient should be counseled about the importance of breaking the itch-scratch cycle.
> 2. Cutting of nails and physically occluding the lesion should be meticulously followed.

PSORIASIS

Mild-to-moderate Skin Involvement

1. *Topical corticosteroids (TCS):* Mild-to-superpotent depending on the anatomical location, thickness of lesion, duration of the lesions, etc. TCS may be combined with salicylic acid in ointment base on very thick hyperkeratotic lesions especially on palmoplantar area or lotion base for thick lesions on scalp.
2. Topical calcipotriene ointment, cream or solution. To start with calcipotriene may be combined with TCS to reduce inflammation.
3. Topical tar ointment for skin or lotion for scalp and hairy skin.
4. *Topical anthralin:* Preferably as short contact therapy on localized skin lesions
5. Topical tazarotene with or without TCS
6. *Topical tacrolimus or pimecrolimus:* In intertriginous or facial lesions
7. UVB NB or PUVA in refractory cases.

Severe Involvement

1. <10% BSA (body surface area) involved (sensitive area/refractory)
   - Superpotent TCS + Calcipotriol/Tazarotene/Anthralin
   - If not response add UVB NB
   - If not response add PUVA/PUVASOL
   - If not response add aprelimast
   - If not response add UVB NB + Acitretin
   - If not response add methotrexate (if contraindicated add cyclosporine/biologics).
2. >10% BSA involved
   - UVB NB
   - If not response add PUVA/PUVASOL
   - If not response add UVB NB + Acitretin
   - If not response add MTX (If contraindicated add cyclosporine/biologics).
   - Biologics: Ixekizumab. Secukinumab, adalimumab

Difficult Situations

1. *Childbearing age:* UVB NB /PUVA/Cyclosporine/Biologics
2. *Pregnancy:* UVB NB/Cyclosporine/Oral corticosteroids/Biologics
3. *Hepatic dysfunction and alcoholics:* UVB NB/Cyclosporine/Aprelimast
4. *In HIV diseases:* UVB NB/UVB NB+ Acitretin/Aprelimast.
5. *Psoriatic arthritis*: Referral to rheumatologist/methotrexate, aprelimast, oral jak inhibitor (tofacitinib), biologics

(British Association Dermatology Guidelines, BJD 2005)

Difficult Psoriasis: Choice of Biologics

- Acute phase/Pustular Ps (generalized)/Erythrodermic/Indoor admitted patients: Infliximab/Ixekizumab
- Chronic plaque/severe/refractory patients not willing to undergo IV infusion by

admission/traveling frequently/had H/o tuberculosis or exposure: Etanercept/Adalimumab/Ixekizumab

Rotational Therapy

- *Objects:* To minimize cumulative toxicity of individual drugs and to prevent resistance
- *Examples:* PUVA → MTX → Retinoids.

Combination Therapy

- *Aims:* To enhance response, to reduce side effects by lowering individual doses
- *Examples:* TCS + calcipotriol/phototherapy
  - Acitretin+ phototherapy
- Contraindicated combinations:
  - Acitretin + Cyclosporine
  - PUVA/UVB + Cyclosporine
  - PUVA+ Methotrexate
  - Adalimubab + methotrexate

Sequential Therapy

- Objects: To clear psoriasis by potent agent initially
- Maintain remission by safer, less effective agents
- Example: Cyclosporine followed by Retinoids + PUVA.

> **PRACTICAL HINTS**
> 1. In stable psoriasis slow but steady therapeutic response is more desirable than drastic suppressive therapy.
> 2. Superpotent topical steroids should be used judiciously only for shorter duration on localized areas followed by less potent steroid. If required superpotent TCS may be used once or twice in a week for maintenance.
> 3. Methotrexate would be restricted when situation really demands. It should not be used casually only to satisfy patients or for prompt response.
> 4. In fertile age group female patients, if systemic retinoids are to be prescribed it is better to start isotretinoin for teratogenicity of much lesser duration.
> 5. Methotrexate-dependancy can be gradually weaned off by UVB NB therapy.

PSEUDOFOLLICULITIS BARBAE

1. Shaving should be stopped till inflammation resolves.
2. The embedded hair shaft is removed by inserting a sterile needle under the hair loop. A toothbrush rubbing in a circular motion can also be used for the same purpose.
3. Topical azelaic acid should be prescribed to reduce bacterial colonization and post-inflammatory hyperpigmentation.
4. 5% benzoyl peroxide alone or in combination with topical 1% clindamycin is also effective.
5. Systemic antistaphylococcal antibiotics are sometimes essential to enhance healing.
6. Topical retinoids can be used as adjunctive treatment.
7. Intralesional triamcinolone (2.5 mg/mL) is sometimes required for persistent papule. Care is to be taken to avoid atrophy.
8. Shaving may be resumed once lesions heal.
9. Use of eflornithine hydrochloride 13.9% cream reduces hair growth and may prevent relapse.
10. Depilatory creams can also be tried.
11. In recurrent cases despite above measure shaving needs to be stopped.
12. Laser hair removal by Nd:YAG Laser is safe in type III to V skin and offers permanent cure from pseudofolliculitis. Diode Laser and IPL are also effective though safety is not warranted in Indian skin.

> **PRACTICAL HINTS**
> 1. Proper shaving instructions are to be given to prevent recurrence.
> 2. Laser hair removal is the only curative option.

PYODERMA GANGRENOSUM

1. Patient should be oriented about available treatment modalities, their adverse effects and slow response of the disease to treatment.
2. Bed rest and pain control is essential in the initial phase of severe disease. Associated anemia should be corrected.
3. In acute stage wound care principle:
    i. Potassium permanganate (1:2,000) solution wash reduces exudation. Tepid normal saline wash is another alternative.
    ii. Wound is smeared with 1% silver sulphadiazine cream.
    iii. A nonadhesive dressing is held in place firmly by a crepe bandage. Care should be taken not to put it too tight.
4. Vegetative or small ulcerative lesion can be treated with local measures.
    i. Class 1 or 2 topical steroid applied on the periphery of an active PG lesion can induce healing.
    ii. Intralesional triamcinolone (5–10 mg/mL) twice weekly at the edge of a lesion can induce healing.
    iii. Topical tacrolimus is an option for peristomal and early PG.
5. In larger lesion, multiple lesions, aggressive spread, lesion unresponsive to topical measures and disease associated with significant morbidity systemic therapy is chosen. Options are:
    i. Oral prednisolone 0.5–1.5 mg/kg/day is started and continued till the lesion shows sign of healing. Then slow tapering is initiated.
    ii. Use of pulse steroid is not recommended in steroid unresponsive cases. In this condition, use cyclosporine at a dose of 3–6 mg/kg/day either alone or in combination with prednisolone.
    iii. In steroid responsive cases where prolong therapy is suspected a steroid sparing agent is introduced. Choices are in the form of dapsone (50–200 mg/day orally), or minocycline (100–200 mg/day orally in 2 divided doses), or clofazimine (100 mg 3 times daily orally).
    iv. Methotrexate is helpful in patients with IBD.
    v. Mycophenolate mofetil and azathioprine can be used alone or in combination with systemic steroid. Any consensus related to their use has not been formed yet. Owing to the severe adverse effects of these agents, a case-to-case basis decision should be taken.
    vi. Same principle is maintained in the use of biologicals (infliximab, etanercept, adalimumab) in PG.
6. Skin grafting is not recommended due to pathergy, but cultured keratinocyte autograft and bovine collagen matrix are useful. Disease activity should be kept minimum using step 6.
7. Gradient support hosiery is helpful in lower extremity PG.
8. *Follow-up:* Ulcerative PG lesions are relapsing in nature. Follow-up protocol is to be decided upon
    i. Initial response to therapy.
    ii. Presence of associated illness.
    iii. Cost.
9. Prevention protocol includes:
    i. Avoidance of trauma.
    ii. In planned operation in a patient with severe PG following guidelines should be followed:
        - Systemic corticosteroid during and after (2 weeks or more) surgery
        - Use of subcuticular suture

iii. Surgeon should be warned about development of peristomal PG in patients suffering from Crohn's disease and PG.

> **PRACTICAL HINT**
> The management of PG is initiated with a battery of investigation to assess the general health status of the patient and to find out any associated underlying disease.

ROSACEA

1. Aggravating factors like hot and spicy food, red wine and sunlight should be avoided.
2. A gentle broad-spectrum ultraviolet A and ultraviolet B sunscreen should be applied. Use of umbrella and broad-brimmed hat as well as restricted daytime outdoor activity should be stressed.
3. Harsh cosmetic ingredients like camphor, menthol and sodium lauryl sulfate should not be used.
4. A soap-free cleanser is preferred for cleansing.
5. Topical barrier repair emollient use is mandatory particularly in dry and sensitive skin.
6. Cosmetic camouflage with a green tint is recommended.
7. For erythematotelangiectatic subset
    - 10% sodium sulfacetamide-sulfur cleanser in the morning followed by cosmetic camouflage with moisturizing sunscreen is advised.
    - At night a metronidazole (0.75 or 1%), topical minocycline, topical ivermectin or azelaic acid (15%) formulation is preferred.
    - For moderate-to-severe flushing oral tetra- cycline (500 mg twice daily), doxycycline (100 mg od), minocycline (100 mg od) or isotretinoin (0.5 mg/kg body weight/day) is effective.
    - Vascular lasers and IPL are effective in reducing redness and telangiectasia.
    - Topical tretinoin can be used as maintenance therapy.
8. For papulopustular subset
    - Morning application includes any one from topical metronidazole, azelaic acid, sodium sulfacetamide-sulfur or benzoyl peroxide clindamycin combination, topical ivermectin or topical minocycline along with a sunscreen.
    - At night any one of the morning products that was not used in morning is applied.
    - For moderate-to-severe flushing oral tetracycline (500 mg twice daily), doxycycline(100 mg od), minocycline (100 mg od) or isotretinoin (0.5 mg/kg body weight/day) is effective.
    - Topical isotretinoin is used for maintenance
9. For phymatous subset
    - Benzoyl peroxide-clindamycin combination is most effective among topical therapy.
    - Oral tetracycline doxycycline, minocycline or isotretinoin is used depending on severity.
    - Surgical intervention according to need.
10. For ocular subset
    - Skin care as step 7.
    - 10% sodium sulfacetamide ophthalmic ointment is helpful.
    - Oral tetracycline, if topical management fails.
    - Ophthalmologist's opinion should be sought.

> **PRACTICAL HINTS**
> 1. To reduce irritation of tretinoin barrier emollients are prior applied.
> 2. In phymatous subset isotretinoin should be started after surgery.

SARCOIDOSIS

Cutaneous Sarcoidosis

1. Corticosteroids: systemic for generalized or scarring lesions; intralesionally 3 mg/mL or potent topical corticosteroids for limited lesion
2. Hydroxychloroquine 100 mg twice daily
3. *Methotrexate:* Low dose
4. Oral minocycline or doxycycline
5. *Others:* Anti-TNF α-blockers, thalidomide.

Systemic Sarcoidosis

Indications of systemic corticosteroids:
1. Active ocular disease
2. Active pulmonary disease
3. Cardiac arrhythmia
4. CNS involvement
5. Hypercalcemia.

> **PRACTICAL HINTS**
> 1. Treatment depends on the type and extent of the lesions present.
> 2. Even when dealing a case of cutaneous sarcoidosis every attempt is to be taken to exclude systemic involvement.

SCABIES

1. Permethrin 5% cream applied from neck-to-toe (head-to-toe in pediatric cases and when involvement of those areas seen in an adult) for 8–14 hours and repeated in 7 days is the mainstay of therapy. It is a pregnancy category B drug, but not recommended in infant under 2 months of age.
2. 1% lindane lotion is around 89% curative but increased resistance is being reported. Nonetheless the drug is toxic and not recommended in children below 2 years, in pregnancy and lactation.
3. Topical ivermectin or topical spinosad may be alternative
4. Crotamiton and precipitated sulfur are of limited efficacy.
5. Oral ivermectin 200 µg/kg body weight given 7–10 days apart is highly effective, safe and recommended along topical agents in resistant or crusted cases.
6. To prevent recurrence all close contacts to be treated with a topical scabicide.
7. Clothing and bedlinen used in last 5 days before treatment should be hot washed or dry cleaned.
8. The associated pruritus in scabies may last for 4 weeks and proper patient counseling is required. Otherwise treatment failure is suspected.
9. Pruritus can be controlled by oral antihistamines, topical corticosteroids or in severe cases with a short course of systemic steroid.
10. Associated pyoderma should be treated with systemic antibiotic.

> **PRACTICAL HINTS**
> 1. Lindane is ineffective, if applied on crusted lesion. So treatment of pyoderma is essential before lindane application.
> 2. Permethrin should be applied on bone dry skin for proper efficacy.
> 3. Lesions of nodular scabies may remain for indefinite period particularly in genitalia. Potent topical or intralesional steroid is indicated.

SYSTEMIC SCLEROSIS (SSC): CUTANEOUS MANAGEMENT

Raynaud's Phenomenon

1. Behavioral therapy
2. To avoid cold exposure
3. *Calcium channel blockers:* Nifedipine
4. *Angiotensin II receptor blocker:* Losartan
5. IV alprostadil (prostaglandin E1) in refractory case

6. Oral iloprost, a prostacycline analogue
7. Oral sildenafil or tadalafil

Cutaneous Ulcers

1. Topically applied growth factors like PDGF
2. Bosentan (oral endothelin receptor antagonist approved for SSC-related pulmonary hypertension).

Cutaneous Sclerosis

1. Methotrexate (MTX) or mycopheolate mofetil for progressive and diffuse skin involvement.
2. MTX for patients who also have arthritis or myositis
3. MMF for patients also with interstitial lung disease
4. For resistant cases: IVIG, rituximab, or tocilizumab
5. Cyclophosphamide should better be reserved for progressive skin involvement in patients who are refractory to treatment with either MTX or MMF or who have severe rapidly progressive skin thickening.

Calcinosis Cutis

1. Oral minocycline
2. MTX
3. Infliximab
4. Rituximab
5. Surgical removal for patients with significant pain and disability

> **PRACTICAL HINTS**
> 1. Vasodilators used in Raynaud's phenomenon should not excessively lower the systemic blood pressure which can further reduce the blood flow to the fingers.
> 2. Mechanical debridement in cutaneous ulcer in scleroderma is contraindicated as the ulcer bed often lies very close to the underlying bone.

SEBORRHEIC DERMATITIS (SD)

1. Seborrheic dermatitis (SD) of infant has excellent prognosis. But in adults the disease is recurrent in nature. This nature should be explained to the guardian or the patient at the beginning of therapy.
2. In infant SD should be managed as below:
   a. *Scalp:* The purpose is to remove of crust/scale, reduce fungal growth and inflammation. Following drugs can be used either alone or in combination:
      i. 3% salicylic in olive oil
      ii. Warm olive oil compress
      iii. Class 5/6 topical steroid for a short period
      iv. Topical antifungal shampoo: Maximum experience is with 2% ketoconazole or shampoo. The recommended regimen is twice weekly with a 5 minutes contact period. The shampoo should be applied to involved facial skin. Povidone iodine shampoo is also effective.
      v. Mild baby shampoos are helpful in early cases.
      vi. Systemic antibiotic is used in suspected secondary bacterial infection.
   b. *Intertriginous area:* Options are
      i. Low potent topical corticosteroids
      ii. Topical antifungal cream
      iii. Combination of above two
3. The adult SD is managed as below:
   a. *Scalp:* The principal is same as infantile SD. Available modalities are:
      i. Selenium sulfide 2.5% shampoo. Irritation and bleaching is use limiting side effect. Contact period is 5–10 minutes. Used 2–3 times/week it is equally effective as ketoconazole.
      ii. Ketoconazole 2% shampoo
      iii. Zinc pyrithione shampoo

iv. Ciclopirox 1% shampoo
v. Salicylic acid
vi. Topical glucocorticoid (class 5–7)
vii. Topical calcineurin inhibitors like tacrolimus (additional antifungal activity) and pimecrolimus.
viii. Vitamin D3 analog (calcipotriol, calcitriol or tacalcitol)
ix. Avoid hair oil, soap, hair tonic, etc.
b. *Face:* Recommendations are
i. Avoid greasy ointment and soap.
ii. Topical ketoconazole 2% cream
iii. Topical corticosteroid (class 5–7)
iv. Topical calcineurin inhibitor
v. Vitamin D3 analog
vi. Topical roflumilast
vii. Topical crisaborole
c. *Seborrheic blepharitis:* Modalities are
i. Hot compress and gentle debridement
ii. Baby shampoo to remove crust/scale
iii. Sodium sulfacetamide ophthalmic ointment.
d. *Seborrheic otitis externa:* Modalities are
i. Topical corticosteroids (class 5–7)
ii. Topical calcineurin inhibitors
iii. Aluminium acetate solution.
4. If step 3 fails proceed to either of the following:
a. Systemic antifungal therapy
b. UVB phototherapy: Disease may flare in a few.
c. *Oral isotretinoin:* 0.05–0.1 mg/kg/day for several months can clear resistant cases. Mandatory precaution in childbearing age group.
d. *Systemic corticosteroid:* May be helpful in acute flare. Prednisolone 30 mg/day produces a rapid response. Long-term use is not recommended.

> **PRACTICAL HINTS**
> 1. Combination of topical corticosteroids and salicylic acid may help in removing thick and adherent scales especially in the cases of sebopsoriasis.
> 2. Secondary bacterial infection or associated pediculosis infestation is to be treated accordingly.

STEVENS–JOHNSON SYNDROME/ TOXIC EPIDERMAL NECROLYSIS (SJS/TEN)

1. Suspect diagnosis and confirm clinically, histologically and immunologically but initiate treatment with clinical suspicion.
2. Identification of the implicated drug is essential but difficult in many cases due to multiple drug use. If causative drug cannot be identified, the basic idea is to discontinue all nonessential drugs introduced in last 8 weeks and essential drugs in the high-risk list should be replaced by an alternative.
3. Next step is withdrawal of all suspected drugs and replace them if necessary with suitable noncross-reacting alternative.
4. Prognostic work-up is done with 'SCORTEN'.
5. Basic management includes:
   - *Hemodynamic equilibrium:* Peripheral channel is preferred mode. Fluid balance is maintained like a burn patient.
   - *Temperature regulation:* 28–30°C is the optimal temperature.
   - Nutritional support
   - *Wound care:* Detached or detachable skin should be left in place as biological dressing. Only sloughed or necrotic skin

is removed. Wound is irrigated with potassium permanganate (1:10,000) solution and the denude area is covered with nonadhesive dressing. Collagen dressing can be used. Petrolatum impregnated gauze piece is a cheaper alternative.
- *Prevention of infection*: Prophylactic antibiotic is not recommended. Aseptic care is essential. Routine culture of skin, blood and urine specimen is done for bacteria and fungi in intervals.
- *Eye care*: Referral to ophthalmologist is mandatory. Antibiotic eye drops and ointment, artificial tear supplementation, and mechanical disruption of synechiae are eye-saving.
- *Mouth and genital care*: According to the severity to avoid pain and complication.

6. Specific treatment till date is elusive. The following drugs may have a place:
- *Cyclosporine:* Cyclosporin is more rational systemic drug than others. Oral cyclosporin at the dose of 3 to 5 mg/kg/day should be given in early course of the disease (within 24 to 48 hours of symptoms onset)
- *Etanercept*: for those in whom cyclosporin is contraindicated, a single dose of tumor necrosis factor (TNF) inhibitor etanercept is an alternative option.
- *Systemic corticosteroid*: Role is uncertain, Treatment modality, dose, timing, and duration have not been determined Routine use cannot be recommended.
- *Intravenous immunoglobulin:* In several meta-analyses no clear survival advantage has been found for patients with SJS/TEN with IVIG. The role of IVIG in combination with systemic steroids needs to be further investigated.
- *Plasmapheresis:* Routine use not recommended.

PRACTICAL HINTS

IV fluid replacement depends on the individual requirement. Albumin and colloids should be replaced with crystalloids, as higher mortality rate were reported with the use of albumin.

SPOROTRICHOSIS

1. Cutaneous lesion is primarily treated with any one of the following regimen:
   a. *Saturated solution of potassium iodide:*
      i. Start with 5 drops three times daily which is to be increased to 30–50 drops three times daily.
      ii. Should be taken with orange juice to mask the taste. Milk remains an inferior alternative.
      iii. After resolution of lesion therapy should continue for another 3–4 weeks.
      iv. This drug is inexpensive but has multiple adverse effects.
   b. *Oral itraconazole:*
      i. Given at a dose of 200 mg/day.
      ii. Should be continued for at least 1 week beyond clinical resolution.
      iii. Expensive but tolerable adverse effect profile.
   c. *Oral terbenafine:*
      i. Given at a dose of 250 mg/day.
      ii. Should be continued for at least 1 week beyond clinical resolution.
      iii. Expensive but tolerable adverse effect profile.
2. Patients not responding to oral itraconazole 200 mg daily may be treated with oral itraconazole 200 mg twice daily or terbinafine 500 mg twice daily.
3. Localized heat therapy at 38.5°C is effective. Should be combined with drug therapy.
4. Intravenous amphotericin B is used for systemic infection.

> **PRACTICAL HINT**
> Though self-healing of lesion has been reported with cutaneous sporotrichosis, treatment should be started without delay.

SYPHILIS

1. *Primary, secondary and early latent:*
   Primary therapy: Benzathine penicillin G 2.4 million units IM single dose
   Alternative: Doxycycline 100 mg orally twice daily × 14 days
   Ceftriaxone 1 g IM or IV daily × 10 to 14 days
2. *Latent of unknown duration and late latent:*
   Primary therapy: Benzathine penicillin G 2.4 million units IM once weekly × 3 weeks
   Alternative: Doxycyclin 100 mg orally twice daily × 28 days or Ceftriaxone 2 g daily IM or IV for 10 to 14 days
3. *Neurosyphilis:*
   Primary therapy: Aqueous penicillin G 18–24 million units IV daily (3–4 million units every 4 hourly or continuous infusion) × 10 to 14 days
   Alternative: Procaine penicillin 2.4 million units IM daily plus probenecid 500 mg orally 4 times daily × 10 to 14 day; Ceftriaxone 2 g IV daily × 10 to 14 days
4. Tertiary (excluding neurosyphylis): Benzathine penicillin G 2.4 million units IM once weekly × 3 weeks

> **PRACTICAL HINTS**
> 1. In case of penicillin allergy alternative regimen may be employed or oral desensitization for penicillin therapy may be attempted.
> 2. In neurosyphilis follow-up treatment to be done with 2 additional weekly injections of benzathine penicillin G 2.4 million units IM.
> 3. In tertiary syphilis before therapy neuro-syphilis to be excluded by CSF test.

TINEA INFECTION

1. Treatment of dermatophyte infection is site specific.
2. *In treatment of tinea capitis:*
   i. Topical antifungals like selenium sulfide, povidone iodine, zinc pyrithione or ketoconazole have adjunctive role.
   ii. Systemic antifungals are mainstay therapy. Griseofulvin (20–25 mg/kg/day), fluconazole (6 mg/kg/day), itraconazole (3–5 mg/kg/day) and terbinafine (3–6 mg/kg/day) are available options.
   iii. Duration of therapy is species specific. Prior culture is essential.
   iv. Systemic corticosteroid is used to relieve pain, swelling and resultant scarring. Oral prednisolone 1–2 mg/kg/day is given for first one week of antifungal therapy.
3. *In treatment of tinea barbae:* Follow same principal as tinea capitis. Only adult dosages of antifungals are slight different. They are
   i. Griseofulvin 1,000 mg/day for 2–4 weeks.
   ii. Fluconazole 200 mg/day for 4–6 weeks.
   iii. Itraconazole 200 mg/day for 2–4 weeks.
   iv. Terbinafine 250 mg/day for 2–4 weeks.
4. *In treatment of tinea corporis:*
   i. Topical antifungals applied twice daily for 2–4 weeks are used for localized disease. Drugs include allylamines, imidazoles, butenafine, ciclopirox, tolnaftate.
   ii. Systemic antifungals are used for extensive and inflammatory lesions. Dosage regimen are

- *In adult:*
  - Griseofulvin 500 mg/day for 2-6 weeks
  - Fluconazole 150 mg/week for 4-6 weeks
  - Itraconazole 100 mg/day for 2 weeks
  - Terbinafine 250 mg/day for 2 weeks.
- *In children:*
  - Griseofulvin 10-20 mg/kg/day for 6 weeks
  - Itraconazole 5 mg/kg/day for 1 week
  - Terbinafine 3-6 mg/kg/day for 2 weeks.
5. *In treatment of tinea cruris:* Treatment modality is same as tinea corporis. Inflammation may be more due to maceration. Keeping the area dry is essential. Weight reduction and wearing loose under clothing are important adjunctive measure.
6. *In treatment of tinea pedis:*
   i. Topical antifungals are sufficient for localized noninflammatory interdigital tinea pedis. Same drugs as in tinea corporis with same dosing schedule are prescribed.
   ii. For more extensive, inflammatory or refractory disease systemic antifungals are used.
      - In adult, dosage are
        - Fluconazole 150 mg/week for 3-4 weeks.
        - Itraconazole 200 mg twice daily for 1 week.
        - Terbinafine 250 mg/day for 2 weeks.
      - In children, itraconazole 5 mg/kg/day for 2 weeks.
   iii. Treatment of associated onychomycosis is essential to avoid relapse.
   iv. Maceration and foul smell indicate secondary bacterial infection which is quite common. Antibiotic should be added to the regimen if gram-stain and culture proves superinfection.
   v. Systemic corticosteroid at a dose of 0.5-1 mg/kg/day for 7-10 days is required in bullous tinea pedis.
7. *In treatment of tinea manuum:* Same as tinea pedis.
8. In treatment of onychomycosis:
   i. Topical therapy by ciclopirox or amorolfine nail lacquers is effective when nail matrix has not been involved.
   ii. With matrix involvement systemic agents are required. Choices are
      - Fluconazole 150-300 mg/weekly for 3-12 month (In refractory case, use 450 mg/week)
      - Itraconazole. For fingernails 200 mg daily for 6 weeks. For toenails 200 mg daily for 12 weeks
      - Terbinafine 250 mg/daily for 6 weeks for fingernail and 12 weeks for toenail.

> **PRACTICAL HINTS**
>
> For chronic and recurrent dermatophytosis (CRD) happening during endemic infection especially in India during last decade:
> 1. Topical antifungals should be applied 1 inch beyond margin of the lesions, to continue for 1 month after clinical remission.
> 2. Hygiene maintenance is of utmost importance to get clinical success. Hygiene maintenance include regular washing and ironing of clothes, separate washing of clothes from other family members, avoiding tight and occlusive clothes

TUBERCULOSIS

1. HIV testing is mandatory in all patients of cutaneous tuberculosis before initiation of therapy because seropositive patients may require prolong therapy.
2. Ideally culture and sensitivity is to be done as multidrug resistant tuberculosis is rising. This is not possible in most clinical set-up.
3. Empirical therapy is initiated with 4 drug regimen for first 8 weeks. Dosage protocol as below:
    i. *Rifampicin:* 10 mg/kg/day orally
    ii. *Isoniazid:* 5 mg/kg/day orally
    iii. *Pyrazinamide:* 30 mg/kg/day orally
    iv. *Ethambutol:* 15 mg/kg/day orally or strepto- mycin 15 mg/kg/day IM.
4. Maintenance is continued with 2 drugs for 16–18 month. Dosage are
    i. Rifampicin: 10 mg/kg/day orally
    ii. Isoniazid: 5 mg/kg/day orally
5. Surgical intervention may be used in conjunction with antitubercular chemotherapy in the following:
    i. Small lesion in lupus vulgaris and tuberculosis verrucosa cutis can be excised.
    ii. Scrofuloderma: Reduces morbidity and total duration of chemotherapy.
    iii. Plastic surgery is helpful in mutilating lupus vulgaris.
6. BCG vaccination may be a double-edged sword:
    i. Its protective role is documented.
    ii. Appearance of lupus vulgaris and tuberculids have been reported following vaccination.
    iii. Owing to paucity of such adverse event vaccination is recommended.
7. Cutaneous tuberculosis and HIV:
    i. Drug regimen is similar to non-HIV person.
    ii. Treatment duration is increased to 9 month.
    iii. Incidence of adverse drug reaction is increased.
8. Multidrug resistance tuberculosis: Referral to specialized center.

> **PRACTICAL HINT**
>
> Search for systemic involvement for every case of cutaneous tuberculosis. Therapy is dictated by the internal organ involved.

URTICARIA

1. Identifying the underlying triggering factors, drugs like NSAIDs, etc., or food additives like preservatives, coloring agents or fragrances and to avoid it.
2. Determining the type of urticaria, physical, autoimmune, contact urticaria, delayed pressure urticaria, etc.
3. Goal of the treatment:
    - Relieving the pruritus
    - Decreasing the size and number of lesions

Treatment of Acute Urticaria

- Antihistamines are effective in most cases and recommended as first-line therapy.
- First-generation antihistamines are rapidly acting but they can produce sedation and impaired motor skills as they can cross the blood–brain barrier. Adult patients and parents of child patients should be made aware of the potential side effect.
- These impairments are less evident or not evident with second-generation antihistamines.
- A brief course of oral corticosteroids may be prescribed in antihistamines refractory patients.

Treatment of Chronic Urticaria

Algorithmic Approach

Recommended treatment algorithm for urticaria [(The EAACI/gA92) LEN/EDF/WAO guideline 2022].

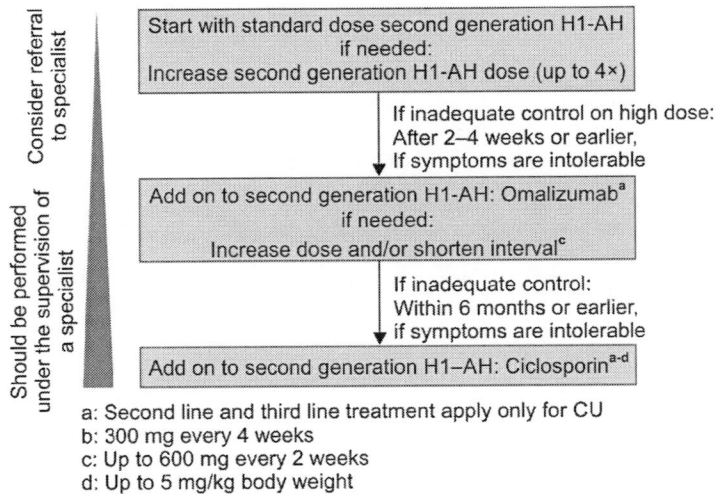

a: Second line and third line treatment apply only for CU
b: 300 mg every 4 weeks
c: Up to 600 mg every 2 weeks
d: Up to 5 mg/kg body weight

This algorithm was voted on after finishing all separate GRADE questions taking into consideration the existing consensus. It was decided that omalizumab should be tried before ciclosporin since the latter is not licensed for urticaria and has an inferior profile of adverse effects. In addition: A short course of glucocorticosteroids may be considered in case of severe exacerbation.

Figure is based on expert consensus and achieved 70% agreement in the consensus conference

Recommended Step Care Approach by American Guideline (AAAAI, ACAAI 2014)

Step 1:
- Monotherapy with second-generation antihistamines
- Avoidance of triggers (e.g., NSAIDs) and relevant physical factors if physical urticaria/angioedema syndrome is present.
- Begin treatment at step appropriate for patient's level of severity and previous treatment history.
- At each level of step-approach, medication(s) should be assessed for patient tolerance and efficacy.
- Step-down in treatment is appropriate at any step, once consistent control of urticaria/angioedema is achieved.

Step 2:
- One or more of the following:
- Dose advancement of second-generation antihistamines used in Step 1
- Add another second-generation antihistamine.
- Add H2-antagonist.
- Add leukotriene receptor antagonist.
- Add first-generation antihistamine to be taken at bed time

Step 3:
Dose advancement of potent antihistamine (e.g., hydroxyzine or doxepin) as tolerated

Step 4:
- Add an alternative agent
- Omalizumab or cyclosporine
- Other anti-inflammatory agents, immunosuppressants, or biologics

Recommended Step Care Approach by British Association of Dermatologists (2021)

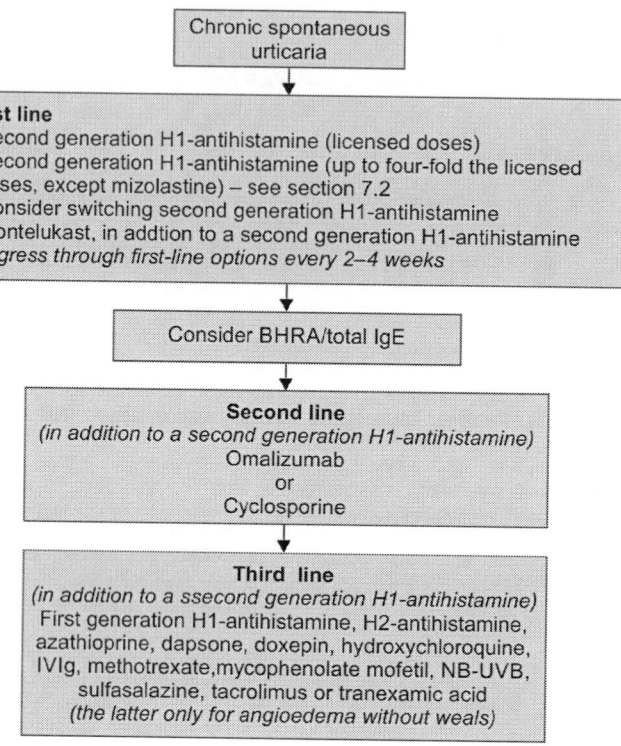

Uticaria Refractory to Antihistamines: Algorithm

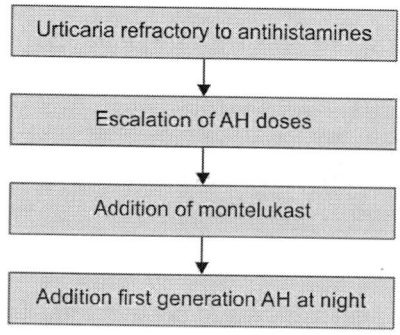

Sources:
1. AAAI, ACAAI, and Joint Council of Allergy, Asthma, and Immunology 2014.
2. Sabroe RA, Lawler F, Grattan CEH, Ardern-Jones MR, Bewley A, Campbell L, et al. Guidelines for the management of people with chronic urticarial. Br J Dermatol. 2022;186:398-413.

Uticaria Totally Refractory to Antihistamines: Algorithm

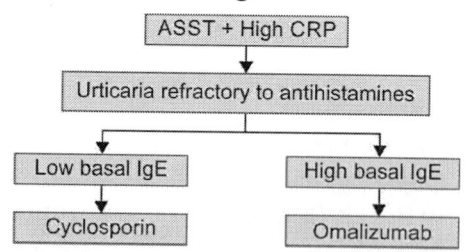

Source: Sanchez-Borges M, Ansotegui IJ, Baiardini I, Bernstein J, Canonica GW, Ebisawa M, et al. The challenge of chronic utricaria part 1: Epidemiology, immunopathogenesis, comorbidities, quality of life, and management. World Allergy Organ J. 2021;14(6): 1005-33.

> **PRACTICAL HINTS**
> 1. Each and every urticaria case demands individualized assessment and management.
> 2. Before starting systemic corticosteroids in acute urticaria especially in children one should exclude any underlying infection.
> 3. No treatment would be ever successful in any treatment of urticaria until the precipitating factors are identified and withdrawn. In fact, many chronic spontaneous urticaria are indeed not idiopathic one. Even in established cases of autoimmune urticaria strict avoidance of NSAIDs are very much rewarding in many cases.

VASCULITIS

Initial evaluation should pinpoint the caliber of the predominantly involved blood vessel and the level of systemic involvement. Mainly the small vessel vasculitis group involving skin with or without systemic involvement is managed by dermatologist. There is no consensus management protocol. Following are the options:

A. For cutaneous involvement only:
   1. *General measures:*
      a. Bed rest
      b. Avoidance of cold and prolong standing.
      c. *Cause elimination:* Withdrawal of suspected drug and treatment of infective focus.
   2. *Pharmacological therapy*
      a. H1 antihistamines
      b. Nonsteroidal anti-inflammatory drugs
      c. Colchicine
      d. Hydroxy chloroquine
      e. Pentoxifylline
      f. Dapsone
   3. If no improvement, following drugs may be introduced.
      a. Systemic corticosteroid
      b. Mycophenolate mofetil
      c. Azathioprine
      d. Methotrexate
      e. Cyclosporine
      f. Hydroxychloroquine (in urticarial vasculitis)
      g. Cyclophosphamide
      h. IVIG
      i. Plasmapheresis
   (Systemic corticosteroid is the preferred agent. Others are used in steroid unresponsive cases or when steroid needs to be stopped or reduced due to adverse effects.)
   4. For ulcerated lesion:
      a. Low dose weekly methotrexate
      b. Systemic steroid
      c. Thalidomide
B. For systemic involvement step 3 drugs may be used from the beginning.

> **PRACTICAL HINTS**
> 1. Underlying infection is to be ruled out before starting systemic immunosuppressives.
> 2. Cutaneous PAN can be treated with NSAIDs or with systemic steroids.
> 3. Hypersensitivity vasculitis is usually self-limited but irreversible damage to kidney may take place.

VIRAL WARTS

1. *Keratolytics:* 5 to 20% salicylic acid, or 17% salicylic acid, 17% lactic acid in flexible collodion
2. *Chemical cautery:* 60 to 80% trichloroacetic acid (TCA)
3. Light electrodessication and curettage
4. Cryosurgery with liquid nitrogen
5. CO_2 laser or pulsed dye laser
6. *Imiquimod:* Not much studied.

> **PRACTICAL HINTS**
> 1. Combined approach is more effective in refractory cases than monotherapy.
> 2. Before doing any destructive procedure all attempts should be taken to minimize scar. Patient's counseling is important for this regard.
> 3. In children, conservative treatment is to be undertaken with reassurance to the patients, otherwise deep permanent scar may ensue.

> 2. Before diagnosing idiopathic vitiligo appropriate history taking and clinical examination should be done to rule out chemical leukoderma. In case of chemical leukoderma therapy regimen would be of same line with that of idiopathic vitiligo. However, strict avoidance of contributing chemicals should be done to prevent further progress of the lesions and for adequate control over the disease.

VITILIGO

Limited Area

1. Topical corticosteroids (class 3)
2. Topical tacrolimus/pimecrolimus especially in facial lesions
3. Topical ruxolitinib
4. Targeted phototherapy
5. Topical paint PUVA/PUVAsol
6. Topical bath PUVA
7. UVB NB or PUVA in refractory lesions
8. Skin grafting in stable, nonresponding localized lesions
9. Covermark.

Extensive Area

1. UVB NB or PUVA
2. Short course of systemic steroids: Only in rapidly spreading vitiligo in younger age group
3. Sunscreen.

> **PRACTICAL HINTS**
> 1. Provoking factors like sun exposure, recurrent herpes labialis should be properly taken care of.

Vitiligo Surgery

Surgical interventions are an alternative therapeutic option in patients with stable vitiligo that is resistant to conventional medical approaches.

Patient Selection

- Age of patient: Younger patients tend to have more effective repigmentation
- Patient expectations: Proper counselling
- Disease stability: No new lesions and no progression of existing lesions for atleast 2 years
- Size and location of the vitiligo patch
- The proposed method of surgery
- Proposed donor site

Poor Candidates

- Significant fingertip involvement
- Periorificial distribution
- Acrofacial distribution
- Isolated scalp leukotrichia
- Patients who are not concerned with their vitiligo
- Unrealistic expectations toward results

Types of Surgery

Types of surgery	Prospects	Constraints
MKTP (melanocyte keratinocyte transplant procedure) (non-cultured)	Large, irregular areas can be treated. 84% repigmentation	Requires specialized training, personnel and equipment
Cultured melanocyte transplantation	Large, irregular areas are treated. 75–84% repigmentation	• Requires increased time for culture, special and training, personnel and equipment • Risk of melanoma
Punch grafting	Readily available, does not require additional equipment or training 75–84% repigmentation	Poor cosmetic effect (cobblestoning), typically needs adjuvant UV treatment
Blister grafting	Readily available, good color matching/cosmetic result 80–91% repigmentation	• Time consuming (5 hours for blister formation alone) • Painful
Split thickness grafting	Treat large areas 87% repigmentation	Milia formation at recipient site (poor cosmetic effect)

MKTP (Melanocyte Keratinocyte Transplant Procedure)

MKTP is a non-cultured cellular grafting technique.

- Appears to be the most effective procedure in stable/segmental vitiligo
- It is an autologous transplantation of epidermal cells from normal skin to depigmented skin

Important Steps in MKTP

1. Donor site is prepared by split thickness skin graft
2. At the recipient site CO_2 laser or dermabrasion is done until pin point bleeding occurs
3. Epidermal cells separated from dermis by trypsinization to form a cell suspension
4. Cell suspension spread topically on dermabraded skin

Repigmentation can be seen as early as 2 weeks, but typically in the first 2 months

Maximum time for repigmentation:
- Is within 18 months
- No additional surgery is recommended for the vitiliginous lesions within this period

Follow-up adjuvant therapies may be needed:
- UV treatment (sunlight, NB-UVB, excimer)
- Topical corticosteroids/calcineurin inhibitors
- Oral minipulse with dexamethasone/betamethasone
- Antioxidants

CHAPTER 2

Systemic Drugs

SYSTEMIC CORTICOSTEROIDS

Glucocorticoids are the cornerstone of dermatological therapy because of their anti-inflammatory and immunosuppressive properties. They have a basic four ring structure of cholesterol with one pentane and three hexane rings. Systemic steroids are synthetic derivatives of natural steroid cortisol, produced by adrenal glands. Different systemic steroids have different potencies, glucocorticoid and mineralocorticoid actions and duration of action.

Classification

	Glucocortico-steroid potency	Mineraloco-rticoid potency	HPA Suppression	Span of action (in hours)	Plasma half-life (in minutes)	Glucocortico-idequivalent dose (mg)
Short-acting						
Cortisone	0.8	0.8		8–12	80–118	25
Hydrocortisone	1	1	1	8–12	90	20
Intermediate-acting						
Prednisone	4	0.25	4	24–36	60	5
Prednisolone	4	0.25		24–36	115–200	5
Methylprednisolone	5	0	4	24–36	180	4
Triamcinolone	5	0	4	24–36	78–188	4
Long-acting						
Dexamethasone	25–30	0	17	36–54	100–300	0.75
Betamethasone	25–40	0		36–54	100–300	0.6

Indications

Autoimmune bullous dermatosis
- Pemphigus vulgaris
- Bullous pemphigoid
- Cicatricial pemphigoid
- Gestational pemphigoid
- Linear IgA bullous dermatosis
- Epidermolysis bullosa acquisita
- Erythema multiforme major
- Controversial use—Stevens–Johnson syndrome/toxic epidermal necrolysis

Autoimmune connective tissue disorders
- Lupus erythematosus
- Dermatomyositis
- Mixed connective tissue disorders
- Eosinophilic fasciitis
- Relapsing polychondritis
- Systemic sclerosis (selective cases)
- Morphea (generalized)

Vasculitis
- Cutaneous
- Systemic

Neutrophilic dermatosis
- Pyoderma gangrenosum
- Sweet syndrome
- Behcet's disease

Dermatitis
- Contact dermatitis
- Atopic dermatitis (flare)
- Photodermatitis
- Exfoliative erythroderma

Papulosquamous disorders
- Lichen planus

Miscellaneous
- Type 1 and type 2 reactions in leprosy
- Sarcoidosis
- Severe urticaria/angioedema
- DRESS

- Arthropod bites
- Androgen excess (hirsuitism/recalcitrant acne vulgaris)
- Postherpetic neuralgia prevention (controversial use)

Oral mini pulse
- Vitiligo Alopecia areata (progressive with >50% scalp involvement)
- Lichen planus

Intramuscular corticosteroid indications
- Dermatitis: contact dermatitis, nummular eczema
- Papulosquamous disorders: lichen planus
- Urticaria
- Prurigo nodularis

Intralesional injections indications
- Alopecia areata
- Granulomatous cheilitis
- Granuloma annulare
- Hemangiomas
- Hypertrophic lichen planus
- Keloid
- Lichen sclerosus
- Lichen simplex chronicus
- Nodular scabies
- Nodulocystic acne
- Prurigo nodularis

Intravenous pulse therapy indications
- Autoimmune bullous disorders: Pemphigus vulgaris, bullous pemphigoid
- Neutrophilic dermatosis: Pyoderma gangrenosum, sweet syndrome
- Systemic vasculitis

Mechanism of Action

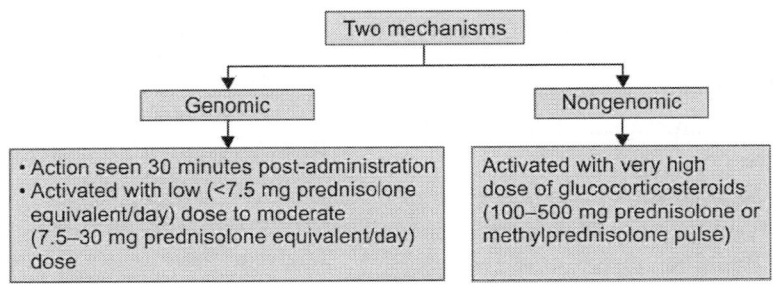

Genomic Mechanism

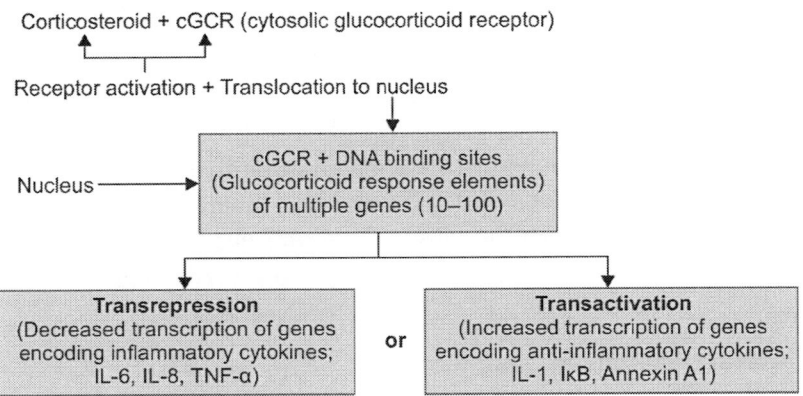

Nongenomic Mechanism

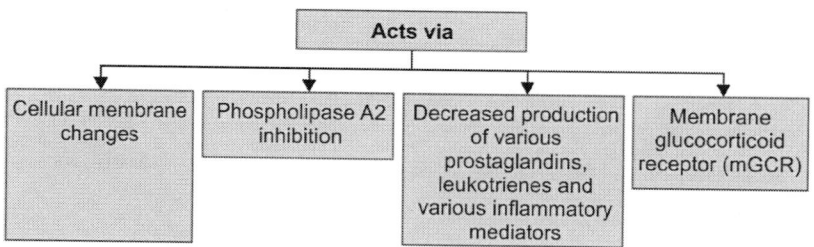

Additional Mechanism of Action

Angiogenic effects: Causes vasoconstriction, decreases angiogenesis and permeability.

Dosage

- Intralesional: 10–40 mg/mL triamcinolone once every 3–4 weekly, methyl prednisolone (depot) 10 mg every 4–8 weeks, hydrocortisone (depot) 25 mg every 4 weeks.
- Intramuscular: 10–40 mg/mL triamcinolone deep IM; longer acting agents like triamcinolone acetonide and methylprednisolone acetate (40–160 mg) to be used 4–6 times/year, chances of HPA axis suppression is high.
- Oral: 2.5 to >100 mg of prednisolone of equivalent. In majority of dermatological disorders an initial dose of 40–60 mg/day in average weight adults or 1 mg/kg/day in children is effective.
- Oral minipulse: Betamethasone or dexamethasone 5 mg as single dose on two consecutive days per week.
- Intravenous and pulse therapy: Methylprednisolone being highly potent with low sodium retaining activity is preferred as pulse therapy in a dose of 500 mg–1 g daily over 2 hours for 1–5 days. Dexamethasone 100 mg IV on 3 consecutive days is also used.

Monitoring

Baseline Checklist (planning for long-term therapy).

History
- Family history of diabetes, hypertension, dyslipidemia, heart disease
- Vaccination history (hepatitis A, B, influenza, tetanus toxoid, varicella zoster, HPV, *Streptococcus pneumoniae*)
- Examination
- BP and body weight measurement
- Eye examination for cataract
- Height and weight plotted on growth chart for children

Laboratory investigations
- Tuberculosis screening: Mantoux test, chest X-ray, interferon-γ-releasing assay
- Triple serology: Hepatitis B, C, HIV
- Fasting blood sugar, HbA1c
- Triglycerides
- Potassium levels
- Measurement of bone density

Follow-up (at 1 month and every 2–3 months)
- Body weight and BP measurements
- Height and weight on growth curve for children
- Eye check up in every 6 months

Laboratory investigations (at 1 month and every 3–4 months)
- Serum electrolytes (mainly potassium)
- Blood sugar (fasting)
- Triglycerides
  - Before stopping therapy: Cortisol levels (AM)

Adverse Effect

Short Term

- Acneiform eruptions
- Increased risk of infections
- Impaired wound healing
- Gastrointestinal intolerance
- Increased appetite, weight gain
- Fluid/sodium retention/hypokalemia
- Hyperglycemia
- Mood fluctuations, anxiety, insomnia
- Muscle weakness
- Amenorrhea

Long Term

Cutaneous

- Atrophy, striae, telangiectasia
- Vascular fragility, purpura Infections
- Acne, acneiform eruptions
- Cutaneous infections (Staphylococcal, herpes)
- Hirsutism

Musculoskeletal

- Osteoporosis
- Osteonecrosis (most common site: proximal femur, used for at least 6–12 months may lead to development)
- Muscle atrophy
- Myopathy
- Growth retardation

Ophthalmologic

- Cataracts
- Glaucoma
- Hemorrhage
- Exophthalmos
- Infection

Gastrointestinal

- Nausea
- Vomiting
- Gastroesophageal reflux
- Peptic ulcer disease
- Intestinal perforation
- Pancreatitis
- Fatty liver changes

Metabolic

- Hyperglycemia
- Hypertension
- Hypokalemia
- Weight gain/obesity/cushingoid changes
- Hypertriglyceridemia
- Hypocalcemia

Neuropsychiatric

- Peripheral neuropathy
- Seizures
- Pseudotumor cerebri
- Epidural lipomatosis
- Mood changes (euphoria/irritability/mania/depression)
- Steroid phobia

Cardiovascular

- Hypertension
- Atherosclerosis
- Peripheral edema

Gynecological

- Amenorrhea

Hematologic

- Leukocytosis
- Eosinopenia
- Lymphopenia

Infections

- Tuberculosis reactivation
- Opportunistic—deep fungal
- Prolonged herpes virus infections

Endocrinal

- HPA axis suppression:
  - Steroid withdrawal syndrome
  - Addisonian crisis.

Pulse IV Therapy

- Cardiac arrhythmia
- Seizures
- Electrolyte abnormality

Intramuscular Therapy
- At injection site: Pain, bleeding, subcutaneous fat atrophy, cold abscess, crystal deposition
- Others: purpura, menstrual abnormalities

Intralesional Therapy
- Immediate: Pain, bleeding, infection (rarely abscess).
- Subsequent: Atrophy, telangiectasia, hypopigmentation, hypertrichosis, stellate pseudoscars, secondary infection.

High risk patients for glucocorticoid toxicity
- Female patients, postmenopausal women and elderly.
- Children
- Patients of autoimmune connective tissue disorders like SLE, dermato/polymyositis, rheumatoid arthritis.
- Liver disorders
- Hypoalbuminemia
- Smokers and alcoholics

Drug Interactions

- Antidiabetics (insulin and oral hypoglycemics): Increase in blood sugar level.
- NSAIDs: Risk of peptic ulcer disease and GI hemorrhage is increased.
- Immunosuppressives (biologics, JAK inhibitors, conventional immunosuppressives like azathioprine, cyclosporine, mycophenolate): Chance of severe infections, myelosuppression.
- Anticoagulants: Anticoagulant effect of warfarin increased.
- Potassium losing diuretics (loop diuretics, thiazides) and inotropic agents (digoxin): Increased risk of hypokalemia.
- Macrolides and azole antifungals: Increase corticosteroid levels through CYP 3A4 inhibition.
- Hormonal contraceptives: CYP3A4 substrates and increase corticosteroid levels.

Drugs reducing corticosteroid levels:
- Rifampicin, phenytoin, carbamazepine, phenobarbital (by induction of CYP3A4)
- Isoniazid
- Cholestyramine: By decreasing absorption

Contraindications

Absolute
- Hypersensitivity
- Herpes simplex keratitis
- Systemic fungal infections

Caution
- Cardiovascular: Hypertension, congestive heart failure, fluid overload
- Psychiatric: Prior psychosis, severe depression
- Infections: Tuberculosis, viral and other active infections
- GI: Peptic ulcer disease, inflammatory bowel disease, diverticulitis
- Musculoskeletal: Osteoporosis, myopathy
- Metabolic: Diabetes mellitus
- Ocular: Cataract, glaucoma
- Vaccinations: Live vaccines to be avoided for at least 1 month in patients receiving high dose of glucocorticoids (prednisolone ≥20 mg or dose equivalent of ≥2 mg/kg body weight in children weighing <10 kg) for >2 weeks. Inactive vaccines can be given 2 weeks prior to starting steroids.

Hypothalamic-Pituitary-Adrenal Axis Suppression and Corticosteroid Tapering
- Basal daily cortisol secretion by adrenal cortex is 20–30 mg/day which is equivalent to about 5–7.5 mg prednisolone daily.
- Dose and duration of glucocorticoid therapy determines the susceptibility to HPA-axis suppression. Doses substantially exceeding the physiological levels for more than 3 weeks can cause mild HPA-axis suppression.
- Chances of HPA-axis suppression is more with long-acting preparations than with short or intermediate acting ones.

- Systemic corticosteroid therapy should continue during periods of stress like trauma, surgery or infection with higher doses needed for up to 3 days during acute stress to avoid acute adrenal crisis.
- Morning cortisol levels may need 6–9 months to return to normal following stoppage of long-term high dose corticosteroid therapy, however, the hypothalamus recovers within 14–30 days.
- Tapering of corticosteroids is essential to help the HPA-axis to recover promptly.
- Tapering schedule for GC when used for > 3–4 weeks

Prednisolone (or equivalent)
- >40 mg/d: reduce 5–10 mg weekly
- 20–40 mg/d: reduce 5 mg weekly
- 10–20 mg/d: reduce by 2.5 mg weekly
- 5–10 mg/d: reduce by 1 mg every 2–3 weeks
- Monitoring of disease activity is essential along with attempts at steroid tapering.

Pregnancy: Category C.

Lactation
- Safe, though small amounts excreted in breast milk doses up to 40 mg/day rarely cause systemic effects in infants.

Children
- Long-term steroid use can lead to growth suppression in children.
- Normal growth in children with 1m2 surface area can be attained with 5 mg of prednisolone per day.

SYSTEMIC IMMUNOSUPPRESSIVE AND IMMUNOMODULATORY AGENTS

Methotrexate

Methotrexate, remains one of the most common anti-metabolite, cytotoxic agents used in dermatology. It has both immunosuppressive and anti-proliferative properties. Structurally it is 4-amino-N^{10}-methylpteroylglutamic acid.

Indications

Approved Indication (FDA)
- Severe psoriasis with or without psoriatic arthritis.
- Sezary syndrome

Unlicensed Indications

Papulosquamous disorders
- Pityriasis rubra pilaris
- Pityriasis lichenoides et varioliformis acuta
- Lichen planus

Immunobullous disorders
- Pemphigus vulgaris
- Bullous pemphigoid
- Mucous membrane pemphigoid
- Epidermolysis bullosa acquisita

Autoimmune connective tissue disorders
- Systemic lupus erythematosus
- Subcutaneous lupus erythematosus
- Dermatomyositis
- Systemic sclerosis
- Morphea

Vasculitis
- Cutaneous small vessel vasculitis
- Cutaneous polyarteritis nodosa
- Kawasaki disease
- Behcet disease

Neutrophilic dermatoses
- Pyoderma gangrenosum

Lymphoproliferative disorders
- Cutaneous T cell lymphoma
- Mycoses fungoides
- Lymphomatoid papulosis

Dermatitis
- Atopic dermatitis

Miscellaneous
- Alopecia areata
- Chronic idiopathic urticaria

- Cutaneous Crohn disease
- Generalized granuloma annulare
- Hailey-Hailey disease
- Keratoacanthoma
- Langerhans cell histiocytosis
- Necrobiosis lipoidica
- Prurigo nodularis
- Reiter disease
- Sarcoidosis
- Scleredema diabeticorum

Pharmacology

Methotrexate is a weak organic acid and can be administered orally, intramuscularly, intravenously and subcutaneously. Mean oral bioavailability is 33% with intramuscular bioavailability around 76%. Milk based food intake can reduce bioavailability in children, though not in adults. It is excreted mainly through kidneys with a terminal half-life of 3–10 hours. Methotrexate is a slow acting drug with full clinical benefit seen in 2–3 months.

Mechanism of Action

- Cytotoxic effects: It competitively inhibits the enzyme dihydrofolate reductase hampering the formation of cofactor tetrahydrofolate. This prevents the synthesis of thymidylate and purine nucleotides need for both DNA and RNA synthesis. A delayed effect occurring 24 hours after methotrexate administration is the partially reversible, competitive inhibition of thymidylate synthetase. The net result is inhibition of the S phase of cell division.
- Immunosuppressive effects: Mediated through DNA synthesis inhibition in immunologically competent cells.
- Anti-inflammatory effects: Inhibition of conversion of AICAR (5-aminoimidazole 4-carboxamide ribonucleotide) to formyl-AICAR by methotrexate results in its intracellular accumulation. This increases local tissue concentration of anti-inflammatory adenosine, which reduces pro-inflammatory cytokines like TNF-α, IL-6,8 and decreases reactive oxygen species. Methotrexate also inhibits methionine synthase, thus decreasing pro inflammatory S-adenyl methionine.

Dosage

- Oral: 7.5–25 mg PO weekly as single dose
- Weinstein Frost regimen: 2.5–7.5 mg every 12 hourly for three doses weekly (8 AM and 8 PM on 1st day and 8 AM on 2nd day).
- Both dosing regimens are equally effective, however split dosing may lessen GI side effects.
- Parenteral: 10–25 mg IM or IV once weekly. 7.5–30 mg in pre pen filled devices are used for subcutaneous injections.

The initial starting dose depends on the patients age, renal function and associated comorbidities. An initial test dose of 2.5–5 mg is given in elderly and patients with renal impairment with a complete blood count and liver function test done after 1 week for early detection of myelosuppression and hepatic injury. In low-risk patients an initial starting dose of 10–15 mg weekly with gradual increments of 2.5 to 5 mg every 2–4 weeks until 25 mg weekly dose is reached with minimal toxicity.

Switching from oral to parenteral route can result in increased bioavailability of the drug, so adequate dose reduction with monitoring of blood parameters for 2 weeks after switching is preferable.

Monitoring

Baseline laboratory monitoring
- CBC with platelet count
- LFT
- Serology for Hep B, C and HIV

- BUN and creatinine
- TB quantiferon gold
- Pregnancy test for women of child bearing potential
- Chest X-ray.

During Therapy

- CBC, platelet count and LFT-1-3 weeks after initiation and after each dose escalation, then monthly for 2-4 months, and then every 3-4 months, if stable.
- Renal function tests: Once or twice yearly
- Fibroscan along with LFT are the primary screening test to assess Methotrexate induced liver injury in patients on long term therapy. Fibroscan is done 1 year after start of therapy and then repeated yearly.
- Other noninvasive test to detect liver fibrosis include NASH Fibrosure, procollagen III, fibrosis 4 (FIB-4), fibrospect II, fibrometer, hepatic USG and Magnetic resonance elastography.
- Liver biopsy, though considered gold standard is rarely needed after 3.5-4 g of cumulative dosage.
- In male patients serum ferritin to exclude hemochromatosis and antimitochondrial antibodies in females to rule out primary biliary cirrhosis.

Risk Factors for Patients Developing Hepatotoxicity on Methotrexate

- Persistent deranged LFT
- History of chronic hepatitis B or C or other liver disease
- Past or present history of excessive alcohol intake
- Family history of inheritable liver disease
- Obesity
- Diabetes mellitus
- Hyperlipidemia
- History of intake of hepatotoxic drugs and chemicals
- No folate supplementation

Adverse Effect

- Hematologic: Bone marrow suppression is the most important acute adverse effect. Leucocyte and platelet counts are reduced maximally within 7-10 days after starting treatment. The main risk factors for pancytopenia are old age, patients with renal disorders, hypoalbuminemia(<3 g/dL), lack of folate supplementation and simultaneous administration of drugs like NSAIDs and trimethoprim-sulfamethoxazole. Folic acid supplementation (1-5 mg/d) helps in preventing myelosuppression. If WBC count is <3,500/mm^3 and platelet count is <1 lakh/mm^3 dose reduction or discontinuation of methotrexate is advised with restart of treatment at lower dose after 2-3 weeks gap following correction of laboratory abnormalities.
- Hepatic effects: Hepatotoxicity with chances of liver fibrosis are significantly more with long term methotrexate therapy. Risk of liver injury is low with cumulative dose <1.5 g. Methotrexate induced liver cirrhosis risk varies between 0-25%. Dose of the drug needs to be reduced if transaminases exceed 2-3 fold the normal values and the drug has to be discontinued if the values are >5 times normal.
- Pulmonary effects: Acute pneumonitis and pulmonary fibrosis, pulmonary toxicity is idiosyncratic.
- GIT effects: Anorexia, nausea, vomiting, diarrhea and ulcerative stomatitis. Ulcerative stomatitis and severe diarrhea need stoppage of treatment. Folate supplementation reduces GI side effects without compromising the efficacy.
- Mucocutaneous effects: Oral ulceration, stomatitis, cutaneous ulceration over lower legs may indicate myelosuppression. Rapid ulceration of methotrexate treated psoriatic plaques also suggest toxicity.

- Methotrexate 'recall reaction' may occur at sites of prior irradiation or recent sunburn. Mild alopecia, acral erythema, epidermal necrosis and vasculitis are other cutaneous side effects.
- Carcinogenic effects: Lymphoma and lymphoproliferative disorders rarely reported, though no statistical evidence of increased risk of malignancy seen with methotrexate use in dermatological disorders.
- Reproductive effects: Category X drug and is to be strictly avoided in pregnancy. Women of reproductive age group should use the drug with proper birth control measures. Men can show reversible oligospermia and should avoid impregnating a woman while on methotrexate. Men are to wait 3 months after stopping the drug and women 1 complete menstrual cycle before attempting conception.
- Opportunistic infections: Pneumocystis pneumonia, histoplasmosis and cryptococcosis have been reported.
- Antidote for Methotrexate toxicity: Leucovorin is the reduced active form of folic acid. Leucovorin is particularly effective in preventing myelosuppression, gastrointestinal toxicity, and neurotoxicity during methotrexate treatment. Leucovorin dose for methotrexate overdose is 10 mg/m^2 orally, IM, or IV every 6 hours, starting immediately after overdose or within 24 hours if delayed methotrexate elimination.

Drug Interactions

- Drugs increasing methotrexate levels and toxicity: Aromatic anticonvulsants (phenytoin), tetracyclines, antipsychotics (phenothiazines), anti-inflammatory drugs (aspirin, NSAIDs), loop diuretics (furosemide), and antiplatelet drugs (dipyridamole).
- Drugs decreasing methotrexate absorption and thus efficacy: Cholestyramine.
- Drugs increasing risk of hepatotoxicity: Retinoids, alcohol.
- Drugs increasing hematologic toxicity: Dapsone, sulfonamides, trimethoprim, cidofovir, zidovudine, azathioprine.
- Immunosuppressives (biologics, JAK inhibitors, conventional immunosuppressants): Increase risk of infections and/or myelosuppression.

Contraindications

Absolute
- Hypersensitivity to methotrexate or components of formulation
- Pregnancy (category X)
- Lactation
- Myelosuppression

Relative
- Renal/hepatic dysfunction
- H/O alcoholism
- Hematological disorders
- Active infection and/or reactivation of infection (tuberculosis)
- Diabetes mellitus
- Obesity
- Recent vaccination with a live vaccine
- HIV infection
- Men and women wanting to conceive.

Pregnancy Category
- Category X

Lactation Category
- Absolutely contraindicated as excreted in breast milk.

Children
Children: Used off label in children with initial dose of 0.2 mg/kg once weekly which can be increased to 0.5 mg/kg (max 25 mg) according to clinical response.

CYCLOSPORINE

Cyclosporine or cyclosporine A (CsA) is a lipophilic and highly hydrophilic cyclic undecapeptide of 11 amino acids, isolated from the soil fungus *Tolypocladium inflatum gams*. Its immunosuppressive properties had been first used in organ transplant recipients to prevent rejection. Subsequently it has been used as an immunomodulator in a number of dermatological disorders.

Indications

Approved indications
- Psoriasis (as intermittent short-term therapy, or rescue therapy for severe flare ups and long term maintenance therapy).
- Severe Atopic dermatitis (adults and children >2 years of age).

Unlicensed indications
- Neutrophilic dermatoses: Pyoderma gangrenosum, Behcet disease
- Chronic idiopathic urticaria (especially auto-immune urticaria)
- Severe adverse cutaneous drug reactions – Stevens-Johnson Syndrome (SJS)/Toxic epidermal necrolysis (TEN)
- Bullous disorders – Pemphigus and its variants, bullous pemphigoid, linear IgA bullous dermatosis, epidermolysis bullosa acquisita.
- Autoimmune connective tissue disorders – Dermatomyositis, SLE, scleroderma
- Papulosquamous disorders – Lichen planus, lichen planopilaris, pityriasis rubra pilaris.
- Granulomatous dermatoses – Granuloma annulare, sarcoidosis
- Alopecia areata
- Photosensitivity dermatoses – Chronic actinic dermatitis
- Prurigo nodularis
- Chronic graft versus host disease.

Mechanism of Action

Cyclosporine + cyclophilin (intracytoplasmic immunophilin) = Cyclosporine-cyclophilin complex

Cyclosporine-cyclophilin complex + calcineurin (calcium dependent serine/threonine phosphatase) inhibits

↓

Dephosphorylation of nuclear factor of activated T cells (NFAT-1).

Calcineurin inhibition by cyclosporin thus leads to reduced action of transcription factor NFAT-1, blocking the production of pro-inflammatory cytokines, and chemokines like interleukin2(IL 2),IL4, interferon γ (IFN-γ), tumour necrosis factor α (TNF-α).

Pharmacology

Absorption of cyclosporine following oral administration depends on the formulation used and patient specific characteristics. The bioavailability of the microemulsion form is 10–54% more than the original non-emulsified form.

The microemulsion form has shown a more rapid response, higher remission rates in the first 8 weeks, and a 10% lower dose to maintain efficacy compared to the nonemulsified formulation.

Peak plasma concentrations occur 2–4 hours after administration and higher serum concentration of cyclosporine is produced when the drug is administered before meals.

Cyclosporine is metabolized by hepatic cytochrome P450 3A4 enzyme (CYP3A4). The elimination half-life is 6–18 hours with more than 90% of the drug undergoing biliary excretion with only 6% being eliminated through urine.

Monitoring

Baseline monitoring

Complete history and physical examination to rule out active infections, hypertension, kidney disease, and malignancy are needed before initiating therapy. Two baseline blood pressure measurements at least a day apart should also be done

Baseline screening	Follow up monitoring
• Two serum creatinine levels at least 1 day apart • CBC with platelet count • Blood urea nitrogen • Electrolytes – potassium, magnesium • Uric acid • Urinalysis with microscopy • Liver function test • Fasting lipid profile	• Blood pressure must be monitored every 2 weeks for first 3 months and if stable then monthly. • CBC with platelet counts at 1 month, then every 2–4 months • Blood urea nitrogen, creatinine, magnesium, potassium-every 2 weeks for 1–2 months, then monthly or every 3 months if stable • LFT – monthly • Urinalysis with microscopy-every monthly if abnormal, otherwise yearly • Fasting lipid profile every 2–4 weeks for 1–2 months, then every 3 months if stable

Dosage

In adults for dermatological indications cyclosporine is used in doses between 2.5–5 mg/kg/day and the pediatric dose is 5–7 mg/kg/d.

Continuous use for up to 1 year is recommended by FDA while worldwide consensus guidelines recommend continuous use for up to 2 years.

Ideal body weight should be used to calculate dosage in obese patients as dose calculations based on actual body weight can lead to excessive dosage.

If serum creatinine remains raised by >30% of baseline over 2 weeks then dose of cyclosporine is to be lowered by 1 mg/kg/d for at least 1 month. If creatinine decreases to <30% above baseline then continue cyclosporine at new dosage. Creatinine persisting above 30% of baseline still, then cyclosporine needs to be stopped. Cyclosporine can be restarted at lower dosage if creatinine returns to within 10% of baseline.

Adverse Effect

Renal

- Nephrotoxicity is one of the most important adverse effects of cyclosporine and renal dysfunction occurs in 25% of patients
- 2 types: 1st type-within 2-3 weeks of starting the drug and is associated with reduced glomerular filtration rate along with hypertension and tubular dysfunction, reversible.
- 2nd type-subclinical chronic nephrotoxicity, irreversible, seen with long term use >6 months.
- Cardiovascular
- Hypertension is usually mild and reversible after dose reduction or discontinuation of cyclosporine.
- Neurologic – most common adverse effects in patients using cyclosporine for less than 2 months.
- Headache, tremor, confusion, paresthesia, hyperesthesia, seizures, psychosis, Pseudotumour cerebri.[12]
- Gastrointestinal: nausea, vomiting, diarrhea, anorexia.
- Mucocutaneous: hypertrichosis (seen in all patients on long term use), gum hypertrophy (>70% patients, more in children), acneiform eruptions, Keratosis pilaris, sebaceous hyperplasia, warts and epidermal inclusion cysts.
- Musculoskeletal: myalgia, lethargy, arthralgia, myopathy in transplant patients on higher doses, osteoporosis.
- Abnormalities in laboratory parameters: hyperkalemia, hypomagnesemia, hyperuricemia, hyperlipidemia, hyperbilirubinemia (rare).

- Malignancy risk: increased risk of malignancies including lymphoma and skin cancers including squamous cell carcinoma, basal cell carcinoma, Kaposi sarcoma and human papilloma virus associated anogenital carcinoma. The risk is more in transplant patients on higher doses of cyclosporine. The incidence of lymphoma is less than 0.2% in dermatology patients on cyclosporine.
- Infections: risk of serious and opportunistic infections like polyoma virus associated nephropathy and JC virus associated progressive multifocal leukoencephalopathy

Drug Interactions

- Drugs inhibiting CYP3A4 system increasing cyclosporine concentrations: Antibiotics (macrolides), Calcium channel blockers, Antifungals (Itraconazole, fluconazole), Antivirals (Ritonavir, indinavir) and Glucocorticoids, Grapefruit juice.
- Drugs stimulating CYP3A4 system decreasing cyclosporine concentrations: Antibiotics (Rifampin, rifabutin), aromatic anticonvulsants (Oxcarbazepine, phenytoin) and terbinafine.
- Drugs increasing the risk of nephrotoxicity when administered with cyclosporine:
  - Antibiotics (fluoroquinolones, aminoglycosides), antimetabolites (melphalan), antifungals (amphotericin B), anti-inflammatory (NSAIDs).
- Drug groups administered with cyclosporine can increase potassium levels:
  - ACE inhibitors, angiotensin II receptor blockers, Potassium sparing diuretics, Potassium supplements.
- Drugs whose renal clearance is affected by cyclosporine thus increasing their levels:
  - Digoxin, Statins, Prednisolone.

Contraindications/cautions

- Hypersensitivity to cyclosporine or components of the formulation (polyoxyethylated castor oil)
- Impaired renal function
- Severe hepatic dysfunction
- Uncontrolled hypertension
- Previous history of malignancy
- Radiation therapy
- Immunocompromised patient
- Active infection
- Patients on phototherapy (PUVA, UV B) as it increases the risk of skin malignancies.

Pregnancy category
- Category C.

Lactation Category
- Acceptable during lactation.
- Children
- Can be used in children with proper monitoring.

AZATHIOPRINE

It is a synthetic purine analog with immunosuppressive, anti-inflammatory and steroid sparing properties.

Indications

Approved
- Pemphigus vulgaris
- SLE
- Dermatomyositis

Unlicensed

Autoimmune bullous disorders
- Bullous pemphigoid
- Mucous membrane pemphigoid

Autoimmune connective tissue disorders
- Generalized Discoid lupus erythematosus
- Refractory subcutaneous lupus erythematosus

Dermatitis
- Atopic dermatitis
- Contact dermatitis, specially parthenium allergic contact dermatitis
- Hand dermatitis

Papulosquamous disorders
- Psoriasis
- Lichen planus (cutaneous and oral)

Vasculitis
- Leukocytoclastic vasculitis
- Wegener granulomatosis
- Polyarteritis nodosa
- Eosinophilic granulomatosis with polyangiitis
- Behcet disease

Photodermatoses
- Chronic actinic dermatitis
- Polymorphous light eruption

Miscellaneous
- Sarcoidosis
- Chronic graft versus host disease
- Persistent erythema multiforme
- Pyoderma gangrenosum

Mechanism of Action

Azathioprine, a pro drug is initially metabolized to 6-mercaptopurine, which is further anabolized by enzyme hypoxanthine-guanine phosphoribosyltransferase (HGPRT) to purine analog 6-thioguanine (6-TG).
- 6-TG inhibits DNA and RNA synthesis and repair resulting in immunosuppression.
- Affects the function of T-cells, B-cells and antigen presenting cells.
- Decreases B-cell mediated antibody production.

Pharmacology

Following oral administration >80% azathioprine is absorbed through GI tract. Peak levels are reached in less than 2 hours and the drug has a half life of 5 hours. It is a prodrug and rapidly metabolized non-enzymatically to methylnitroimidazole and 6-mercaptopurine in red blood cells. 6-mercaptopurine is further metabolized enzymatically to active metabolite 6-thioguanine. Excretion is minimal as azathioprine is practically completely metabolized.

Dose

- Empirical dose: 2–2.5 mg/kg/day in bd dose to be taken with food. It is available as 50 mg tablets.
- Dose recommendations are usually based on erythrocyte TPMT (thiopurine methyltransferase) levels.
- TPMT levels <5 U Contraindicated, 5---13.7 U Up to 0.5 mg/kg/day, 13.7---19 U 1–1.5 mg/kg/day and >19 U Up to 2.5 mg/kg/day. Initially begin with 1–2 mg/kg/day, divided BID, then increase by 0.5 mg/kg/d after 6–8 weeks till a maximum dose of 3 mg/k/d is reached.
- Therapeutic benefits are usually seen in 6–8 weeks.

Monitoring

Baseline
- Physical examination of skin and lymphoreticular system
- Laboratory: CBC with platelet count, LFT, pregnancy test for women of child bearing potential, serum electrolytes, urea, creatinine, urinalysis, Hepatitis B, C and HIV serology, tuberculin test, erythrocyte TPMT assay or TPMT gene test (thiopurine methyltransferase) For Asian and Hispanic NUDT15 (nucleotide diphosphatase) genotype testing is also recommended.

Follow up
- Annual physical examination
- Laboratory: CBC, LFT – biweekly for first 2 months, then 2–3 month intervals

Adverse Effect

- GI: nausea, vomiting, diarrhea-most common adverse effect seen within first 10 days of therapy, pancreatitis (rarely).
- Myelosuppression: serious adverse effect, leucopenia, anemia, thrombocytopenia. Drug to be stopped if WBC < 3,500–4,000 mm^3, hemoglobin < 10 g/dL and platelet count <1 lakh/mm^3.
- Hypersensitivity: idiosyncratic and occurs between 1st and 4th week of starting treatment
- Nonspecific flulike symptoms like fever, malaise, arthralgia, myalgia, headache, nausea, cutaneous manifestations like urticaria, morbilliform, vesiculopustular eruptions, erythema multiforme, Sweet syndrome and erythema nodosum has also been seen
- Malignancy risk: long term use increases the risk of malignancies like non-Hodgkin B cell lymphoma and squamous cell carcinoma of skin.
- Infection: increased risk of infections like verruca vulgaris, dermatophytosis, varicella zoster due to immunosuppression.
- Hepatitis: acute hepatic injury can be hepatocellular with raised transaminases or cholestasis with increase in bilirubin and alkaline phosphatase. Nodular regenerative hyperplasia can occur due to chronic liver injury.
- Pancreatitis: in patients of Crohn's disease.

Drug Interactions

Drugs	Effects
Xanthine oxidase inhibitors (allopurinol, febuxostat)	Increased myelosuppression (due to increase in active metabolites 6–mercaptopurine and 6–thioguanine

Continued...

Continued...

Drugs	Effects
Folate inhibitors (methotrexate, dapsone, trimethoprim, sulfamethoxazole)	Increased myelosuppression
Immunosuppressants (biologics, JAK inhibitors, cyclosporine, MMF)	Increased risk of severe infections and myelosuppression
Angiotensin converting enzyme inhibitors	Leucopenia
TNF inhibitors	Increased risk of T-cell lymphomas
Anticoagulants (warfarin)	Decrease in anticoagulant effects
Vaccines	Live – to be given 1 month before Inactivated – 2 weeks before start

Contraindications/cautions

- Hypersensitivity to azathioprine is an absolute contraindication
- Severe infection
- Very low/absent TPMT levels
- Severe hepatic dysfunction or severe myelosuppression.
- Malignancy
- Pregnancy use with caution

Pregnancy Category: D

Lactation

Compatible but breastfeeding to be done 4 hours after taking azathioprine.

Children: Can be safely used in childhood.

MYCOPHENOLATE MOFETIL

Mycophenolate mofetil is a lymphocyte specific immunosuppressive agent. It is a 2-morpholinoethyl ester of mycophenolic acid (active metabolite) and was first isolated as a fermentation product of *Penicillium stoloniferum*. Though used extensively as prophylaxis for acute organ transplant rejection in dermatology it is used as a steroid sparing agent.

Indications

Unlicensed

- Papulosquamous disorders: Psoriasis vulgaris, Lichen planus, Lichenplanopilaris.
- Dermatitis: Atopic dermatitis, Dyshidrotic eczema, Chronic actinic dermatitis.
- Autoimmune bullous disorders: Pemphigus vulgaris, pemphigus foliaceus, bullous pemphigoid, mucous membrane pemphigoid, paraneoplastic pemphigus, linear IgA bullous disease, epidermolysis bullosa acquisita.
- Autoimmune connective tissue disorders: SLE, SCLE, chronic cutaneous LE, chillblain LE, dermatomyositis, diffuse systemic sclerosis.
- Vasculitis: Wegener granulomatosis, microscopic polyangiitis, eosinophilic granulomatosis with polyangiitis, hypocomplementemic urticarial vasculitis, nodular vasculitis.
- Neutrophilic dermatosis: Pyoderma gangrenosum
- Granulomatous disorders: Sarcoidosis, cutaneous Crohn disease
- Others: Acute and chronic graft versus host disease, recurrent erythema multiforme, necrobiosis lipoidica, chronic urticaria.

Mechanism of Action

- Non competitively inhibits the type II isoform of enzyme inosine monophosphate dehydrogenase, thus preventing inosine and xanthine-5-phosphate from being converted to guanosine 5-phosphate. This prevents de novo synthesis of guanine nucleotides and its incorporation into DNA. De novo purine synthesis is affected in both T and B lymphocytes.
- Changes the expression and processing of cell surface adhesion molecules (E-selectin, VCAM-1), thus decreasing both recruitment and flow of inflammatory cells into areas of inflammation.
- Blocks antibody production by activated B lymphocytes.

Pharmacology

MMF is rapidly absorbed following oral administration and converted to Mycophenolic acid, the active metabolite by esterases in the plasma, liver, and kidney, MPA is inactivated in the liver via glucuronidation. Phenolic glucuronide of MPA (MPAG), is secreted into the bile and recycled to the liver by enterohepatic recirculation. The half-life of MPA is approximately 16 to 18 hours. More than 90% of the administered drug is excreted in the urine as MPAG.

Dosage

- 2–3 g/day in 2 divided doses
- Start with a dose of 500 mg/day at night × 1 week (minimizes GI side effects).
- From week 2: 500 mg twice daily and subsequently increased by 500 mg every 2 to 4 weeks until a maximum dose of 1.5 g twice daily (range 2–3 g daily) is reached or the patient begins to develop intolerance.
- Response to MMF takes at least 6–8 weeks
- Enteric coated Mycophenolate sodium 720 mg in BD dosage has shown similar efficacy to 1,000 mg Mycophenolate mofetil BD.

Monitoring

Baseline	Follow up
Complete physical examination	Complete physical examination every 3–6 months

Continued...

Continued...

Baseline	Follow up
Laboratory	Laboratory (every 2–4 weeks after dose escalation and every 2–3 months once dose is stable
Complete blood count with differential and platelet count	Complete blood count with differential and platelet count
Serum chemistry including creatinine	Serum chemistry including creatinine
Pregnancy test for women of child bearing potential negative test within 1 week before starting treatment and repeat test 8–10 later	Monthly pregnancy testing throughout therapy
Screening for hepatitis B, C, HIV	Liver function test
Liver function test	
Tuberculosis screening-PPD/IGRA	

Adverse Effect

- Gastrointestinal: most common-diarrhea, nausea, vomiting, abdominal cramps, anorexia (dose related).
- Taking the drug with food and BD/TDS dosing, using enteric coated mycophenolate sodium (EC_MPS) lessens GI side effects.
- Genitourinary: urgency, frequency, dysuria, sterile pyuria (these adverse effects decrease after first year of therapy).
- Infections: opportunistic infections (viral, bacterial, fungal and atypical mycobacterial) mainly drugs.
- Hematologic: anemia, leucopenia, thrombocytopenia, agranulocytosis. (dose related, reversible), pure red cell aplasia.
- Neurologic: weakness, fatigue, insomnia, dizziness, tinnitus in children mood lability.
- Mucocutaneous: Oral aphthae (in organ transplant), generalized urticaria, blistering hand dermatitis, alopecia. skin infections (varicella-zoster, tinea).
- Carcinogenicity: lymphoma and lymphoproliferative disorders (mainly in organ transplant patients).

Drug Interactions

Drugs which increase levels of MMF	Drugs which decrease levels of MMF	Drugs whose levels are decreased on coadministration with MMF
- Phenytoin - Salicylates - Xanthines - Acyclovir - Ganciclovir - Valganciclovir - Probenecid	- Cholestyramine - Antacids - Proton pump - Inhibitors - Antibacterials (β-lactams, fluoroquinolones, TMP/SMX, clindamycin, linezolid, metronidazole)	- Levonorgestrel - Nevirapine

Contraindications

Absolute
- Hypersensitivity to the drug
- Pregnancy
- Relative
- Lactation
- Peptic ulcer
- Hepatic, severe renal dysfunction, cardiopulmonary disease.

Pregnancy Category
- Category D.

Lactation
To be avoided

Children
Mycophenolate mofetil has been used safely in children ≥2 years of age.

CYCLOPHOSPHAMIDE

It is an alkylating agent derived from nitrogen mustard used both as an antineoplastic and immunosuppressive agent with steroid sparing effects.

Indications

- Approved
- Advanced stage of mycosis fungoides.
- Hemopoietic malignancies
- Unlicensed Indications

Autoimmune Bullous Disorders

- Pemphigus vulgaris and foliaceus
- Bullous pemphigoid
- Mucous membrane pemphigoid

Vasculitis

- Eosinophilic granulomatosis with polyangiitis
- Leukocytoclastic vasculitis (including Henoch-Schonlein purpura)
- Microscopic polyangiitis
- Polyarteritis nodosa
- Granulomatosis with polyangiitis
- Cryoglobulinemic vasculitis.

Autoimmune connective tissue disorders

- Dermatomyositis
- Scleroderma
- Severe SLE

Neutrophilic dermatoses

- Pyoderma gangrenosum
- Behcet disease
- Erythema elevatum diutinum

Mechanism of Action

It is a cell cycle independent cytotoxic drug whose metabolites cause cross linking of DNA strands, abnormal base-pair formation, cleavage of imidazole ring with depurination and chain split. DNA damage ultimately results in mutagenesis and cell death.

Pharmacology

Oral bioavailability of cyclophosphamide is >75% with peak plasma levels occurring within 1–2 hours. It has a half life of 5–9 hours. Cyclophosphamide is a prodrug and is metabolized by hepatic cytochrome P-450 to 4-hydroxycyclophosphamide and aldophosphamide. Aldophosphamide is broken down within the cells to cytotoxic phosphoramide mustard and acrolein. These metabolites are excreted in urine.

Dosage

- Routine therapy: Oral-1–3 mg/kg/day in single morning dose or divided doses. Patient to be well hydrated to avoid bladder toxicity.
- Pulse therapy: Monthly IV pulse therapy 500–1,000 mg (0.5–1 g/m^2) over 30 minutes to 2 hours has lesser chances of bladder toxicity.

Monitoring

- Baseline monitoring
- History and physical examination.
- Laboratory
  - CBC with platelet count
  - Liver function tests
  - Urinalysis with microscopic examination
  - Blood urea nitrogen and creatinine.
  - Pregnancy testing for females of child bearing potential.

During Therapy

- CBC, platelet count and urinalysis—weekly for 2–3 months, then biweekly after 2–3 months, then monthly after dose stabilization.
  Note: Discontinue if WBC count is < 4,000/mm3 or platelet is <100,000/m^3)
- Serum chemistry and LFT: Initially monthly, then every 3–6 months quarterly.
- Urinalysis: weekly for 2–3 months, then biweekly after 2–3 months, then monthly after dose stabilization. Urinalysis with cytologic examination is indicated when the cumulative dose exceeds 50 g, and every 6 months or on occurrence of hemorrhagic cystitis.

Adverse Effect

- GI: Nausea, vomiting, diarrhea (70–90%), anorexia, stomatitis, liver toxicity in high doses.
- Hematologic: Myelosuppression with leucopenia, thrombocypenia, anemia)
- Genitourinary: hemorrhagic cystitis (caused by acrolein metabolite, concurrent use of mesna protective), dysuria, urgency, microscopic hematuria, vesicourethral reflux, bladder fibrosis.
- Cutaneous: alopecia (anagen effluvium), diffuse hyperpigmentation of skin, nail hyperpigmentation with transverse ridging, irreversible pigmentation bands on teeth, acral erythema.
- Reproductive: azoospermia, amenorrhea, ovarian failure.

Malignancy: increased risk of bladder carcinoma, non-Hodgkin lymphoma, leukemia and squamous cell carcinoma of skin.

Drug Interactions

- Drugs increasing cyclophosphamide levels by reducing metabolism: allopurinol, ciprofloxacin, chlorpromazine, fluconazole.
- Drugs reducing cyclophosphamide levels by increasing metabolism: prednisolone, phenytoin, rifampicin, nevirapine, ondansetron.
- Coadministration of other cytotoxic drugs like chlorambucil and immunosuppressive agents like cyclosporine and azathioprine increases its myelosuppressive, immunosuppressive and carcinogenic effects.

Contraindications

Hypersensitivity to cyclophosphamide or components of formulation

- Pregnancy and lactation, severe myelosuppression
- Severe infection
- Hemorrhagic cystitis

Caution

- History of lymphoproliferative disorder.
- Hepatic and renal dysfunction (reduce dose)
- Elderly (reduce dose)

Pregnancy Category

- Category D

Lactation Category

- To be avoided.

Children

To be avoided as it may cause permanent infertility.

BLEOMYCIN

It is an antineoplastic glycopeptide antibiotic obtained from *Streptomyces verticillus*. Subtypes A2 and B2 of bleomycin are common used clinically.

Indications

Unlicensed indications in dermatology

- Intralesional injections
- Verruca vulgaris: 0.2–1 mL injected per lesion with local anesthesia, hemorrhagic eschar formation after-3 weeks indicates adequate infiltration.
- Non melanoma skin cancer: intralesional bleomycin with local electroporation.
- Cutaneous metastasis: bleomycin with local electroporation.
- Keloid and hypertrophic scars.
- Hemangioma, macrocystic lymphatic malformations: as sclerosing agent
- Corns: after callus pairing.

Mechanism of Action

- DNA-strand scissoring is its main mode of action resulting in cell cycle arrest. Its cutaneous effects include keratinocyte apoptosis, inhibition of collagen synthesis and sclerosis of endothelial cells.

- Pharmacokinetics
- It is administered IV, IM or subcutaneously due to poor oral bioavailability. Bleomycin undergoes both renal and hepatic metabolism. Half life is 2 hours with 50–70% excreted in urine.

Monitoring

- Not required for dermatological usage.

Adverse Effect

- Post intralesional injection: Local pain, burning, erythema, edema, blackening, eschar formation, pigmentary changes.
- Gangrene of fingertips, nail ridging and nail dystrophy. urticaria
- Raynaud's phenomenon
- Flagellate pigmentation
- Sclerotic tissue reactions

Drug Interaction

- Not relevant for intralesional use in dermatology.

Contraindications

- Pregnancy
- Lactation
- Peripheral vascular disease.
- H/o Raynaud's phenomenon
- Bleomycin intolerance.

Pregnancy category: D

Lactation
Avoid in lactation.

Children: Can be used.

Saturated Solution of Potassium Iodide (SSKI)

Potassium iodide(KI) has been used in treatment of various thyroid disorders and its saturated solution is indicated in the treatment of various dermatological conditions. It is prepared by adding KI to hot purified water, using sodium thiosulfate as preservative.

Indications

Unlicensed

- Fungal: Sporotrichosis-lymphocutaneous and cutaneous, subcutaneous mucormycosis.
- Panniculitis
  - Erythema nodosum
  - Nodular vasculitis
  - Subacute nodular migratory panniculitis
- Neutrophilic dermatoses: Sweet syndrome, pyoderma gangrenosum.
- Others: erythema multiforme, Granuloma annulare, granulomatous polyangitis.

Mechanism of Action

Possible immune modulator, suppresses inflammatory oxygen intermediates generation from activated polymorphonuclear neutrophils, thus inhibiting neutrophil migration and toxicity.

Dosage

- Concentration-100 mg/mL of saturated solution
- Sporotrichosis: starting dose is 5 drops (each drop containing 67 mg) 3 times daily in milk or juice. Dose increased by 3–5 drops weekly until a dose of 15 drops thrice daily is reached (maximum 50 drops tds may be needed) with resolution within 2–4 weeks. (0.3 mL = 10 drops from calibrated dropper supplied with SSKI)
- Children: 1.25–2 g (25–50 drops) tds
- Panniculitis: 900 mg/day

Adverse Effects

Dose related with long term treatment.

Cutaneous: acniform eruptions, iododerma, flare-up of dermatitis herpetiformis and pustular psoriasis, development of bullous pemphigoid

Metabolic: reversible hypothyroidism, irreversible hyperthyroidism, goiter, hyperkalemia

GI: nausea, vomiting, abdominal pain, enlarged salivary glands

Monitoring

Baseline
- Previous history of thyroid disease and assessment of thyroid gland size
- T4, TSH, antithyroglobulin and antimicrosomal antibodies
- Pregnancy test in women of childbearing age

Followup
After 1 month: TSH and annual TSH to be repeated.

Drug Interactions
- Coadministration with ACE inhibitors, potassium sparing diuretics, potassium containing medications–risk of hyperkalemia
- Coadministration with amiodarone, lithium, phenazone, sulfones – increased risk of hypothyroidism

Contraindications

Absolute
- Hypersensitivity to iodides

Relative
- Hypothyroidism
- Cardiac disease
- Renal impairment
- Hyperkalemia
- Addison disease

Pregnancy: Category D

Lactation: compatible

ANTIHISTAMINES

Drugs that neutralize the action of histamine by acting as inverse agonists of histamine receptors and downregulating their constitutive activated state.

Traditionally classified as first and second-generation antihistamines.

First Generation Antihistamines

Salient Features
- Ethers derived from imidazole ring structure of histamine.
- Lipophilic, effectively cross blood brain barrier
- Highly sedative as they block CNS stimulatory effects of histamine via H1 receptor.
- Short acting so frequent dosing needed.
- Onset of action within 1–2 hours after ingestion.
- Peak plasma concentration is reached within 2 hours and metabolized by cytochrome P-450 in liver.
- Excretion is mainly renal except diphenhydramine which has minimal renal excretion.
- No evidence of development of tolerance or tachyphylaxis.
- Promethazine and hydroxyzine are category C while the other are pregnancy category B.
- Cetirizine and loratadine can be used in lactation.

Classification of first-generation H1 antihistamines

Class	Agent
Ethanolamines	Clemastine, Carbinoxamine, Dimenhydrinate, Diphenhydramine, Doxylamine, Phenyltoloxamine
Ethylenediamines	Antazoline, Tripelennamine
Alkylamines	Chlorpheniramine, Dexchlorpheniramine, Pheniramine maleate, Triprolidine

Continued...

Continued...

Class	Agent
Piperazines	Hydroxyzine, Cyclizine, Meclizine
Piperidines	Cyproheptadine, Azatadine, Ketotifen
Phenothiazines	Promethazine
Tricyclic dibenzoxepins	Doxepin

Classification of second-generation H1 antihistamines

Class	Agent
Alkylamines	Acrivastine
Piperazines	Cetirizine, Levocetirizine
Piperidines	Loratadine, Desloratadine, Ebastine, Fexofenadine, Mizolastine, Olopatadine, Rupatadine, Bilastine
Phthalazinones	Azelastine

Second Generation H1 Antihistamines

Salient Features

- Less lipophilic and does not actively cross the blood brain barrier
- Less sedative and low potential for cognitive impairment compared to first generation antihistamines.
- Less anticholinergic effects.
- Some are active metabolites of other antihistamines (fexofenadine is an active acid metabolite of terfenadine, cetirizine and desloratadine are metabolites of hydroxyzine and loratadine respectively)
- Onset of action is within 1-2 hours following oral ingestion
- Peak plasma concentration is usually reached within 1-3 hours with cetirizine and olopatadine being fastest (30 minutes)
- Majority metabolized by liver except fexofenadine, cetirizine, levocetirizine, loratadine and mizolastine.
- Cetirizine and levocetirizine are mainly excreted through kidneys and fexofenadine via feces. Others have minimal renal elimination and so their dose adjustment is not required in kidney disorders.
- Bilastine is rapidly absorbed in fasting state and has to be administered at least 1 hour before or 2 hours after meal. Food has no effect on the absorption of cetirizine, desloratadine, ebastine, levocetirizine, mizolastine and fexofenadine.
- Cetirizine, levocetirizine, loratadine and bilastine are pregnancy category B while fexofenadine and desloratadine are category C.

Indications

H1 Antihistamines

- Acute urticaria and chronic idiopathic urticaria
- Acute allergic reactions
- Physical urticaria and dermographism
- Mastocytosis
- Pruritus secondary to:
  - Dermatological disease, e.g., lichen planus, eczema
  - Infestations
  - Medical disorders
  - Idiopathic
- Miscellaneous (other than use in urticaria and pruritus control)
- Acne
- Darier disease
- Eosinophilic fasciitis
- Eosinophilic pustular folliculitis.
- Erythromelalgia
- Generalized lichen nitidus, lichen planopilaris
- Psoriasis.

Dose

Sedating first-generation H_1 antihistamines

Group	Agent	Dosage
Ethanolamine	Diphenhydramine	25–50 mg, 4–6 hourly (adults), 6–12 years-12.5–25 mg, 4–6 hourly, <6 years– 6.25–12.5 mg, 4–6 hourly.
	Clemastine	1–2 mg BID
Ethylenediamine	Tripenelamine	25–50 mg, 4–6 hrly
Piperazine	Hydroxyzine	25–50 mg, 6–8 hourly, <6 years age-25–50 mg daily.
		50 mg HS
Alkylamine	Chlorpheniramine	2–4 mg, 4–6 hourly (adults), 6–11 years-2 mg, 4–6 hourly
Phenothiazine	Promethazine	12.5 mg TID 25 mg HS
Piperadine	Cyproheptadine	4 mg, 6–8 hourly (adults), 7–14 years-4 mg bid/tid.

Nonsedating second generation H1 antihistamines

Azelastine	2-4 mg BID (adults), 0.1% nasal spray; 6–12 years
Cetirizine	10 mg daily, 2–6 years-5 mg daily.
Levocetirizine	5 mg daily (≥ 6 years)
Ebastine	10 mg daily or BID
Fexofenadine	60–180 mg daily
Loratadine	10 mg daily (≥ 6 years)
Desloratadine	5 mg daily (≥ 12 years), 6–12 years-2.5 mg daily, 1–6 years-1.25 mg daily, 6–12 months-1 mg daily.
Mizolastine	10 mg daily (adults)

Mechanism of Action

- Inverse agonist: helps in stabilizing the inactive form of H1 receptors by reversibly binding to it.
- Decreases the proinflammatory cytokines (TNF-α, Il-1β, Il-6, IL-8), expression of cell adhesion molecules(ICAM1-intercellular adhesion molecule1, VCAM-1-vascular cellular adhesion molecule1) and chemotaxis of inflammatory cells
- Inhibit calcium ion channels and cause a reduction in mediator release from both basophils and mast cells.
- Acts on muscarinic, alpha-adrenergic, serotonin receptors.
- Second generation H1 antihistamines bind noncompetitively to H1 receptors with slow dissociation and longer duration of action.

Monitoring

- Monitoring of the adverse effects suffices in most cases.
- Liver transaminase evaluation is recommended when cyproheptadine is used.
- Patient having hepatic/renal impairment requires dose monitoring.

Adverse Effect

- Sedation: Highest with ethanoldiamine and phenothiazine, lowest with alkylamine.
- CNS effects: Dizziness, blurred vision, insomnia, tremor-seen with alkylamine group
- GI effects: Nausea, vomiting, epigastric distress, seen mainly with ethylenediamine group.
- Anticholinergic effects: Dry mouth, postural hypotension, urinary retention, glaucoma seen with ethanolamine group
- Cardiac: arrhythmias.
- Cutaneous: urticaria, petechiae, maculopapular rash, allergic contact dermatitis, fixed drug rash (cetirizine), photosensitivity.

Drug Interactions

- Chlorpheniramine, hydroxyzine, promethazine and diphenhydramine increase the level of drugs metabolized by CYP2D6, such as metoprolol and venlafaxine.
- CNS depression effects may be increased if given with alcohol and benzodiazepines.
- Phenothiazines may rarely block and reverse vasopressor effect of epinephrine.
- Antacids decrease absorption of fexofenadine
- Sedative and antimuscarinic effects of antihistamines are increased by concurrent use of antidepressants (both tricyclic and MAO inhibitors).

Contraindications

- Hypersensitivity to active drug
- Newborn or premature infants (first generation)
- Lactating mothers (first generation)
- Narrow-angle glaucoma: Use antihistamines with least anti cholinergic effects
- Elderly with benign prostatic hypertrophy (can cause urinary retention)

Caution

- Children, especially promethazine to be avoided in children < 2 years of age due to risk of respiratory depression. Children are at risk of developing insomnia and excitability due to first-generation H1 antihistamines.
- Drivers, machine operators, pilots (cause sedation).
- First trimester of pregnancy.
- Renal/hepatic compromise, ischemic heart disease, hypertension, thyroid dysfunction.

Pregnancy

Diphenhydramine, chlorpheniramine, cetirizine or loratadine can be administered in pregnancy.

H2 Antihistamines

Salient Features

- Inverse agonists bind to H2 receptors located in epithelial, endothelial, dermal dendritic cells, mast cells and white blood cells
- Involved in antigen presentation, inflammatory mediator release and also affects cutaneous vascular permeability.
- Reach peak levels 1–2 hours following ingestion with half-life between 2–3 hours. (famotidine up to 8 hours)
- Eliminated mainly through kidneys with 10–35% metabolized by liver by cytochrome P450.
- Include cimetidine, ranitidine, famotidine, nizatidine.
- Ranitidine has presently been withdrawn due to the presence of low levels of an impurity called N-nitrosodimethylamine (NDMA), a probable human carcinogen.
- Tolerance or tachyphylaxis on regular use
- Pregnancy: category B.
- Lactation: considered safe.

Indications

- Acute allergic reactions
- Chronic urticaria (second line)
- Systemic GI symptoms of mastocytosis.

Dose

Famotidine	20–40 mg bid (adults), pediatric: 1–16 years age- 1 mg/kg/day bid
Nizatidine	Age >12 years 150 mg bid

Monitoring

- CBC is warranted to rule out thrombocytopenia and anemia.
- LFT and serum creatinine: modest increase, reversible on withdrawal.

Adverse Effects

- Generally well tolerated than H1 antihistamines with few uncommon adverse effects
- CNS: confusion, dizziness, drowsiness, headache (higher plasma levels)
- GI: nausea, vomiting, diarrhea/constipation, abdominal pain, increased transaminases and rarely hepatitis.
- Gynecomastia with decreased libido, reduction in sperm count in men and galactorrhea in women with cimetidine.
- Hematologic: thrombocytopenia, anemia.
- Cutaneous: alopecia, urticarial vasculitis.

Drug Interactions

- Narcotics, β blockers, tricyclic antidepressants, SSRIs (CYP2D6 substrates): serum levels increased, can cause toxicity.
- Warfarin, theophylline, melatonin (CYP1A2 substrates): increased levels and likely to cause toxicity.
- Phenytoin, esomeprazole, thalidomide (CYP2C19 substrates): can increase drug levels and possible toxicity.
- Statins, cyclosporine, benzodiazepines, calcium channel blockers, warfarin, rifampin, dapsone (CYP3A4 substrates): drug levels are increased with more chances of toxicity.

Contraindications

Hypersensitivity to the drug or components of formulation.

ANTILEUKOTRIENES

Leukotrienes (LTs) are proinflammatory mediators derived from arachidonic acid through the 5-lipoxygenase pathway. They are of two types—cysteinyl and noncysteinyl LTs.

Montelukast and zafirlukast are cysteinyl leukotriene receptor antagonists.

Mechanism of Action

Cysteinyl leukotrienes (LTC4, LTD4, and LTE4) bind to cysteinyl leukotriene receptors (CysLT1 and CysLT2). Cysteinyl leukotriene receptors mediate bronchoconstriction, vascular permeability, eosinophil recruitment, and chronic inflammation. Montelukast and zafirlukast are antagonists to cysteinyl leukotriene CysLT1 receptors only.

Indications

Approved
Montelukast
- Chronic asthma and prophylaxis along with prevention of exercise-induced bronchoconstriction.
- Relieve seasonal and perennial allergic rhinitis symptoms.

Zafirlukast

Approved
- Chronic asthma.

Unlicensed
Dermatological indications of both montelukast and zafirlukast.
- Atopic dermatitis.
- Chronic urticaria.
- Acne vulgaris.
- Granuloma annulare.
- Bullous pemphigoid.
- Psoriasis.
- Pruritus associated with Sjogren-Larssons syndrome (SLS).

Montelukast

Pharmacokinetics

It is rapidly absorbed following oral administration with a bioavailability of 64%.

Montelkast is more than 99% bound to plasma proteins. It is metabolized in liver by CYP3A4 and 2C8 and its plasma half-life is 3–6 hours. The metabolites are excreted via bile.

Monitoring

Clinicians should monitor patients for mood or behavioral changes including suicidal thoughts and other neuropsychiatric signs.

Dose

- 10 mg single dose in the evening (≥ 15 years of age)
- 5 mg single dose (6–14 years)
- 4 mg single dose tablet or 4 mg oral granules (2–5 years)
- 4 mg oral granules (6–23 months).

Adverse Effects

- Common: upper respiratory infection, fever, headache, pharyngitis, cough, abdominal pain, diarrhea, otitis media, influenza, rhinorrhea, sinusitis, otitis.
- Neuropsychiatric: depression, aggression, suicidal ideation, insomnia, anxiety, and nightmares.
- Gastrointestinal: nausea, diarrhea, vomiting, abdominal pain, dyspepsia, pancreatitis.
- Ocular: conjunctivitis.
- Cutaneous: pruritus, eczema, atopic dermatitis, angioedema, urticaria, skin rash, bruising, erythema multiforme, erythema nodosum, toxic epidermal necrolysis, and Stevens-Johnson syndrome.
- Musculoskeletal signs: arthralgia, myalgia
- Hypersensitivity manifestations: anaphylaxis, eosinophilic infiltration of the liver.

Drug Interactions

Cytochrome P450 enzyme inducers like rifampicin and phenobarbital: decrease montelukast levels, clinical monitoring required.

Contraindications

- Hypersensitivity to the drug or any component of the formulation.
- Phenylalanine-containing formulations to be used with caution in Phenylketonuria patients.

Pregnancy: Category B.

Lactation: no special precautions required.

Children: can be safely used in infants also.

Zafirlukast

Pharmacokinetics

Zafirlukast is rapidly absorbed following oral administration reaching peak plasma concentration approximately 3 hours after the oral ingestion. Its bioavailability decreases by 40% when administered with food and so should be taken 2 hours after or 1 hour before meals.

Zafirlukast requires 2–6 weeks for optimal efficacy with an average half-life of 10 hours.

It is 99% bound to plasma proteins and is mainly metabolized by CYP2C9 enzyme in liver. Majority of the drug is excreted in feces with 10% in urine.

Monitoring

LFT: monitoring at periodic intervals to detect hepatic injury.

Dosage

20 mg bd pediatric dose (5–11 years) 10 mg bd.

Adverse Effects

- Neuropsychiatric: headache, dizziness, neuropathy, hallucinations, insomnia, depression, and abnormal dreams.
- GI: nausea, vomiting, diarrhea, dyspepsia, abdominal pain.
- Hepatic: transaminase elevation, symptomatic hepatitis, hyperbilirubinemia, fulminant hepatitis, and progressive hepatic failure.
- Musculoskeletal: myalgia, back pain, arthralgia, malaise.
- Cutaneous: alopecia, bruising, pruritus, urticaria, angioedema, and rashes.

- Hematologic: agranulocytosis, eosinophilia, thrombocytopenia.
- Reproductive: menorrhagia.
- Respiratory tract infections.

Drug Interactions

- It is a substrate and weak inhibitor of CYP2CP9.
- Warfarin: Zafirlukast increases half-life of warfarin resulting in increased international normalized ratio (INR) requiring careful monitoring of warfarin effects.
- Erythromycin and theophylline reduces mean plasma levels of zafirlukast.
- Aspirin: increases plasma levels of zafirlukast by 45%.
- Tizanidine: administered with zafirlukast could result in hypotension, potentially increasing the risk of falls and fractures.

Contraindications

- Hypersensitivity to the drug or any active or inactive (povidone, lactose, titanium dioxide, or cellulose) component of the formulation.
- In cirrhosis and hepatic impairment due to increased risk of hepatic failure.

Pregnancy Category: B

Lactation: limited data, according to international guidelines can be used during breastfeeding.

SYSTEMIC ANTIBACTERIAL AGENTS

β-lactam group includes Penicillin's, cephalosporins, monobactams, and carbapenems

First-generation (isoxazolylpenicillins)
- Natural penicillin G, penicillin V
- antimicrobial spectrum against Gram positive cocci and rods, Gram-negative cocci, and anaerobes

Second-generation agents (aminopenicillins)
Also effective against Gram-negative bacilli.

Third generation: extended-spectrum penicillins (carboxypenicillins)

Fourth generation: penicillins (ureidopenicillins) are both parenteral and exhibit antipseudomonal activity

Indication

Antibacterial Indications

- Staphylococcal and Streptococcal Infections
- extensive impetigo and ecthyma,
- Early stages of erysipelas
- Empiric therapy of SSSS should include a penicillinase resistant penicillin in combination with clindamycin, while awaiting culture results

Sexually Transmitted Diseases

Syphilis and chlamydial infections

Others

Erysipeloid, scarlatina, cutaneous anthrax, Lyme disease, actinomycosis, lis teriosis, gas gangrene, gingivostomatosis, and leptospirosis (Weil disease)

Mechanism of Action

1. Attachment to specific penicillin-binding proteins (which vary in their affinities for different β-lactam antibiotics);
2. Inhibition of bacterial cell wall peptidoglycan synthesis; and
3. Disinhibition of cell wall autolysis.

Pharmacology

- Gastrointestinal (GI) absorption can be optimized by administration 1 hour before or after a meal.
- The elimination half-lives for most penicillins are short (<1.5 hours).

Adverse Effects

- Hypersensitivity reactions–including urticaria, morbilliform eruptions, anaphylaxis.
- Cross-reaction potential

Drug Interactions

- Probenecid blocks the secretion of penicillins in the distal renal tubules, so, concomitant administration of these two drugs increases the serum levels and duration of action of the penicillins.
- When amoxicillin or ampicillin is used concomitantly with allopurinol, there is an increased risk of morbilliform drug eruption, and when tetracyclines are used together with penicillins, the bactericidal effect of penicillins is decreased.
- β-lactams may alter the anticoagulant effects of warfarin, warranting closer monitoring of international normalized ratio (INR).

Pregnancy Category: B

Lactation: Safe

Children: Safe

Cephalosporins

It is derived from *Cephalosporium acremonium*. The two-ring combination of cephalosporin gives the cephalosporin structure inherent resistance to β-lactamase enzymes.

Indication

- Skin and soft tissue infection (SSTI), such as impetigo, folliculitis, furuncles, carbuncles, acute bacterial paronychia, cellulitis, ecthyma, erysipelas, and postoperative wound infections.
- Severe infections, such as complicated cellulitis and necrotizing fasciitis require intravenous (IV) antibacterial agents

Mechanism of Action

Same as beta lactams

Pharmacology

- Cefaclor, cefadroxil, and cephalexin are best absorbed from an empty stomach, whereas the bioavailability of cefuroxime is increased when taken with food.
- The half-life of most parenterally administered cephalosporins varies between 0.5 and 2 hours.
- 6–8 hours half-life of ceftriaxone permits once-daily dosing.

Adverse Effects

Hypersensitivity reactions and cross-reaction potential

Nausea, vomiting, or diarrhea, vaginal candidiasis, hematopoietic changes, mental and sleep disturbance, and transaminitis

First-Generation	Second-Generation	Third-Generation	Fourth-Generation	Fifth-Generation
• Cefadroxil • Cefazolin • Cephalexin	• Cefaclor • Cefprozil • Cefuroxime axetil Cefuroxime Cefotetan • Cefoxitin	• Cefixime • Cefdinir • Cefotaxime Cefpodoxime • Ceftazidime Ceftibuten Cefditorenc Ceftriaxone	• Cefepime • Cefpirome	• Ceftaroline • Ceftobiprole

Drug Interactions

- Disulfiram-like reactions with alcohol ingestion
- It inhibits production of vitamin-K clotting factors, resulting in prolongation of INR in patients on warfarin
- Probenecid competes with renal tubular secretion, thus increasing and prolonging their plasma levels
- Nephrotoxicity, when coadministered with aminoglycosides or potent diuretics
- Oral contraceptives

Pregnancy Category: B

Lactation: Safe

Children: Safe

β-Lactam and β-Lactamase Inhibitor Combinations

As clavulanate, sulbactam, and tazobactam, when combined with a β-lactam antibiotic, inhibit β-lactamase produced by Enterobacteriaceae, S. aureus, and Gram-negative anaerobes, thereby restoring the spectrum activity of the β-lactams.

Other Cell Wall Synthesis Inhibitors

Glycopeptides

- Vancomycin
- Teicoplanin
- Oritavancin
- Dalbavancin
- Telavancin

Indication

Treatment of skin and soft tissue infection (SSTI) caused by MRSA

Mechanism of Action

- It forms noncovalent complexes with precursors of bacterial peptidoglycan, a contrasting mechanism to that of the β-lactam agents.
- Spectrum-Gram-positive bacteria (important use in MRSA), enterococci.

Pharmacology

- Vancomycin and teicoplanin are administered parenterally given their minimal intestinal absorption.
- Teicoplanin has a longer half-life and is less nephrotoxic.

Adverse Effects

- Cutaneous reactions and hypersensitivity.
- Red man syndrome and shock secondary to histamine release may follow rapid infusion of vancomycin.
- Toxic epidermal necrolysis (TEN)
- Drug-induced linear IgA bullous dermatosis (LABD).
- Dose-related hearing loss
- Nephrotoxicity.
- Others: fever, neutropenia, thrombocytopenia, and phlebitis.

Drug Interaction

Vancomycin may enhance the activity of nondepolarizing muscle relaxants.

Pregnancy: Category C

Lactation: Safe

Children: Safe

Macrolides

- Erythromycin
- Azithromycin
- Clarithromycin
- Roxithromycin
- Fidaxomicin

Indication

- Treatment of SSTI including pyodermas, abscesses, infected wounds, infected ulcers, and erysipelas.

- Erythrasma, anthrax, erysipeloid, chancroid, and lymphogranuloma venereum.
- Erythromycin is the treatment of choice for early Lyme disease (erythema migrans) in children under 8 years of age
- Azithromycin is effective for acne, rosacea, pityriasis lichenoides, confluent and reticulated papillomatosis, donovanosis, cat-scratch disease, toxoplasmosis, and Mediterranean spotted fever.
- Single dose of azithromycin is effective for treatment of uncomplicated urethritis or cervicitis caused by *N. gonorrhoea* or *C. trachomatis*.
- Clarithromycin is effective in leprosy, as well as the atypical mycobacterial skin infections.

Pharmacology

- Erythromycin is vulnerable to gastric acid inactivation and must be taken on an empty stomach.
- Azithromycin and clarithromycin are more stable in gastric acid than erythromycin, increasing their absorption.
- Clarithromycin is well absorbed with or without food, but azithromycin absorption is decreased with food and should be taken 1–2 hours before a meal.

Mechanism of Action

- Bind to 50s subunit of bacterial ribosome, inhibiting RNA dependent protein synthesis
- Anti-inflammatory properties.

Adverse Effects

General

- Nausea, abdominal pain, and diarrhea
- Acute generalized exanthematous pustulosis (AGEP).
- Cholestatic hepatitis and exacerbate myasthenia gravis.

Specific

- Erythromycin-QTc prolongation and torsades de pointes
- Clarithromycin-metallic or bitter taste, fixed drug eruption, leukocytoclastic vasculitis and hypersensitivity reactions
- Azithromycin-irreversible deafness, angioedema, photosensitivity, and hypersensitivity.
- Infants-hypertrophic pyloric stenosis.
- Pregnancy-erythromycin cause maternal hepatotoxicity, cardiotoxicity

Drug Interactions

- Erythromycin, clarithromycin are CYP3A4 inhibitor
- Azithromycin minimally inhibits CYP3A4 isoenzymes, and so can be safely coadministered with other drugs.
  1. Carbamazepine and phenytoin
  2. Theophylline
  3. Certain benzodiazepines (i.e., triazolam, midazolam).
  4. Warfarin, with potential for severe bleeding complications
  5. Cyclosporine, with potential for renal toxicity and hypertension.
  6. Drugs with potential for QTc prolongation and torsades de pointes, (terfenadine, astemizole, cisapride, and pimozide; all but pimozide have been withdrawn from the market).
  7. Some HMG-CoA reductase inhibitors or 'statins' (i.e., atorvastatin, simvastatin, lovastatin), enhancing their risk for rhabdomyolysis.
  8. Coadministration with ergot alkaloids (dihydroergotamine, ergotamine, etc.) can lead to ergotism and is contraindicated.
  9. Clarithromycin may reduce the absorption of zidovudine (AZT) by 20% and may also reduce the serum levels of didanosine (ddI).

10. Clarithromycin may significantly increase linezolid serum concentrations when co-administered.
11. Macrolide-induced digoxin toxicity has been described, because of alterations in gut flora or P-glycoprotein.

Pregnancy category: B (Clarithromycin C)

Lactation: compatible

Children: should be used with caution

FLUOROQUINOLONES

- 1st generation- Nalidixic acid, cinoxacin, flumequine, oxolinic acid, piromidic acid, pipemidic acid, rosoxacin
- 2nd generation- Lomefloxacin, norfloxacin, ciprofloxacin, ofloxacin, fleroxacin, pefloxacin, rufloxacin
- 3rd generation- Levofloxacin, sparfloxacin, temafloxacin, grepafloxacin, balofloxacin, pazufloxacin, tosufloxacin
- 4th generation- Moxifloxacin, gemifloxacin, trovafloxacin, gatifloxacin, clinafloxacin, garenoxacin, sitafloxacin, prulifloxacin, finafloxacin

Indication

- Because of high drug levels in the skin and appendages, oral fluoroquinolones (FQ) are ideal agents for treating uncomplicated skin and soft tissue infections (uSSTI) caused by gram-negative bacteria, such as folliculitis, abscesses, cellulitis, infected ulcers (especially diabetic), Gram-negative toe web-space infections and wound infections.
- Donovanosis and chancroid
- Cutaneous anthrax
- Acne vulgaris
- Pseudomonas spp ("hot-tub folliculitis")
- Gram-negative folliculitis

Mechanism of Action

- Interfere with bacterial DNA replication via inhibition of DNA gyrase (bacterial topoisomerase II) +/-topoisomerase IV.
- First-and second-generation quinolones (ciprofloxacin, ofloxacin and nalidixic acid) only target DNA gyrase → only effective against Gram-negative organisms Third and fourth generation quinolones (levofloxacin, moxifloxacin, sparfloxacin and gatifloxacin) target both topoisomerase forms (IV > II) → increased Gram-positive (GP) coverage, but decreased Gram-negative (GN) coverage.
- Ciprofloxacin, ofloxacin and levofloxacin have some activity against atypical mycobacteria
- Spectrum–GP (target is topoisomerase IV) and GN (target is DNA gyrase)

Pharmacology

- Oral bioavailability of FQ is excellent and minimally affected by food.
- Metal ions co-administered in high concentration, such as in antacids or vitamin/mineral supplements, impair FQ absorption
- Half-lives of individual FQ vary from 3–13 hours.
- Except for moxifloxacin, FQ are excreted renally.

Adverse Effects

- Nausea, vomiting, and diarrhoea.
- Headaches, dizziness, agitation, and sleep disturbance, to severe reactions, including seizures, psychosis, hallucinations, and depression.
- Exacerbate muscle weakness in patients with myasthenia gravis
- Hypersensitivity and photosensitivity reaction

- Phototoxic reactions, including pseudoporphyria and photo-onycholysis
- Altered cardiac conduction, prolonged QTc interval, ventricular dysrhythmia, risk of aortic aneurysms and rupture

Drug Interactions

- FQ show decreased bioavailability when administered with calcium-, aluminum-, or magnesiumcontaining antacids.
- Decreased GI absorption of FQ has also been noted with coadministration of sucralfate and iron-or zinc-containing products.
- Theophylline metabolism is reduced by ciprofloxacin and norfloxacin, via hepatic CYP isozyme 1A2.
- The metabolism of caffeine is similarly inhibited, and patients should reduce caffeine intake while taking FQ.
- Decrease in warfarin and cyclosporine metabolism.

Pregnancy category: C

Lactation: Contraindicated

Children: Not recommended for routine use in children under 18 years of age.

Tetracyclines (TCN)

It includes Tetracycline, Doxycycline and Minocycline. The TCNs are divided into:
1. the short-acting TCN (half-life 6–12 hours);
2. intermediate-acting demeclocycline (half-life 16 hours); and
3. the long-acting drugs doxycycline (half-life 18–22 hours) and minocycline immediate-release (IR, half-life 11–22 hours), and minocycline ER formulations

Indication
- Acne vulgaris
- Rosacea
- Immunobullous dermatoses
- Granulomatous dermatoses like cutaneous sarcoidosis, Melkersson-Rosenthal syndrome, confluent and reticular papillomatosis, prurigo pigmentosa, oral lichen planus, acne keloidalis.
- Pyoderma gangrenosum
- Aphthous stomatitis
- Community-acquired MRSA infections
- Rickettsial disease, vibrio-vulnificus infections
- Spirochete infections-syphilis, Lyme's disease
- Sexually transmitted diseases like lymphogranuloma venereum caused by *C. trachomatis*
- Atypical mycobacterial infections
- Leprosy (minocycline)
- Second-line therapy (in penicillin-allergic patients) for cutaneous actinomycosis.

Mechanism of Action

- It is bacteriostatic and inhibit bacterial protein synthesis by binding to the 30S subunit of the bacterial ribosome.
- Anti-inflammatory properties include:
  - Inhibition of the production of neutrophil chemoattractants by P. acnes (i.e., peptide chemotactic factor, lipase);
  - Inhibition of neutrophil migration in vitro and in skin window studies in vivo;
  - Inhibitory activity against granuloma formation in vitro, likely because of protein kinase C inhibition;
  - Inhibition of multiple matrix metalloproteinases (MMP), which are involved in dermal matrix degradation of both collagen and elastic tissue;
  - Downregulation of cytokines involved in the innate immune response; and
  - A possible scavenger effect against reactive oxygen species (ROS).
  - **Spectrum**-Various GP and GN skin infections, including MRSA and those

caused by Chlamydia spp., Rickettsia spp., Mycoplasma spp., atypical mycobacteria, spirochetes and Lyme disease

Pharmacology

- TCNs are lipophilic, reaching high concentrations in skin and nails.
- TCNs (especially TCN) are better absorbed in the fasting state.

Adverse Effects

- Nausea, abdominal discomfort.
- 'Pill esophagitis,' are notably more common with doxycycline than with other TCNs.
- Acute Vestibular Side Effects.
- Benign Intracranial Hypertension/pseudotumor cerebri
- Photosensitivity
- Dyspigmentation-blue to grey to brown, black bones', 'black or green roots' of teeth, and blue-gray to gray darkening of crowns.
- Hypersensitivity Reactions-Serum sickness-like reactions (SSLR)
- Autoimmune adverse reactions (autoimmune hepatitis, systemic lupus-like reactions, and anti-cytoplasmic antibody [ANCA] vasculitis)
- Stevens-Johnson syndrome, DRESS. Lupus-Like Syndrome

Drug Interaction

TCNs may potentiate the pharmacologic effects and toxicity of warfarin, lithium, theophylline, digoxin, methotrexate, and insulin.

Pregnancy category: D

Lactation: moderate to high risk.

Children:
- **Old**: TCN should be avoided (apart from life-threatening infections) in children younger than 9 years of age
- **New**: The American Academy of Pediatrics permits use of doxycycline for less than 21 days in children of all ages.

Trimethoprim Sulfamethoxazole/cotrimoxazole

Fixed dose ratio of 1 part TMP to 5 parts SMX.

Indication

- Alternative agent for acne vulgaris and for uSSTI because of community acquired Methicillin resistant Staph aureus (CA-MRSA)
- Hidradenitis suppurativa
- Granuloma inguinale
- Atypical mycobacterial infections
- Cutaneous nocardiosis, including actinomycetoma.
- Cat-scratch disease.
- Aeromonas species infections.
- Chronic melioidosis (Burkholderia pseudomallei)

Mechanism of Action

- Dihydrofolate reductase inhibitor (trimethoprim) and dihydropteroate synthetase inhibitor (sulfamethoxazole) → decreased tetrahydrofolic acid → decreased bacterial nucleic acid and protein synthesis.
- Spectrum: Various GP cocci (MRSA, *Enterococcus faecalis* and *S. pyogenes*), *H. influenzae*, *Pneumocystis jirovecii*, *Nocardia* spp., Chlamydia, and various GN

Pharmacology

Both TMP and SMX are well absorbed orally (70-100%), with half-lives of 8-10 hours and 10-12 hours, respectively,

Adverse Effects

- Nausea, vomiting, loss of appetite, diarrhea, cephalgia, dizziness, and tinnitus

- Hypersensitivity reactions
- Hematologic toxicity-agranulocytosis, thrombocytopenia, neutropenia, hypoprothrombinemia, aplastic anemia (very rare), and pure red cell aplasia (very rare). Hemolytic anemia may occur in patients with glucose-6-phosphate dehydrogenase (G6PD) deficiency.
- Metabolic disturbances-hyperkalemia.
- Pulmonary infiltrates and upper respiratory symptoms
- Pustular skin eruptions, drug-induced Sweet's syndrome.
- Cholestatic hepatitis, nephrolithiasis and interstitial nephritis.

Drug Interactions

1. Increase dapsone serum levels
2. Severe hyperkalemia when used concomitantly with an ACE inhibitor or and AR blockers
3. Increase the risk of blood dyscrasias in patients on methotrexate via multiple mechanisms: combined inhibition of folic acid synthesis (methotrexate inhibits dihydrofolate reductase and thymidylate synthetase) and inhibition of protein binding by TMP-SMX.
4. Increase phenytoin serum levels predisposing patients to phenytoin toxicity.
5. Inhibit the metabolism of warfarin leading to increased anticoagulant effect and risk of bleeding.
6. Toxic delirium has been reported in individuals who have received amantadine and TMP.
7. Reversible nephrotoxicity has also been reported in renal transplantation recipients, receiving cyclosporine and TMP-SMX; avoidance of coadministration is suggested, as TMP-SMX (especially IV) can reduce cyclosporine serum levels, increase serum creatinine levels.
8. Renal insufficiency is a risk factor for many of the drug interactions involving TMP-SMX.

Pregnancy category: D

Lactation: Moderate to high risk

Children: Not recommended children below 2 months of age

Lincosamides

Clindamycin

Clindamycin is a lincosamide antibiotic derived from lincomycin that has increased antibacterial activity and is better absorbed than its parent drug

Indication

- USSTI, primarily those caused by staphylococci, cellulitis, folliculitis, furunculosis, carbuncles, impetigo, ecthyma, and hidradenitis suppurativa.
- Deep soft tissue infections, including streptococcal myositis, necrotizing fasciitis, and C. perfringens infection, may also be treated with this agent. Infected diabetic foot ulcers.

Mechanism of Action

- It binds to 50S subunit of bacterial ribosomal RNA → decreased ribosomal translocation and protein synthesis.
- Spectrum: GP cocci (*Staphylococcus spp.* and *Streptococcus spp.*) and anaerobes (*Bacteroides spp.* and *Clostridium perfringens*), but not usually GN (except *Capnocytophaga canimorsus*)

Pharmacology

- Clindamycin is metabolized in the liver by CYP3A4, with a plasma half-life of 2.4–3.0 hours.

- The plasma half-life is extended in adults with severe renal or hepatic failure requiring dose adjustment.

Adverse Effects

- Diarrhea, nausea, vomiting, and elevated transaminases
- Cutaneous-Morbilliform eruptions are most commonly reported, less common hypersensitivity reactions, including acute generalized exanthematous pustulosis, erythema multiforme, DRESS, Sweet syndrome and urticaria

Drug Interactions

- Clindamycin has been shown to have neuromuscularblocking properties that may enhance other neuromuscular agents, such as tubocurare and pancuronium.
- CYP3A4 inducers like rifampin can significantly decrease clindamycin concentrations.

Pregnancy category: B

Lactation: Compatible

Children: Safe

OXAZOLIDINONES

Linezolid

It is a synthetic oxazolidinone antibiotic.

Indications

- Skin infections because of staphylococcus or streptococcus, including uSSTI caused by *S. aureus*, CA-MRSA, or susceptible *S. pyogenes*.
- Linezolid should be considered for treatment of CAMRSA in patients who have failed oral doxycycline, minocycline, TMP-SMX, clindamycin/rifampin, or vancomycin.

Mechanism of Action

- Oxazolidinones inhibit protein synthesis by binding to the 23S portion of the 50S ribosomal subunit; owing to a unique binding site, there is no cross-resistance with other antimicrobial agent, Production of exotoxins by Gram-positive bacteria is also reduced.
- Spectrum: Linezolid has a broad spectrum of activity, including as MRSA, vancomycin-resistant *Staph. aureus* (VRSA), penicillin-resistant *S. pneumoniae*, and vancomycin-resistant enterococci (VRE).

Pharmacology

- Linezolid is 100% bioavailable, with serum half-life of 5–7 hours.
- Its metabolism is unaffected by the CYP system.
- No dosage adjustments are generally needed with renal or hepatic impairment.

Adverse Effect

- Hematologic effects: Myelosuppression, including anemia, leukopenia, pancytopenia, and reversible thrombocytopenia
- Neurologic effects: Serotonin syndrome characterized by cognitive dysfunction, hyperpyrexia, hyperreflexia, and incoordination

Drug Interactions

- Concomitant use with MAO inhibitors, SSRI, Tricyclic antidepressants, sympathomimetic agents (e.g., pseudoephedrine), vasopressive agents (e.g., epinephrine, norepinephrine), and dopaminergic agents (e.g., dopamine, dobutamine) can cause serotonin syndrome.

Pregnancy category: C

Lactation: Not recommended

Children: Safe

SYSTEMIC ANTIFUNGAL

The availability of modern antifungal agents has greatly improved the treatment of a wide range of superficial and systemic dermatomycoses.

Classification

1. **Antifungal antibiotics:**
   A. Polyenes: Amphotericin B, Nystatin.
   B. Heterocyclic benzofuran: Griseofulvin
   C. Echinocandins: Caspofungin, micafungin and anidulafungin
2. **Antimetabolite:** Flucytosine
3. **Azoles:**
   A. Imidazole: Ketoconazole
   B. Triazole: Fluconazole, Itraconazole, Isavuconazole, Voriconazole, Posaconazole, Ravuconazole, Albaconazole
   C. Tetrazole: Oteseconazole
4. **Allylamine:** Terbinafine

MOA	Antifungal agents
Fungal cell wall synthesis inhibition	Caspofungin
Bind to fungal cell membrane ergosterol and form pores	Amphotericin B, Nystatin
Inhibition of ergosterol and lanosterol synthesis	Terbinafine
Inhibition of ergosterol synthesis	Azoles
Inhibition of nucleic acid synthesis	5-Flucytosine
Disruption of mitotic spindle and fungal mitosis	Griseofulvin

TERBINAFINE

Terbinafine is an allylamine antifungal.

Indications

- Approved: Tinea capitis and onychomycosis.
- Unlicensed: Tinea corporis, cruris, seborrheic dermatitis.

Mechanism of Action

- Inhibits squalene epoxide leading to accumulation of squalene and subsequent deficiency of ergosterol leads to fungistatic action, accumulation squalene leads to fungicidal action.
- Terbinafine is delivered to the stratum corneum by passive dermo-epidermal diffusion, through sebum and through incorporation of drug from migrating basal keratinocytes.

Pharmacology

- Has oral bioavailability of 40% due to significant fast-pass metabolism (CYP2C9, 1A2, 3A4, 2C8, 2C19).
- Tablets are not affected by food. Renal 70%; clearance decreased 50% in renal impairment or hepatic cirrhosis.
- In patients with renal insufficiency (serum creatinine >3.4 mg/dL, or creatinine clearance <50 mL/min), terbinafine clearance is decreased by about 50%.

Dosage

- Above 2 years and below 20 kg–62.5 mg
- Above 2 years and between 20 and 40 kg–125 mg
- Above 2 years and above 40 kg–250 mg

Monitoring

Liver function tests should be performed in all patients before prescribing terbinafine for courses of at least 3–4 weeks continuously (serum transaminase tests: alanine aminotransferase [ALT], AST).

Adverse Effects

- Cutaneous morbilliform eruption and, less commonly, urticaria, pruritus, alopecia, or dermatitis. Additional cutaneous reactions

include SJS, TEN, AGEP, flares of pustular or other forms of psoriasis, and subacute cutaneous lupus erythematosus.
- Systemic
  - GIT: Nausea, vomiting, elevated liver enzymes
  - CNS: Headaches, taste and visual disturbances
  - Blood: Transient decreases in absolute lymphocyte count, and rarely, neutropenia.

Drug Interaction

Terbinafine is as a CYP2D6 inhibitor, so it increases level of opioids, betablockers, tricyclic antidepressants, pimozide and amiodarone.

Contraindication

Hypersensitivity to terbinafine or components of formulation, Chronic or active hepatic disease, psoriasis.

Pregnancy category: B

Lactation: Safe

Children: Contraindicated ≤2 years

ITRACONAZOLE

Itraconazole is a triazole antifungal.

Indications

- Approved: Onychomycosis, oropharyngeal and esophageal candidiasis, histoplasmosis, blastomycosis, aspergillosis.
- Unlicensed: Tinea corporis, cruris, Tinea imbricata, seborrheic dermatitis, pityriasis versicolor, subcutaneous mycosis like sporotrichosis, chromoblastomycosis, Majocchi's granuloma, HIV-associated eosinophilic folliculitis, vaginal candidiasis, chronic mucocutaneous candidiasis.

Mechanism of Action

- It inhibits the CYP-dependent enzyme lanosterol 14-demethylase, with resultant inhibition of the conversion of lanosterol to ergosterol. Because of this mechanism of inhibition, these drugs are associated with a fungistatic action.
- Itraconazole is delivered to the skin mainly as a result of passive diffusion from the plasma to the keratinocytes, with strong drug adherence to keratin.

Pharmacology

- Itraconazole is excreted in sebum. Therefore, it is eliminated as the stratum corneum renews itself, and when the hair and nails grow out. Itraconazole may persist in the stratum corneum for 3–4 weeks after discontinuation of therapy.
- It undergoes fast-pass metabolism with oral availability of 55% and highest plasma levels achieved with full meal or fasted with cola beverage.
- Metabolized in liver by CYP3A4; active metabolite is hydroxyl-itraconazole.

Dosage

- Pediatric dose: 3–5 mg/kg.
- Adult: 100 mg po daily for 2 weeks – or – 200 mg po daily for 1 week.

However, duration can be extended depending on clinical severity of infection.

Monitoring

Liver function tests should be performed in all patients before prescribing and after 1 month of treatment.

Adverse Effects

- Cutaneous Morbilliform eruption, pruritus, urticaria, alopecia, Stevens-Johnson syndrome (rarely).
- Systemic
  - GIT: Anorexia, nausea, vomiting, abdominal pain, hepatic dysfunction.
  - Fatigue, headaches, dizziness, Fever, edema.

- Hypokalemia.
- Neutropenia (rarely).
- Rarely causes congestive heart failure, pulmonary edema, anaphylaxis, peripheral neuropathy.

Contraindication

Hypersensitivity to itraconazole or components of formulation, Chronic or active hepatic disease.

Drug Interaction

- It interferes with CYP3A4. Thus, it increases the level of cyclosporine, simvastatin, atorvastatin, lovastatin (risk myopathy, rhabdomyolysis), Benzodiazepines—Alprazolam, triazolam, midazolam (risk excessive sedation), Antipsychotics—Pimozide (risk QT prolongation, torsades de pointes), Dapsone (risk hemolysis, agranulocytosis), Warfarin (2nd most important substrate pathway after CYP1A2) risk bleeding.
- Rifampin, rifabutin, rifapentine causes CYP3A4 induction with resultant decrease in itraconazole drug levels and loss of efficacy.

Pregnancy category: C

Lactation: Contraindicated

Children: Contraindicated

Fluconazole

It is a triazole antifungal.

Indication

- Approved: Vaginal candidiasis, oropharyngeal and esophageal candidiasis, cryptococcal meningitis, prophylaxis in transplant patients receiving chemotherapy and/or radiation therapy.
- Unlicensed: Tinea corporis, cruris, seborrheic dermatitis, pityriasis versicolor.

Mechanism of Action

It inhibits the CYP-dependent enzyme lanosterol 14-demethylase, with resultant inhibition of the conversion of lanosterol to ergosterol. It is fungistatic.

Pharmacology

- It undergoes little first-pass hepatic metabolism, much of dose is excreted as unchanged parent drug; so oral bioavailability is >90%.
- The drug accumulates in the stratum corneum through sweat and by direct diffusion through the dermis and epidermis. Excretion in the sebum may be more limited.

Dosage

Pediatric dose is 6 mg/kg/week for tinea corporis, cruris and 6 mg/kg/day for capitis.

Monitoring

Liver function tests should be performed in all patients before prescribing.

Adverse Effects

- **Cutaneous** Morbilliform eruption, exfoliative dermatitis (rarely).
- **Systemic** Nausea, vomiting, abdominal pain, diarrhea, hepatotoxicity, Headache.

Contraindication

Hypersensitivity to fluconazole or components of formulation, Drug interactions involving QT prolongation.

Drug Interaction

- It interferes with CYP3A4 along with CYP2C9.
- The most notable CYP2C9 interactions with the azoles are coadministration of fluconazole with warfarin, which can lead to significant increases in international normalized ratio (INR) values and excessive anticoagulation.

- Other involving 2C9 pathway include rosuvastatin, fluvastatin, doxepin, phenytoin and valproate.

Pregnancy category: D

Lactation: Safe

Children: Safe

GRISEOFULVIN

Indication

Approved

Tinea capitis, corporis, cruris, pedis and onychomycosis.

Unlicensed

Lichen planus.

Mechanism of Action

Disruption of mitotic spindle and fungal mitosis

Pharmacology

- Its affinity for keratin is low.
- Absorption is significantly enhanced by administration with or after a fatty meal.
- It undergoes hepatic metabolism, major metabolites are 6-demethylgriseofulvin and its glucuronide conjugate.

Dosage

T. corporis, cruris	T. pedis, manuum, unguis, capitis	Pediatric dose
500–1,000 mg daily	750–1,500 mg daily	15–20 mg/kg daily (usual maximum 1 g); use higher range of 20–25 mg/kg daily for tinea capitis
375–500 mg daily	500–750 mg daily	10–15 mg/kg/day (maximum usually 750 mg/day)

Adverse Effects

- Headache and gastrointestinal disturbances common.
- Cutaneous: Fixed drug eruptions, photosensitivity, petechiae, pruritus, exfoliative dermatitis, urticaria/angioedema, and serum sickness-like reactions. It can also precipitate or exacerbate lupus erythematosus or porphyria.

Monitoring

During prolonged griseofulvin therapy, periodic assessment of renal, hepatic, and hematopoietic functions should be performed.

Pregnancy category: X

Lactation: Not recommended

Children: Safe.

VORICONAZOLE

- Voriconazole is a triazole antifungal agent which inhibits ergosterol synthesis in fungal cell membranes.
- It has a broad spectrum of activity against all *Candida species* (including strains resistant to fluconazole), *Aspergillus* spp., *Scedosporium* spp., and *Fusarium* spp.

Indications

Approved

- Esophageal candidiasis
- Aspergillosis
- Systemic candida infection (non-neutropenic and disseminated candidiasis)

Adverse Effects

- Transient and reversible visual disturbances
- Fever; headache; abdominal pain; chills
- Asthenia; back pains; chest pain; face edema

- Flu-like syndrome
- Hypotension; thrombophlebitis; phlebitis
- GI disturbances (e.g., nausea, vomiting, diarrhea); jaundice; cheilitis; cholestatic jaundice; gastroenteritis
- Blood dyscrasias; purpura; peripheral edema; facial edema
- Hypokalemia; hypoglycemia
- Dizziness; hallucinations; confusion; depression; tremor; agitation; paraesthesia
- Rash; pruritus; photosensitivity; alopecia; exfoliative dermatitis
- Acute kidney failure; hematuria; infusion related reactions.
- Increased LFT and serum creatinine; prolongation of QT interval.

Contraindications

- Hypersensitivity
- Lactation.

Pregnancy: Category D

Lactation: Not recommended

Children: Not recommended

POSACONAZOLE

- Blocks the synthesis of ergosterol, a key component of the fungal cell membrane, through the inhibition of the enzyme lanosterol 14 alpha-demethylase and accumulation of methylated sterol precursors.
- Posaconazole has activity against *Candida* spp., *Aspergillus* spp., *Coccidioides immitis*, *Fonsecaea pedrosoi*, and some species of *Fusarium* and Zygomycetes.
- Approved indications include Onychomycosis caused by dermatophytes, Tinea corporis/cruris, Tinea pedis, Tinea capitis, Aspergillosis (prophylaxis – immunocompromised patients), Systemic candida infection (prophylaxis-immunocompromised patients).

Adverse Effects

- Fever, headache, rigors, fatigue, edema
- Dizziness, weakness, blurred vision
- Diarrhea, nausea, vomiting, abdominal pain, constipation
- Anorexia, anemia
- Febrile neutropenia, thrombocytopenia
- Petechiae, thrombotic thrombocytopenic purpura
- Electrolyte imbalance
- Bacteremia, herpes simplex, cytomegalovirus infection
- Increased LFT's and bilirubin; increased serum creatinine; adrenal insufficiency.

Contraindication

Hypersensitivity

Pregnancy: Category C

Lactation: Not recommended

Children: Not recommended

SYSTEMIC ANTIVIRAL AGENTS

The first antiviral developed was idoxuridine about 60 years ago and since then more than 30 systemic antiviral drugs have been approved for the treatment of various viral infections.

Classification

I. Antihuman herpes virus (anti-HHV) drugs: acyclovir, famciclovir, valacyclovir
II. Anti-CMV drugs: Foscarnet, ganciclovir, cidofovir
III. Anti-retroviral drugs.

Acyclovir

Acyclovir is a synthetic purine nucleoside analogue which is a derivative of acycloguanosine.

Indication

Approved

- Herpes simplex infection—primary episode, recurrent episodes, suppressive

therapy, in both immunocompetent and immunocompromised patients.
- Varicella zoster infection—chickenpox, herpes zoster, in both immunocompetent and immunocompromised patients.

Unlicensed
- Recurrent Erythema Multiforme
- Eczema herpeticum
- Herpetic whitlow
- Neonatal herpes

Mechanism of Action

The active moiety is acyclovir triphosphate. It is a potent inhibitor of viral DNA polymerase thus inhibiting viral DNA synthesis. Acyclovir is first converted to acyclovir monophosphate by viral thymidine kinase, and then to acyclovir triphosphate in presence of cellular kinase. Viruses which are deficient in thymidine kinase will not respond to acyclovir.

Pharmacology

- It has an oral bioavailability of 15–30%.
- Plasma half-life is of 1.3–1.5 hours.

Dosage

In immunocompetent patients:
- Primary HSV infection: 400 mg 3 times/day for 7 days
- Recurrent HSV infection: 400 mg 3 times/day for 7 days
- Chickenpox: 20 mg/kg 4 times up to 800 mg/dose for 5–7 days.
- Herpes zoster: 800 mg 5 times/day for 7 days.

In immunocompromised patients:
- Primary HSV infection: 200–400 mg 5 times/day for 10 days
- Recurrent HSV infection: 400 mg TID/day for 7–10 days

- Chickenpox (children): 10 mg/kg IV 8 hourly for 7–10 days
- Herpes zoster: 800 mg 5 times/day for 7 days.

Monitoring

- Monitor urea and creatinine only in renal failure patients on oral acyclovir.
- IV administration requires monitoring for such as malaise, inflammation or phlebitis at the infusion site, nausea, vomiting, Steven-Johnson syndrome, transaminitis, nausea, vomiting, diarrhea, headache, abdominal pain, aggression/confusion, agitation, alopecia, anaphylaxis, anemia, angioedema, anorexia, ataxia, coma, disseminated intravascular coagulation (DIC), dizziness and fatigue.

Adverse Effects

Systemic
- Hypersensitivity
- Headache, nausea, malaise
- Rash, sweating, hypotension, vomiting
- Reversible crystalluria-induced nephropathy due to intravenous acyclovir.

Cutaneous

Morbilliform eruptions, Stevens-Johnson syndrome, urticaria, injection site reactions, angioedema.

Drug Interaction

Mycophenolate (mofetil and sodium) serum levels are increased by acyclovir.

Contraindication

- Hypersensitivity to the drug, prodrug or any component.
- Dose adjustment required in patients with renal impairment, those taking any nephrotoxic medication.

Pregnancy Category: B

Lactation: Safe

Children: Safe

Valacyclovir

- Valacyclovir (VACV) is an oral prodrug of acyclovir. This 1-valyl ester of ACV has a bioavailability 3 to 5 times greater than that of oral ACV. In the oral form, it is nearly as potent as intravenous ACV.
- The mechanism, clinical spectrum, and adverse effects are similar.

Dosage

- Herpes simplex—primary: 1000 mg BID for 10 days.
- Herpes simplex—recurrences: 500 mg twice daily for 3 days
- Herpes simplex—suppression 1000 mg daily suppressive dose (single dose) if 10 or more HSV recurrences each year.
- HZ—acute treatment: 1000 mg 3 times daily for 7 days.
- Primary varicella—20 mg/kg 3 times daily up to 1000 mg/dose for 5 days.

Drug Interaction

Same as acyclovir.

FAMCILOVIR (FCV)

FCV is the oral prodrug of penciclovir (PCV), an acyclic nucleoside.

Indications

Approved

- Herpes simplex Infection: Primary episode, recurrent episodes, suppressive therapy, immunocompromised patients (such as HIV infections).
- Varicella-Zoster infections: Herpes zoster, immunocompromised patients (such as HIV infections).

Unlicensed

Other subsets of herpes simplex infections, primary varicella.

Mechanism of Action

Like ACV, PCV must be phosphorylated to PCV triphosphate to be pharmacologically active.

Pharmacology

- PCV triphosphate has a much longer intracellular half-life (10–20 hours in HSV-infected cells and 7 hours in VZV-infected cells) than ACV triphosphate.
- Oral FCV has a 77% bioavailability.
- Famciclovir is converted to penciclovir by deacetylation and oxidation in liver and intestine. Plasma half-life of penciclovir is 2 hours.

Dosage

- Herpes simplex—250 mg TID for 10 days
- Herpes simplex—recurrences 125 mg BID for 5 days
- Herpes simplex—suppression 250 mg BID
- HZ—acute treatment 500 mg TID for 7 days.

Monitoring

Liver function test.

Adverse Effects

Hypersensitivity, headache, nausea and vomiting.

Drug Interaction

No significant drug interaction.

Contraindication

Hypersensitivity famciclovir or formulation.

Pregnancy Category: B

Lactation: Safe

Children: Unknown

FOSCARNET

It is a synthetic non-nucleoside analogue. It is an analogue of pyrophosphate.

Indication

Approved
- Cytomegalovirus (CMV) and CMV-associated ophthalmic retinitis in individuals diagnosed with AIDS and who are unable to tolerate ganciclovir.
- Salvage therapy for patients with drug-resistant CMV who have failed ganciclovir.

Unlicensed
Acyclovir resistant HSV infection.

Mechanism of Action

It noncompetitively inhibits DNA polymerase by preventing the cleavage of pyrophosphate without the activation by cellular or viral kinase. It does not require phosphorylation for its antiviral activity and is therefore active against viruses that are resistant to acyclovir, famciclovir.

Pharmacology

- Plasma half-life is approximately 3.3–4.0 hours.
- Due to its accumulation in bone, it exhibits a prolonged urinary excretion half-life of 87.5 hours.

Dosage

40 mg/kg 8 hourly for 10–42 days or until healed.

Monitoring

- Baseline:
  - 24-hour creatinine clearance, ECG, and baseline electrolyte measurements.
  - Complete blood count
  - Serum electrolytes
- During therapy:
  - Weekly evaluation of calcium, potassium, sodium, magnesium, and phosphorus levels.

Adverse Effects

- Proteinuria
- Nephrogenic diabetes insipidus
- Increased creatinine level
- Hypokalemia, hypocalcemia, hypomagnesemia
- Headache, fatigue, fever, seizures
- Anemia, low WBC
- In males, meatal irritation and ulceration (foscarnet ulcers), about 2 weeks after beginning of treatment.

Drug Interaction

- Concomitant administration of cidofovir with foscarnet should be avoided due to the increased risk of additive nephrotoxicity.
- Pimozide should not be used with foscarnet, as both can exacerbate QT prolongation, increasing the risk of serious cardiac arrhythmias.
- Pentamidine: Use with foscarnet requires caution due to the potential for hypocalcemia and renal impairment.

Contraindication

Patients with severe hypersensitivity reactions such as angioedema or a history of anaphylactic reactions to it.

Pregnancy category: C

Lactation: Unknown

Children: Not recommended

ANTIPARASITIC

These drugs are used to treat infections by parasitic worms.

Classification

1. Benzimidazoles: Albendazole, mebendazole, thiabendazole
2. Vinyl pyrimidine: Pyrantel pamoate
3. Piperazine: Diethylcarbamazine (DEC)
4. Macrocyclic lactone derivative: Ivermectin
5. Imidazole thiazole: Levamisole
6. Salicylamides: Niclosamide
7. Heterocyclics: Praziquantel

ALBENDAZOLE

Albendazole is [methyl 5-(propylthiol)-2-benzimidazolecarbamate] chemically. It has both anthelminthic and antiprotozoal activity.

Indications

- Approved—Neurocysticercosis
- Hydatid disease
- Unlicensed indications:
  - Cutaneous larva migrans
  - Crusted scabies as monotherapy or in combination with topical 10% crotamiton and 5% salicylic acid.
  - Infestations by by *A. lumbricoides, T. trichiura, E. vermicularis, Ancylostoma duodenale, Necator americanus Taenia* spp. and *S. stercoralis, Giardia*.

Mechanism of Action

It inhibits tubulin polymerization which results in the loss of cytoplasmic microtubules which immobilizes and then kills the susceptible organism.

Pharmacology

Albendazole is poorly absorbed after oral administration with increased bioavailability following intake with fatty meal. Anthelminthic action is due to the active metabolite sulfoxide which attains maximum concentration after 2.5 hours. It is 70% protein bound with half-life of 8 hours. The drug is metabolized by the liver with biliary elimination being the major route of elimination.

Monitoring

Baseline

Ocular examination at start of therapy to identify retinal lesions.

Laboratory

- CBC, LFT at start of each treatment cycle
- Pregnancy test

Follow up

CBC and LFT every 2 weeks during therapy.

Dosage

- Cutaneous larva migrans: Albendazole 400–800 mg daily for 3–5 days.
- Crusted scabies: 800 mg per day oral albendazole for three consecutive days as monotherapy or per week for 3 cycles along with 10% crotamiton and 5% salicylic acid.

Adverse Effects

- Hematological: Bone marrow suppression, aplastic anemia, agranulocytosis.
- Gastrointestinal: Hepatotoxicity, GI discomfort, diarrhea
- Headache
- Dizziness
- Cutaneous: Anagen effluvium, erythema multiforme, Stevens-Johnson syndrome.
- Hypersensitivity reaction: Rash, pruritus, urticaria.

Drug Interactions

- Cimetidine (CYP 450 inhibitor)—suppresses metabolism of albendazole and increases bioavailability.
- Anticonvulsants (carbamazepine, phenytoin)—decrease serum concentration of albendazole.

- Dexamethasone—increase plasma levels of albendazole by up to 50%.
- Antimalarials (aminoquinolines): Decrease serum concentration of albendazole.

Contraindication

- Hypersensitivity to drug or components of formulation.
- During pregnancy and lactation
- Hepatic impairment

Pregnancy: Category C

Lactation: Data regarding excretion of drug in breast milk is limited.

Children: Dose in halved in children <2 years of age.

THIABANDAZOLE

It is a broad-spectrum anthelmintic. It is chemically 2-(4-thiazolyl)-1/-/-benzimidazole.

Indication

Approved
- Strongyloidiasis
- Cutaneous larva migrans
- Visceral larva migrans

Unlicensed
- Trichinosis
- Hookworm infestation with *N. americanus* and *A. duodenale*
- Trichuriasis
- Ascariasis

Mechanism of Action

It inhibits the helminth-specific enzyme fumarate reductase.

Pharmacology

It is absorbed rapidly after oral dosing and reaches peak within 1 to 2 hours. It should be chewed before swallowing. It undergoes hepatic metabolism and is excreted by the kidney.

Monitoring

CBC, LFT, urea, creatinine, urine examination at intervals to monitor for adverse effects.

Dosage

Depends on body weight, maximum daily dose is 3 g.
1. Strongyloidiasis—two doses per day for 2 successive days.
2. Cutaneous larva migrans—two doses per day for 2 successive days.
3. Visceral larva migrans—two doses per day for 7 successive days.

Adverse Effects

- GI: Anorexia, abdominal pain, hepatotoxicity.
- Ocular: Abnormal sensation in eyes, xanthopsia, blurred vision.
- Central nervous system: dizziness, drowsiness, giddiness, headache, numbness, hyperirritability, convulsions, collapse, confusion, depression, floating sensation, lack of coordination.
- Mucocutaneous: Drying of mucous membranes, Sicca syndrome, erythema multiforme, Stevens–Johnson syndrome.
- Genitourinary: Hematuria, enuresis, malodor of the urine, crystalluria.

Drug Interaction

Increase in caffeine and theophylline levels when used concurrently.

Contraindication

- Hypersensitivity to drug.
- Prophylactic use in worm infestation to be avoided.

Pregnancy: Category C.

Lactation: No data regarding excretion of drug in breastmilk.

Children: Not to be used in children weighing <30 pounds (lb).

IVERMECTIN

Ivermectin is a semisynthetic antihelminthic derivative of the avermectins, derived from the fermentation products of *Streptomyces avermitilis*.

Indications

Approved
- Intestinal strongyloidiasis
- Onchocerciasis

Unlicensed
- Scabies
- Pediculosis
- Demodicosis
- Cutaneous larva migrans
- Lymphatic filariasis

Mechanism of Action

It selectively binds to γ-aminobutyric acid (GABA) gated chloride channels found in the invertebrate nerve and muscle cells with increased cell membrane permeability and hyperpolarization of nerves and muscles followed by paralysis and death of parasites.

Pharmacology

Peak serum level after oral administration is reached around 4 hours. Half life is about 18 hours. Primarily hepatic metabolism by cytochrome P-450 and excreted in feces over 12 days. High fatty meal increases bioavailability of the drug.

Monitoring

Laboratory

CBC, LFT—as elevation of transaminases and leucopenia can occur on treatment.

Dosage

- 150–400 μg/kg.
- Scabies: Single oral dose of 200 μg/kg, can be repeated in 7–10 days as it is not ovicidal.
- Crusted scabies: 3, 5 or 7 doses.
- Lice: Single 400 μg/kg dose given on day 1 and day 8.
- Cutaneous larva migrans: 12 mg on first day and repeated the next day.

Adverse Effects

Mazzotti type reaction—systemic inflammatory reaction consisting of fever, urticaria, lymphadenopathy, arthralgia and cardiovascular instability in patients treated for onchocerciasis.
- General: Headache, Myalgia.
- GI: Diarrhea, nausea, vomiting, constipation, anorexia, abdominal pain
- Neuropsychiatric: Dizziness, somnolence, vertigo, tremor
- Cutaneous: Pruritus, rash, urticaria
- Tachycardia, facial edema, orthostatic hypotension
- Anaphylactoid reactions.

Drug Interactions

- Anticoagulants (warfarin): Increase anticoagulant effect.
- CYP 3A4 inducers (rifampicin, phenobarbital): Alter ivermectin GI disposition by P-glycoprotein mediated intestinal transport.

Contraindication

- Hypersensitivity to ivermectin or components of formulation.
- Lactation
- Children <15 kg

Pregnancy: Category C

Lactation: Not to be used.

Children: Avoid in children <5 years of age and weighing <15 kg.

ANTILEPROTICS

Dapsone, rifampicin and clofazimine are the three main antiprotic drugs used in the treatment of leprosy.

Dapsone

Dapsone (4,4'-diaminodiphenyl sulfone) is structurally related to sulfonamides and has antimycobacterial and anti-inflammatory action.

Indications

Approved

1. Acne vulgaris
2. Leprosy
3. Dermatitis herpetiformis

Unlicensed

- Autoimmune bullous disorders
  - Linear Ig A dermatoses,
  - Chronic bullous dermatosis of childhood,
  - Bullous eruption of systemic lupus erythematous
  - Bullous and cicatricial pemphigoid
  - Pemphigus vulgaris, pemphigus foliaceus
  - Epidermolysis bullosa acquisita
- Neutrophilic dermatoses:
  - Erythema elevatum diutinum
  - Sweet syndrome
  - Subcorneal pustular dermatosis
  - Pyoderma gangrenosum
  - Behcet syndrome
- Vasculitis: leukocytoclastic vasculitis, urticarial vasculitis.

Others

- Subacute cutaneous lupus erythematosus
- Panniculitis
- Granuloma faciale
- Relapsing polychondritis
- Pustular psoriasis
- Delayed pressure urticaria
- Granulomatous rosacea
- Brown recluse spider bites.

Mechanism of Action

It impairs microbial synthesis of folate from para-aminobenzoic acid by competitive inhibition of the enzyme dihydropteroate synthetase.

It has anti-inflammatory effects—by suppressing neutrophil chemotaxis and myeloperoxidase activity and preventing release of inflammatory mediators. Dapsone also inhibits formation of 5-lipoxygenase products in neutrophils and macrophages.

Pharmacology

Dapsone is a lipid soluble, water insoluble compound, readily absorbed from the gut with good bioavailability (70–80%) and a relatively long half-life (14–18 hours) allowing once daily dosing. Peak plasma levels are reached in 2–6 hours with plasma protein binding being 70–90%. It is metabolized by N-acetylation and N-hydroxylation. N-hydroxylation occurs in liver by CYP450 enzymes with production of hydroxylamine metabolite.

Monitoring

Baseline

History of any pre-existing cardiorespiratory, gastrointestinal, neurologic and renal disorders.

Laboratory

- CBC
- Renal and liver function tests
- Serum electrolytes
- G6PD level (quantitative) Wolverton's
- Urinalysis

Follow up

History and examination for methemoglobinemia and peripheral neuropathy at every visit.

Laboratory

- CBC: Every week for 4 weeks then fortnightly for next 12 weeks.
- Reticulocyte count as necessary to assess response to hemolysis.
- Methemoglobin levels should be checked if there are signs or symptoms to suggest methemoglobinemia.
- RFT and LFT: Weekly for first month, then monthly for 2 months, subsequently every 3-4 months. Every fortnightly for first 3 months then every 3-4 months (ROOK 2024).
- Urinalysis: Every 3-4 months.

Dosage

50-200 mg/day. WHO recommended dose for leprosy is 100 mg daily for adults. Minimum dose requirement is 1-2 mg/kg/day.

Adverse Effects

- Pharmacologic
- Hemolytic anemias and methemoglobinemia
- These are dose dependent side effects. Dapsone hydroxylamine has strong oxidizing properties which can cause severe hemolysis and methemoglobinemia in individuals with G6PD deficiency.

Idiosyncratic

- Hematologic: Agranulocytosis, leucopenia.
- CNS: Peripheral neuropathy (more commonly motor than sensory), psychosis, headache, insomnia.
- Dapsone hypersensitivity syndrome.
- Ocular: Optic neuritis, optic atrophy and macular infarction (rare).
- GI: Gastrointestinal upset, anorexia, nausea, vomiting.
- Dapsone hypersensitivity syndrome/DRESS—usually within 4-6 weeks of starting treatment.
- Hepatic: Hepatitis, cholestatic jaundice
- Cutaneous: Morbilliform eruption, erythroderma and toxic epidermal necrolysis.

Drug Interaction

- Concentration of dapsone reduced by: Rifamycins, aromatic anticonvulsants, griseofulvin.
- Concentration of dapsone increased by: Trimethoprim, methotrexate, probenecid, cimetidine with increased risk of adverse effects.
- Antimalarials: Increased risk of hemolysis specially in G6PD deficient patients.
- Colchicine: Risk of agranulocytosis.

Contraindication

- Known hypersensitivity to dapsone
- Severe G6PD deficiency
- Advanced cardiovascular or pulmonary disease
- Severe anemia
- Acute porphyria

Pregnancy: Category C

Lactation: Can be used in nursing mothers but can cause mild hemolytic anemia in infants.

Children: Safe in children.

RIFAMPIN AND OTHER RIFAMYCINS

The rifamycins includes rifampin, rifapentin and rifabutin.

Rifampin/Rifampicin

Rifampicin is a semisynthetic derivative of rifamycin B, an antimicrobial agent produced by *Streptomyces mediterranei*. It is a broad spectrum antimicrobial used widely in dermatology.

Indications

- Infections
  - Mycobacterial infections
- Cutaneous tuberculosis
- Leprosy
- Atypical mycobacterial infection
  - Bartonella infection

Cat-scratch disease, bacillary angiomatosis and peliosis hepatitis caused by *Bartonella henselae*.

- Methicillin sensitive *Staphylococcus aureus* infections.
- Others: Cutaneous leishmaniasis, rhinoscleroma, meningococcal and *Haemophilus influenza* prophylaxis, recurrent and recalcitrant folliculitis to eliminate the carrier state.
  - Pruritus associated with primary biliary cirrhosis,
- Chronic inflammatory dermatoses—hidradenitis suppurativa, folliculitis decalvans, dissecting cellulitis of scalp.

Mechanism of Action

Rifampicin acts by binding to bacterial DNA dependent RNA polymerase causing 'steric occlusion' which prevents RNA transcription. Rifampicin has a broad spectrum of activity that includes mycobacteria, including *M. tuberculosis* and *M. leprae*, staphylococci, *Neisseria meningitidis* and *N. gonorrhoeae* and *H. influenzae*.

A high level of activity against atypical mycobacterial mainly *M. kansasii* and *M. marinum* has been seen.

Pharmacology

- Rifampin is available as oral or IV use. Absorption improves when taken in empty stomach.
- Rifampin is a potent inducer of multiple CYP isoforms which results in increased hepatic metabolism.

Monitoring
Adverse Effects

1. Orange—red discoloration of body fluids (i.e., urine, sweat, tears, breast milk).
2. GI side effects—epigastric distress, nausea, vomiting and diarrhea.
3. CNS symptoms-headache, drowsiness, ataxia, dizziness, inability to concentrate and fatigue.
4. Flu like syndrome
5. Liver toxicity—transaminitis, serious hepatotoxicity.
6. Hypersensitivity reactions—urticaria, rash, pemphigoid reaction, erythema multiforme, acute generalized exanthematous pustulosis, Stevens-Johnson syndrome, toxic epidermal necrolysis, DRESS syndrome.
7. Deep venous thrombosis.

Dose

600 mg daily for adults and 10 mg/kg/day (600 mg maximum) for children.

Drug Interactions

Rifampin is a potent inducer of multiple CYP isoforms, including CYP1A2, 2C9, 2C19, 2D6, and 3A4.

- Rifampin increases clearance of oral contraceptive hormones leading to decrease efficacy.
- It decreases anticoagulant effects of warfarin leading to reduce efficacy.
- It reduces antifungal activity of azole antifungal agents leading to persistence of infection.
- It decreases serum levels of several HMG CoA-reductase inhibitors like atorvastatin, simvastatin and lovastatin leading to loss of cholesterol control.

Contraindications

- Hypersensitivity to the drug or its derivative
- Hepatic derangements.

Pregnancy: Rifampin and rifapentine are both pregnancy category C and rifabutin is pregnancy category B.

Lactation: Breastfeeding not to be stopped in women on rifampicin.

Children: Safe in children with dosing based on body weight.

CLOFAZIMINE

Clofazimine, an orange colored iminophenazine dye is an antimycobacterial agent. Clofazimine along with dapsone and rifampicin is a part of multidrug leprosy treatment regimen.

Indications

Approved
Leprosy and other mycobacterial infection.

Unlicensed
Neutrophilic dermatoses:
- Pyoderma gangrenosum
- Sweet syndrome

Granulomatous cheilitis

Lobomycosis

Mechanism of Action

1. Antimicrobial effects—clofazimine selectively binds to deoxyribonucleic acid guanine residues present in higher concentration in mycobacteria. It also inhibits respiratory chains in mitochondria. It is bactericidal against *M. leprae*.
2. Immunological effects—mild immunosuppressive effect mainly by altering the functions of monocytes and neutrophils. It inhibits T lymphocyte activation and proliferation.

Pharmacology

Clofazimine is highly lipophilic and is deposited in lipid rich tissues mainly in the reticuloendothelial system. The drug reaches peak levels in 1–6 hours with a long half-life of 70 days. Bioavailability ranges from 20–705 with predominantly hepatic metabolism and excretion in small amounts through urine, sweat, sebum and tears. Food increases absorption of Clofazimine.

Dosage

50 to 300 mg daily. In MB-MDT (multibacillary—muti drug treatment) it is given orally in a dose of 50 mg daily, with a supervised dose of 300 mg on a monthly basis.

Adverse Effects

Cutaneous
- Reversible orange-brown discoloration of the skin, beginning within 2 to 4 weeks of initiation.
- Generalized xerosis

Systemic
- GI: Abdominal cramping, nausea and diarrhea.
- Crystal deposition within small bowel may rarely cause fatal enteropathy.
- Splenic infarction and eosinophilic enteritis.

Monitoring

Baseline
Examination: For symptoms and signs of GI disorders.

Laboratory
Serum electrolytes, LFT.

Periodic monitoring of LFT if dose is more than 100 mg daily.

Drug Interactions

- CYP3A4 inhibitors (azole antifungals, certain protease inhibitors): increase Clofazimine levels with risk of toxicities.

- CYP3A4 inducers: could potentially decrease Clofazimine levels, reducing its therapeutic efficacy.
- Drugs prolonging QT intervals: clofazimine cause increase risk of arrhythmias.
- Photosensitizing agents: risk of phototoxic reactions.

Contraindications

Absolute
- Hypersensitivity to clofazimine.

Relative
- During pregnancy and lactation
- Pre-existing gastrointestinal disease or individuals prone to electrolyte disturbances.

Pregnancy: Category C

Lactation: better to avoid

Children: safely used in children with dose adjusted to body weight.

ANTITUBERCULAR DRUGS

The first line antitubercular drugs used in the treatment of cutaneous tuberculosis are isoniazid, rifampicin, pyrazinamide and ethambutol.

The initial phase of treatment is for 2 months with all four drugs followed by a continuation phase of 4 months with isoniazid and rifampicin.

Isoniazid

Small water soluble molecule and a synthetic isonicotinic acid derivative.

Mechanism of Action

It is a prodrug activated by mycobacterial catalase—peroxidase (KatG). Isonicotinoyl radical from isoniazid interacts with mycobacterial NAD and NADP and inhibits synthesis of mycolic acid leading to bacterial cell death. Isoniazid specifically inhibits InhA, the enoyl reductase from *Mycobacterium tuberculosis*, by forming a covalent adduct with the NAD cofactor. It is bactericidal against actively growing both intracellular and extracellular *Mycobacterium tuberculosis*.

Pharmacology

It is rapidly absorbed orally reaching peak blood levels in 1–2 hours. Isoniazid is to be taken in empty stomach. Plasma protein binding is <10% and is metabolized by the liver mainly by acetylation and dehydrazination. The half-life in fast acetylators is 1 to 2 hours while in slow acetylators it is 2 to 5 hours. Isoniazid and its metabolites are mainly excreted in the urine.

Monitoring

Baseline
History and clinical examination of symptoms and signs of pre-existing liver disease.

Laboratory
LFT before starting treatment.

Follow-up
LFT at periodic intervals along with clinical evaluation of symptoms and signs of liver damage.

Dosage

- Adults: 5 mg/kg once daily with maximum of 300 mg.
- Children: 10 to 20 mg/kg once daily (maximum 300 mg)

Adverse Effects

- CNS: peripheral neuropathy, convulsions, toxic encephalopathy, optic neuritis and atrophy, toxic psychosis.
- Gastrointestinal: nausea, vomiting, epigastric distress, pancreatitis.

- Hepatic: elevated serum transaminases and bilirubin.
- Hematologic: agranulocytosis, hemolytic, sideroblastic or aplastic anemia; thrombocytopenia; eosinophilia.
- Hypersensitivity reactions: in first 6–7 weeks.
- Metabolic and endocrine: pyridoxine deficiency, pellagra, hyperglycemia, metabolic acidosis, gynecomastia.

Drug Interaction

- A potent inhibitor of CYP3A and CYP2C19 and a weak inhibitor CYP2D6.
- Anticonvulsants (carbamazepine and phenytoin): inhibits hepatic metabolism resulting in increased plasma concentration with chances of toxicity.
- Antacids (aluminum hydroxide): decreases gastrointestinal absorption of isoniazid.
- Cycloserine: increased cycloserine CNS side effects such as dizziness or drowsiness.
- Rifampin: combination increases risk of hepatotoxicity.
- Acetaminophen, corticosteroids, diazepam, oral anticoagulants, primidone and theophyllines: inhibits their metabolism with resultant increase in efficacy and toxicity.

Contraindications

Hypersensitivity to the drug or components of the formulation.
Severe hepatic dysfunction.
- Pregnancy: Category A.
- Lactation: can be used in nursing mothers.
- Children: safe in children.

PYRAZINAMIDE

It is a synthetic pyrazine analog of nicotinamide.

Indication

Tuberculosis

Mechanism of Action

Poorly understood Pyrazinamide (PZA) is metabolized via pyrazinamidase (PZAse) within the cytoplasm to pyrazinoic acid, the active form of the drug. PZA and its analog, 5-chloro-PZA, may inhibit the fatty acid synthetase I enzyme of *M. tuberculosis*. PZA is a bacteriostatic drug and is active in acidic environment.

Pharmacology

Pyrazinamide is well absorbed from the GI tract and attains peak plasma concentrations within 2 hours. Bioavailability exceeds 90%. It is widely distributed throughout the body. Pyrazinamide is approximately 10% bound to plasma proteins. Its half-life is 9 to 10 hours. The drug is hydrolyzed in the liver to its major active metabolic, pyrazinoic acid and 70% of drug is excreted in urine.

Monitoring

Baseline
History of preexisting liver disease or those at increased risk for drug related hepatitis should be followed closely.

Laboratory
Serum uric acid, LFT

Follow-up
Laboratory test at periodic intervals if suggestive clinical signs and symptoms develop during treatment.

Dosage

20 to 25 mg/kg/day (maximum 2 g) orally once or in two divided doses.

Adverse Effects

- General: fever, dysuria, mild arthralgia, myalgia.
- Hepatotoxicity.
- GI: nausea, vomiting and anorexia.

- Hyperuricemia and acute episodes of gout.
- Hematologic: thrombocytopenia and sideroblastic anemia.

Drug Interactions

No significant drug interaction.
- Used with caution with other hepatotoxic drugs.

Contraindications

- Hypersensitivity to the drug.
- Severe hepatic dysfunction
- In acute gout.

Pregnancy: Category C.

Lactation: breast feeding should not be stopped in lactating mothers.

Children: safe in children.

ETHAMBUTOL

It is a water soluble and heat stable bacteriostatic antimycobacterial drug.

Indication

- *M. tuberculosis*
- Disseminated *M avium intracellulare*
- *M. kansasii* infection

Mechanism of Action

- Inhibits arabinosyltransferase enzyme III, which in turn disrupts the assembly of mycobacterial cell wall.

Pharmacokinetics

Ethambutol is rapidly absorbed after oral administration upto 80% reaching peak plasma levels within 2–4 hours. It is widely distributed throughout the body with only 20–30% plasma protein bound. 80% of the drug is excreted through kidneys and the rest through feces. Half-life is 3.3 hours.

Dosage

15 to 25 mg/kg/day (maximum 1600 mg)

Monitoring

Baseline

History of any pre-existing visual or ophthalmic complaints at treatment initiation.
Ophthalmologic evaluation: should include visual acuity, color vision, contrast sensitivity, and visual field test.

Laboratory

CBC, LFT, urea, creatinine

Follow-up

Ophthalmologic examination every 2 months.
CBC, LFT, urea, creatinine at periodic intervals at clinician's discretion.

Adverse Effects

- Ocular: optic neuritis with decreases in visual acuity, constriction of visual fields, central and peripheral scotomas, and loss of red-green color discrimination.
- Drug fever, malaise
- Cutaneous: pruritus, dermatitis.
- Joint pain
- GI upset, abdominal pain, nausea, vomiting, anorexia.
- Neuropsychiatric: mental confusion, disorientation, peripheral neuropathy and possible hallucinations.

Drug Interactions

Neurotoxic medications—concurrent administration of ethambutol with other neurotoxic medications may increase the risk for neurotoxicity like optic and peripheral neuritis.

Contraindications

- Hypersensitivity to drug or its excipients.
- Optic neuritis (unless absolutely essential)

Pregnancy: Category A

Lactation: breast feeding should not be discontinued.

Children: used with caution in infants as they are incapable of reporting visual changes accurately.

Special Notes

Treat latent tubercular infection before starting biologics or JAK inhibitors.

Rifampicin daily for 4 months, 3 months combination therapy of INH and Rifampicin, 3 months of once-weekly regimen of INH plus rifapentine are some of the short course CDC recommended regimens If short course regimens are not feasible, then 6 months or 9 months INH are alternatives.

ANTIRETROVIRAL DRUGS

Antiretroviral drugs are used to treat retroviral infections, mainly HIV. Highly active anti-retroviral therapy is a treatment regimen combing three or more antiretroviral drugs to suppress HIV replication and disease progression. Presently there are more than 30 antiretroviral drugs belonging to different classes, blocking different steps in HIV life cycle and viral replication. according to their mechanism of action.

Classification

Class	Examples
Entry inhibitors (CD4: directed post-attachment inhibitors)	Ibalizumab (IBA)
Fusion inhibitors	Enfuvirtide (T-20)
Entry inhibitor Chemokine receptor antagonists (CCR5 antagonists)	Maraviroc (MVC)
Nucleoside/nucleotide reverse transcriptase inhibitors (NRTIs/NtRTI)	Zidovudine (ZDV/AZT), Lamivudine (3TC), Didanosine (ddI), Abacavir (ABC), Emtricitabine (FTC), Tenofovir disoproxil fumarate (TDF), Tenofovir alafenamide (TAF)

Continued...

Continued...

Class	Examples
Non-nucleoside reverse transcriptase inhibitors (NNRTIs)	Nevirapine (NVP), Efavirenz (EFV), Etravirine (ETR), Rilpivirine (RPV), Delavirdine (DLV), Doravirine (DOR)
Protease inhibitors (PIs)	Lopinavir (LPV)/ritonavir (RTV/r), Saquinavir (SQV), Indinavir (IDV), Nelfinavir (NFV), Darunavir (DRV), Atazanavir (ATV), Tipranavir (TPV), Fosamprenavir (FPV)
Integrase inhibitors/integrase strand transfer inhibitors (INSTIs)	Raltegravir (RAL), Dolutegravir (DTG), Bictegravir (BIC), Cabotegravir (CAB)
Capsid inhibitors	Lenacapavir (LEN)

ART initiation: Start as early as possible after being detected HIV positive.

Goals of Antiretroviral therapy (ART).
- Decrease morbidity and mortality associated with HIV/AIDS.
- Prevent HIV transmission to others
- Reduce HIV viral loads
- Improve immune function
- Decrease drug resistance
- Improve quality of life.

Monitoring in case of ART

Monitoring at the start of treatment

Routine investigations	Special investigations

• Complete blood count (CBC) with differential
• Renal function test
• Liver function test
• Fasting lipid profile
• Fasting glucose and HbA1C
• Urinalysis
• Hepatitis B serology
• Hepatitis C screening
• Pregnancy test
	• HIV specific investigations:
	  – CD4 count
	  – HIV viral load
	• Drug specific investigations:
	  – Resistance testing
	  – HLA-B 5701 testing
	  – Tropism testing

Follow-up monitoring

Every 3 to 6 Months	• CD4 count for the first 2 years of antiretroviral therapy or if viremia develops • Renal function test • Liver function test • CBC with differential • Fasting glucose and HbA1C if abnormal before
Every 6 Months	• Urinalysis if on bictegravir/emtricitabine/TAF or efavirenz/emtricitabine/TDF • HIV viral load

Every 12 Months	• After 2 years:
	  – CD4 count: 300–500 → then every 12 months
	  – CD4 > 500 → monitoring is optional.
	• Hepatitis B serology may be repeated unless the patient is immunized.
	• Screen for hepatitis C if the patient is at risk.
	• Fasting lipid profile
	• Fasting glucose and HbA1C
	• Urinalysis
	• QuantiFERON tuberculosis test

Entry Inhibitors

Ibalizumab is a monoclonal antibody approved for treatment of HIV1 infection in adults.

It blocks the entry of HIV-1 virus into CD4 cells without affecting normal immune function, as it is a CD4-directed post-attachment inhibitor.

Mechanism of Action

Ibalizumab prevents conformational changes within CD4 T cell and HIV glycoprotein gp120 complex resulting in inhibition of interaction of gp120 with CXCR4 and CCR5 coreceptors along with rearrangement of gp41 domain. This prevents viral fusion with CD4 cells and its entry.

Pharmacology

The half-life of ibalizumab is 3 to 3.5 days. It is metabolized by CD4 receptor internalization without any effect on liver and kidney metabolism.

Indications

Used in the treatment of multidrug resistant HIV-1 infection.
- Adult dose: First dose (single loading dose), 2000 mg IV infused over at least 30 min. Maintenance doses, 800 mg IV every 2 weeks infused over at least 15–30 min.

Adverse Effects

Diarrhea, dizziness, nausea, and rash

Fusion inhibitors

Enfuvirtide

It is a 36 amino acid synthetic peptide, derived from C-terminal heptad repeat 1 region of HIV-1 glycoprotein subunit gp41.

Mechanism of Action

It blocks the formation of a six helix bundle core responsible for fusion of the virus with host cell.

Pharmacology

The bioavailability of enfuvirtide is 84% and it is 94% plasma protein bound mainly to albumin. Its half-life is 3.8 hours.

Dose

90 mg subcutaneously bd for adults. Children 6–16 years-2 mg/kg subcutaneously bd (max. 90 mg).

Adverse Effects

- Injection site reactions like erythema, induration, nodules and cysts, edema and hemorrhage.
- Peripheral neuropathy
- Decreased appetite

- Eosinophilia
- Increased risk of bacterial pneumonia.

Contraindications

Hypersensitivity reactions (<1%): rash, fever, nausea and vomiting, chills, rigors hypotension, and/or elevated serum liver transaminases.

Pregnancy: Category B

Lactation: avoid during lactation.

MARAVIROC

It is a CCR 5 receptor antagonist and acts as an entry inhibitor.

Mechanism of Action

Maraviroc selectively attaches to the human chemokine receptor CCR5 present on CD4 cell membranes, preventing the interaction of HIV-1 gp120 and CCR5 required for CCR5-tropic HIV-1 cellular entry.

Pharmacology

Maraviroc is rapidly absorbed orally with an absolute bioavailability of 33% following a 300 mg dose. The peak plasma concentrations are reached in 0.5–4 hours after a single dose. It is mainly metabolized by cytochrome CYP3A4 enzyme and is 76% plasma protein bound.

Dose

150–600 mg bd (dosage changes according to concomitant use of drugs which are CYP3A4 inducers or inhibitors).

Monitoring

- Prior coreceptor tropism assay to determine whether it can be used.
- Periodic LFT.

Drug Interactions

It is a substrate of CYP3A4 and P-glycoprotein Pharmacokinetics of maraviroc are regulated by inhibitors and inducers of these enzymes and transporters.

Adverse Effects

Fever, dizziness, cough, abdominal pain, upper respiratory tract infections, musculoskeletal symptoms.

Contraindications/cautions

- Pre-existing hepatic dysfunction as it can cause hepatotoxicity.

Pregnancy: Category B

Lactation: not recommended.

NUCLEOSIDE AND NUCLEOTIDE REVERSE TRANSCRIPTASE INHIBITORS (NRTIs/NtRTI)

These are the earliest class of approved antiretroviral drugs which inhibit the viral enzyme reverse transcriptase, thus preventing the virus from making DNA copies of its RNA. They are active against both HIV1, HIV2 and other retroviruses.

Zidovudine is no longer commonly used in developed countries due to the availability of better tolerated nucleoside analogues. Use of stavudine, didanosine and zalcitabine has also been discontinued due to their adverse effects and availability of safer alternative drugs.

Mechanism of Action

They are prodrugs, which are phosphorylated by intracellular kinases to active triphosphate forms. The triphosphate form is taken up by DNA resulting in chain termination.

Pharmacology and Dosage of NRTI/NtRTIs

Drug	Bioavailability	Protein binding	Half-life	Metabolism	Excretion	Dose
Abacavir	83%	49%	1.5 hours	Hepatic	Renal: 82.2% Feces: 16%	Adults: 300 mg bd/600 mg od, Pediatric: ≥ 3 months age 8 mg/kg bd
Lamivudine	80–85%	< 36%	5–7 hours	Cleared unchanged by kidneys, hepatic metabolism is low (5–10%)	Renal > 70%	Adults: 300 mg od/150 mg bd, Pediatric: < 4 weeks 2 mg/kg bd, < 50 kg- 4 mg/kg bd
Tenofovir disoproxil fumarate	25%	< 1%	17 hours	Phosphorylated to active diphosphate, no cytochromal P450 enzymes involved	Renal	Adults: 300 mg od Pediatric: 2–<18 years: 8 mg/kg od
Emtricitabine	93% capsule 75% oral solution	< 4%	10 hours	Limited metabolism	Renal 86%	200 mg od (capsule) 240 mg od (oral solution)
Zidovudine	60–70%	34–38%	1.1 hours	Hepatic conjugated to inactive 5'-O-glucuronide metabolite	Renal 74%	Adult: 300 mg bd Pediatric: 4 to < 9 kg: 12 mg/kg bd ≥9 to <30 kg: 9 mg/kg bd ≥30 kg: 300 mg bd

Adverse effects, interactions and contraindications

Drug	Adverse Effects	Interactions	Contraindications
Abacavir	Nausea, vomiting, diarrhea, headache, fever, fatigue, hypersensitivity reactions, musculoskeletal pain, pancreatitis, skin rash, lipoatrophy, hyperlipidemia, lactic acidosis	• Opioids (Methadone): ↓ the level of methadone • Anti-obesity (Orlistat): orlistat decrease the level or efficacy of abacavir • Antiviral (Ganciclovir): risk or severity of cytopenia can be increased	Hypersensitivity, HLA-B*5701 allele carriers
Lamivudine	Headache, nausea, vomiting, diarrhea, abdominal pain, peripheral neuropathy, paresthesia, oral ulcers, pancreatitis, lactic acidosis, aplastic anemia	• NRTI (Abacavir) combination may decrease lamivudine efficiency. • INSTI (Bictegravir): increase lamivudine levels. • Antimalarial (Tafenoquine): may increase lamivudine levels by inhibition of renal transport.	Hypersensitivity, lactation
Tenofovir disoproxil fumarate	Nausea, vomiting, diarrhea, abdominal pain, asthenia, nephrotoxicity, Fanconi syndrome (long term toxicity)	• NRTI (Didanosine): Co-administration causes 40–60% increase in systemic exposure to didanosine with increased risk of adverse events. • Antivirals (acyclovir, valacyclovir, ganciclovir), • Antibiotics (aminoglycosides)and high-dose or multiple NSAIDs: increase serum concentrations of tenofovir with increased risk of nephrotoxicity • Protease inhibitor (Atazanavir) increases tenofovir levels	

Continued...

Continued...

Drug	Adverse Effects	Interactions	Contraindications
Emtricitabine	• Headache, muscle weakness, arthralgia, fatigue, fever, abdominal pain, nausea, vomiting, diarrhea, depression, anxiety, insomnia, rhinitis, cough, and pharyngitis. • Cutaneous: discoloration of tongue, arms, lips, and nail beds, hyperpigmentation of palms and soles	The potential for CYP450 mediated interactions involving emtricitabine with other drugs is low.	Hypersensitivity to drug

Zidovudine	• Nausea/vomiting, diarrhea, headache, myalgias, insomnia, myelosuppression, peripheral myopathy, hepatotoxicity, lactic acidosis
	• Mucocutaneous: nail hyperpigmentation, Stevens-Johnson syndrome
		• Trimethoprim can inhibit renal elimination resulting in increased concentrations of zidovudine.
		• Probenecid increases side effects of zidovudine, likely from either decreased excretion and/or metabolism
		• Hematologic/Bone Marrow Suppressive/ Cytotoxic Agents:
		  – Coadministration of ganciclovir, interferon alfa, ribavirin, or cytotoxic agents may increase the hematologic toxicity of zidovudine.
		  – Concomitant use of zidovudine with doxorubicin and stavudine should be avoided due to antagonistic effect
			Hypersensitivity lactation

Pregnancy

Abacavir: Category C

Lamivudine: Category C

Tenofovir: Category B

Emtricitabine: Category B

Zidovudine: Category B

NONNUCLEOSIDE REVERSE TRANSCRIPTASE INHIBITORS (NNRTI)

They are the second class of reverse transcriptase inhibitors and are structurally different from NRTIs.

Nevirapine, delavirdine and efavirenz are first generation NNRTIs, while etravirine, rilpivirine and doravirine are second generation with higher genetic barrier to developing resistance. Delavirdine is no longer used because of its adverse effects, multiple drug interactions and low genetic barrier to drug resistance.

Mechanism of Action

NNRTIs are non-competitive inhibitors of the enzyme reverse transcriptase. Their attachment to reverse transcriptase results in a hydrophobic pocket formation proximal to the catalytic site. The pocket termed as NNRTI pocket, forms a new spatial configuration of the substrate binding site decreasing polymerase activity. The end result is slow DNA synthesis and reduced viral replication. NNRTIs do not act against HIV-2 reverse transcriptase.

Pharmacology and Dosage

Drug	Bioavailability	Protein binding	Half-life	Metabolism	Excretion	Dose
Nevirapine	>90%	60%	25–30 hours	Hepatic Induces CYP3A4 and 2B6	Urine: 80% Feces: 10%	Adult: 200 mg od for 14 days followed by 200 mg bd Pediatric: 150 mg/m$_2$ od for 14 days then bd
Efavirenz	40–45%	99.5%	52–76 hours	Hepatic CYP3A4 substrate	Feces: 16–61% Urine 14–34% with <1% unchanged	Adults ≥40 kg: 600 mg od Pediatric: 10–<15 kg: 200 mg od 15–<20 kg: 250 mg od 20–<25 kg: 300 mg od 25–<32.5 kg: 350 mg od 32.5–<40 kg: 400 mg od
Etravirine	Not known	99.9%	41 hours	Hepatic via CYP2C19, 3A4, and 2C9	Fecal	10 kg to < 20kg: 100 mg bd 20–< 25 kg: 125 mg bd 25–<30 kg: 150 mg bd ≥30 kg 200 mg bd
Rilpivirine	Unknown	99.7%	13–28 weeks	Hepatic By CYP3A4	85% feces 6.1% urine	Age ≥ 12 years and weight ≥35 kg: 25 mg od
Doravirine	64%	76%	15 hours	Hepatic via CYP3A4 and 3A5	Feces: 90% Urine: 10%	100 mg od

Adverse effects, drug interactions and contraindications of NNRTIs

Drug	Adverse effects	Interactions	Contraindications
Nevirapine	• Mucocutaneous: rash (20%), Stevens-Johnson syndrome, toxic epidermal necrolysis, severe stomatitis • Others: fever, headache, abdominal pain, joint pain, edema, jaundice	• Not to be used with atazanavir • Drugs that induce or inhibit CYP3A4 may require dose adjustments or are to be used with caution.	• Hypersensitivity, severe hepatic impairment
Efavirenz	• Dizziness, insomnia, nightmares, confusion, headache, nausea, vomiting, hyperlipidemia, rash	• Drugs undergoing metabolism through CYP2B6, 3A4, 2C9, and 2C19 may require dose adjustment or are to be used with caution • Contraindicated: dasabuvir, grazoprevir, ritonavir, and voriconazole.	• Hypersensitivity, severe hepatic impairment, lactation
Etravirine	• Rash, blurred vision, burning, numbness, tingling, or painful sensations, dizziness, headache, nervousness, tachycardia, Stevens–Johnson syndrome	• Increases the metabolism of CYP3A4 and CYP2C19 substrates • Increase serum concentration of Efavirenz • Decrease serum concentration of statins and phosphodiesterase 5 inhibitors • Protease inhibitors (darunavir, saquinavir, lopinavir, ritonavir) decrease serum concentration of etravirine	• Hypersensitivity, lactation, hereditary galactose intolerance, lactase deficiency or glucose-galactose malabsorption

Continued...

Continued...

Drug	Adverse effects	Interactions	Contraindications
Rilpivirine	Depression, insomnia, headache and rash	• Not to be used with other NNRTI • Drugs that induce or inhibit CYP3A4 may affect the plasma concentrations of rilpivirine. • Drugs that increase gastric pH may decrease plasma concentration.	Hypersensitivity, severe hepatic insufficiency, lactation
Doravirine	Nausea, dizziness, headache, fatigue, diarrhea, abdominal pain, and abnormal dreams	• Drugs inducing CYP3A4 decrease plasma concentration of doravirine Anticonvulsants: carbamazepine, oxcarbazepine, phenobarbital, phenytoin • Androgen receptor inhibitor: enzalutamide • Antimycobacterials: rifampin, rifapentine Cytotoxic agent: mitotane	Hypersensitivity, children, lactation

Pregnancy category

Nevirapine: Category B.

Efavirenz: Category D

Etravirine: Category B.

Rilpivirine: Category B.

Doravirine: Category B.

PROTEASE INHIBITORS

These are antiretroviral drugs that block the HIV protease enzyme and thus prevent mature virus formation which are unable to infect CD4 cells.

HIV protease inhibitors are classified as first-generation or second-generation protease inhibitors. The first-generation protease inhibitors which were initially effective for treating HIV have started developing viral resistance due to mutations in the active site of the HIV protease enzyme. First-generation protease inhibitors include saquinavir, ritonavir, nelfinavir, indinavir, and amprenavir. Second-generation protease inhibitors have greater potency against HIV infection and include lopinavir, fosamprenavir, darunavir, tipranavir and atazanavir. Indinavir, amprenavir, fosamprenavir and tipranavir are minimally used now.

Mechanism of Action

Protease inhibitors are competitive inhibitors which on binding to HIV protease prevent the proteolytic cleavage of viral polypeptide precursors into functional units for viral capsid formation. They act against both HIV 1 and HIV 2.

Pharmacokinetics and dosage

Drug	Bioavailability	Protein binding	Half-life	Metabolism	Excretion	Dose
Atazanavir	60–68%	86%	7 hours	Hepatic by CYP3A4	79% feces, 13% renal	300 mg with ritonavir (RTV) 100 mg as booster od

Continued...

Continued...

Drug	Bioavailability	Protein binding	Half-life	Metabolism	Excretion	Dose
Darunavir (DRV)	37% (alone), 82% (with ritonavir)	95%	15 hours	Hepatic by CYP3A4	Feces: 79.5% Renal: 13.9%	800 mg with ritonavir 100 mg od Pediatric: Darunavir and Ritonavir Dose bd 3 Years—<12 Years and Weight ≥10 kg 20–<30 kg: DRV 375 mg + RTV 100 mg 30–<40 kg: DRV 450 mg + RTV 100 mg ≥40 kg: DRV 600 mg+RTV 100 mg
Saquinavir	4%	97%	7–12 hours	Hepatic by CYP3A4	81–88% feces Renal: 1–3%	Saquinavir 100 mg + RTV 100 mg Not approved in < 16 years
Nelfinavir	70 to 80% with food	> 98%	3.5–5 hours	Hepatic by CYP3A4	Feces: 87% Urine: 1–2%	1250 mg bd/750 mg tds Pediatric: no longer recommended due to inferior potency compared to other drug regimens
Lopinavir	25% when used alone Increases with concurrent RTV use	>98%	5–6 hours	Hepatic by CYP3A4	Feces: 82% Urine: 10.4%	Lopinavir 400 mg + RTV 100 mg bd 800 mg + RTV 200 mg od
Ritonavir	Not determined	98–99%	3–4 hours	Mainly as unchanged drug in plasma Hepatic by CYP3A4 and CYP2D6	Feces: 86% Urine: 11%	• Initial dose: 300 mg bd increase by 100 mg bd every 2 to 3 days to maintenance dose of 600 mg bd • Booster: 100–400 mg bd • Pediatric: Initial 250 mg/m^2 bd increase by 50 mg/m^2 bd every 2 to 3 days to maintenance dose • 350 to 400 mg/m^2 bd (max. 600 mg)

Adverse effects, interactions and contraindications

Drug	Adverse effects	Interactions	Contraindications
Atazanavir	• Common: hyperbilirubinemia, rash, hypercholesterolemia, hyperamylasemia, jaundice, nausea, cough, fever • Severe: Stevens-Johnson syndrome, erythema multiforme, angioedema, cholecystitis, pancreatitis, interstitial nephritis, nephrolithiasis diabetic ketoacidosis, and AV block	• Drug which are inhibitors or substrates of CYP3A4, CYP 1A2, CYP2C9 can cause serious interactions with atazanavir. • Include: warfarin, diltiazem, triazolam, oral midazolam, pimozide, cisapride, simvastatin, lovastatin, oral contraceptives, phosphodiesterase 5 inhibitors, and tenofovir • To be used with caution or avoided.	• Hypersensitivity, infants < 3 months of age

Continued...

Continued...

Drug	Adverse effects	Interactions	Contraindications
Darunavir	• Common: Diarrhea, nausea, rash, headache, abdominal pain, vomiting, dizziness, insomnia, asthenia, fatigue • Others: Hepatotoxicity, hyperglycemia, hypertriglyceridemia, hypercholesterolemia, lipodystrophy, SJS, TEN, peripheral neuropathy	• Drugs which induce inhibit CYP3A4 have significant interactions with darunavir • Phosphodiesterase 5 inhibitors: increases plasma concentration • Sedative/hypnotics: concentration increased (contraindicated with oral midazolam, triazolam) • Estrogen based contraceptives: efficacy reduced • Narcotic analgesics: reduced plasma levels • Statins (lovastatin, simvastatin): risk of rhabdomyolysis • Antidepressants (paroxetine, amitriptyline): increase antidepressant concentration.	• Hypersensitivity, severe hepatic impairment, lactation
Saquinavir	Common: nausea, vomiting, diarrhea, fatigue, pneumonia, lipodystrophy and abdominal pain.	• Being a potent inhibitor of CYP3A4 it increases the concentration of drugs primarily metabolized by CYP3A. • Coadministration with drugs that induce CYP3A4 decreases plasma concentrations of saquinavir and reduced efficacy. • Antiarrhythmics: risk of cardiac arrhythmias • Antimycobacterial (Rifampicin): increased hepatotoxicity • Statins (Lovastatin, Simvastatin): risk of myopathy including rhabdomyolysis • Neuroleptics (Pimozide): cardiac arrhythmias • PDE5 Inhibitors (Sildenafil): increased side effects • Sedative/Hypnotics: increased sedation	• Hypersensitivity, severe hepatic impairment, congenital or acquired QT prolongation, complete AV block, recalcitrant hypokalemia, hypomagnesemia, lactation
Nelfinavir	Diarrhea, nausea, flatulence, abdominal pain, leucopenia, mouth ulcers, pancreatitis, dermatitis, maculopapular rash, arthralgia, myalgia, abnormal liver function tests, hyperglycemia, hypertriglyceridemia, nephrolithiasis	• Drugs which induce/inhibit CYP3A and 2C19 have significant interactions with nelfinavir • Antimycobacterials (rifampicin): decrease nelfinavir concentration • Anticonvulsants (phenytoin): decrease nelfinavir concentration • PDE5 inhibitors: increase adverse effects • Proton pump inhibitors: decrease nelfinavir concentration • Antidepressants (trazodone): increase adverse effects of trazodone • Immunosuppressants (cyclosporine, tacrolimus): concentration of both nelfinavir and immunosuppressants increased • Statins (Lovastatin, Simvastatin): risk of myopathy including rhabdomyolysis • Oral contraceptives: decreased efficacy of OCPs • Antimycobacterials: (Rifampicin): reduce nelfinavir concentrations • Other protease inhibitors (Saquinavir): concentration of saquinavir increased	• Hypersensitivity, • Severe hepatic impairment, lactation

Continued...

Continued...

Drug	Adverse effects	Interactions	Contraindications
Lopinavir/ Ritonavir combination	• Common: nausea, diarrhea, rash, abdominal pain, hyperlipidemia, elevated liver transaminases • Others: headache, arthralgia, weakness, hyperuricemia flatulence, neutropenia, lipodystrophy, nephrolithiasis	• Concomitant administration of drugs which are CYP3A4 inducers and/or major substrates require dose adjustment or monitoring of adverse effects • Antimycobacterial (rifampin): decrease virologic response • GI motility agent(cisapride): life threatening cardiac arrhythmias • HMG-CoA Reductase Inhibitors (lovastatin, simvastatin): risk of myopathy including rhabdomyolysis. • Alpha 1—Adrenoreceptor antagonist (alfuzosin): risk of hypotension • Sedative/Hypnotics (midazolam, triazolam): increased sedation or respiratory depression • PDE5 enzyme inhibitor(sildenafil): increased side effects	• Hypersensitivity • Severe hepatic dysfunction • Lactation

Pregnancy

Atazanavir: Category B

Darunavir: Category C

Saquinavir: Category B

Nelfinavir: Category B

Lopinavir/Ritonavir: Category C

INTEGRASE INHIBITORS/INTEGRASE STRAND TRANSFER INHIBITORS (INSTIS)

Integrase inhibitors are antiretroviral drugs that prevent HIV infection by blocking viral integrase enzyme.

First-generation INSTIs are raltegravir (RAL) and elvitegravir (EVG). Development of resistance to first generation INSTIs have resulted in the development of second generation integrase inhibitors dolutegravir, bictegravir, and cabotegravir which are structurally different from the first generation drugs and are effective against many of the first generation INSTI resistant mutants.

Elvitegravir is not used singly nowadays but in combination with emtricitabine, tenofovir and cobicistat (a CYP3A inhibitor which increases the pharmacokinetic properties of antiretrovirals).

Mechanism of Action

These drugs inhibit the enzyme HIV integrase, thus preventing the incorporation of viral DNA into the host genomic DNA. This prevents HIV-1 provirus formation and transmission of infection.

Pharmacology and dosage

Drugs	Bioavailability	Plasma protein binding	Half-life	Metabolism	Excretion	Dose
Raltegravir	Absolute bioavailability not confirmed	83%	7–12 hours	Hepatic by glucuronidation	Fecal: 50–74% Urine: 7–14%	Adults: 400 mg bd Pediatric: • 10–14 kg: 75 mg bd • 14–20 kg: 100 mg bd • 20–28 kg: 150 mg bd • 28–40 kg: 200 mg bd • >40 kg: 300 mg bd

Continued...

Continued...

Drugs	Bioavailability	Plasma protein binding	Half-life	Metabolism	Excretion	Dose
Dolutegravir	Not determined	>98.9%	14 hours	Hepatic glucuronidation by UGT1A1	Feces: 53% Urine: 31%	50 mg od/bd (in INSTI resistant cases) Pediatric: • 3 kg to <6 kg: 5 mg od • 6 kg to <10 kg: 15 mg od • 10 kg to <14 kg: 20 mg od • 14 kg to <20 kg: 25 mg od • ≥20 kg: 30 mg od
Bictegravir	Not determined	>99%	17.3 hours	Hepatic by CYP3A and UGT1A1	Feces: 60.3% Urine: 35%	• Fixed dose combination of 3 drugs • 50 mg of bictegravir (BIC) +200 mg of emtricitabine (FTC)+ 25 mg of tenofovir alafenamide
Cabotegravir	Not determined	>99.8%	41 hours (oral) 5.6–11.5 weeks IM	Hepatic glucuronidation by UGT1A1	Feces: 58.5% Urine: 26.8%	• Adults and children ≥12 years of age and weight ≥ 35 kg: 30 mg + 25 mg of rilpivirine od for at least 28 days. • Injection once monthly regimen: One-time initiating injection • Initiate on last day of current ART therapy or oral lead-in (if used) • Cabotegravir 600 mg (3 mL) IM + Rilpivirine 900 mg (3 mL) IM

Adverse effects, interactions and contraindications

Drug	Adverse effects	Interactions	Contraindications
Raltegravir (RAL)	• Common: insomnia, headache, dizziness, nausea, abdominal pain, dyspepsia, back pain and fatigue	• Drugs decreasing RAL concentration: antacids, antimycobacterials (rifampicin), anticonvulsants (carbamazepine, phenobarbital, phenytoin) So dose of RAL needs to be increased. Concomitant use of anticonvulsants better to be avoided	• Hypersensitivity, lactation
Dolutegravir (DTG)	• Headache, nausea, diarrhea, insomnia dizziness, abnormal dreams, depression, fatigue, abdominal pain or discomfort, flatulence, rash, itching, increase in liver enzymes, increase in creatine phosphokinase	• Drugs decreasing DTG concentrations thus needing dose escalation: antacids, antimycobacterials (rifampicin), anticonvulsants (carbamazepine, phenobarbital, phenytoin): decrease DTG levels • Antiarrhythmics (dofetilide, disopyramide): increase concentration of antiarrhythmics • Hypoglycemics (metformin): concentration increased, monitor for adverse effects of metformin	• Hypersensitivity, severe hepatic impairment, lactation

Continued...

Continued...

Drug	Adverse effects	Interactions	Contraindications
Bictegravir (BIC)	Diarrhea, nausea, headache, fatigue, abnormal dreams, dizziness, insomnia, depression	• Drugs decreasing BIC concentrations: antacids, antimycobacterials (rifabutin, rifampicin—better to avoid), anticonvulsants (carbamazepine, phenobarbital, phenytoin–better to avoid), dexamethasone • Antiarrhythmics (dofetilide) increased concentration • Hypoglycemics (metformin): concentration increased, monitor for adverse effects of metformin	Hypersensitivity, severe hepatic and renal impairment
Cabotegravir (CAB)	Injection site reactions, fever, fatigue, headache, musculoskeletal pain, nausea, sleep disorders, dizziness, rash, abdominal pain, increased CPK, lipase and hepatic transaminases	• Antacids: reduce plasma concentration of oral CAB • Antimycobacterial (rifabutin): decrease levels of both oral and IM CAB • Anticonvulsants (carbamazepine, phenobarbital, phenytoin): decrease levels of CAB, to avoid usage	Hypersensitivity, lactation

Pregnancy

Raltegravir: Category C

Elvitegravir: Category B

Dolutegravir: Category B

Bictegravir: Category B

Cabotegravir: Category B

POST-EXPOSURE PROPHYLAXIS

- Post-exposure prophylaxis (PEP) refers to taking anti-HIV drugs soon after a possible exposure to HIV to prevent HIV acquisition.
- It works by stopping viral replication and preventing the development of persistent infection during the brief interval between viral entry into the body and the development of established infection.
- The first dose of PEP should be administered ideally within 2 hours (but preferably within the first 72 hours) of exposure and the risk evaluated as soon as possible.
- Anyone with a known or suspected exposure to HIV should be offered PEP.

Recommended PEP regimen (NACO 2021)

Age of the exposed person	PEP Regimen	Alternate Regimen
Children: Age < 6 years Weight < 20 kg	AZT + 3TC + LPV/r (Dosage according to weight band)	If Hb <9 g/dL: ABC + 3TC + LPV/r (Dosage according to weight band)
Children: Age > 6 years Weight > 20 kg	AZT + 3TC (Dosage as per weight band) + DTG (50 mg) once daily	If Hb <9 g/dL: ABC + 3TC (dosage according to weight band) + DTG (50 mg) once daily
Adolescents and Adults (Age >10 years and weight >30kg)	TDF (300 mg) + 3TC (300 mg) + DTG (50 mg) (FDC: Once daily)	TDF (300 mg) + 3TC (300 mg) (FDC: once daily) + LPV (200 mg)/r (50 mg) (two tablets twice daily) OR TDF (300 mg) + 3TC (300 mg) + EFV (600 mg) (FDC: Once daily)

Pre-Exposure Prophylaxis (PrEP)

- Part of integrated HIV prevention strategy.
- To be used by individuals who are HIV negative but are at high risk of acquiring infection through either sexual route of iv drug abuse.
- Persons benefiting from PrEP include:
- Sexual partner of individual who is HIV positive and nor virally suppressed on treatment.
- Recent or probable future inconsistent use of condoms for vaginal or anal sex;
- Recent sexually transmitted infection (STI) in last 6 months
- Recent PEP use for sexual exposure to HIV, especially for individuals who have used PEP more than once.

WHO-recommended PrEP products (2024)
1. Oral PrEP: Tenofovir disoproxil fumarate (TDF) 300 mg + emtricitabine (FTC) 200 mg OR TDF 300 mg + lamivudine (3TC) 300 mg tablets
   - Event-driven PrEP (ED-PrEP): PrEP for a single event (for example, sex on only one day), or for infrequent "single" events that are weeks or months apart.
   - Daily oral PrEP: If exposure to HIV continues for more than one day—if an individual prefers to continue to take oral PrEP daily rather than stopping and restarting—they should take one dose of oral PrEP every day for as long as they desire and until at least two days after the last potential exposure.
2. DVR (25 mg dapivirine impregnated silicone vaginal ring)—long-acting, user-controlled, non-systemic, HIV prevention product: to be worn for 24 hours prior to exposure to HIV. The DVR is designed to be worn continuously in the vagina for one month until it is replaced with a new ring.
3. Injectable CAB-LA (600 mg cabotegravir extended-release injectable suspension)—long-acting injection schedule:

- First injection: month 0.
- Second injection: one month (+/– 7 days) after the first injection.
- Third and subsequent injections: two months (+/– 7 days) after the previous injection.

Antiretroviral drugs of various classes are used in combinations as fixed dose or separately to treat HIV.

As per NACO guidelines 2021, the basic principle for first-line ART for treatment-naive adult and adolescent patients is to use a triple drug combination from two different classes of anti retrovirals. The first-line ART consists of a NRTI backbone, preferably Non-thymidine (Tenofovir plus Lamivudine) and one INSTI, preferably Dolutegravir.

- The preferred first-line ART regimen for all HIV patients >10 years of age and weight >30 kg is:
  - Tenofovir (TDF 300 mg) + Lamivudine (3TC 300 mg) + Dolutegravir (DTG 50 mg) regimen (TLD) as FDC in a single pill once a day.

In special situations, where this preferred first line regimen can't be used, alternative effective drug regimens are used.

ANTIMALARIALS

The most commonly used antimalarials (Hydroxychloroquine & Chloroquine) are 4-aminoquinolines and derivatives of quinine, Quinine is an alkaloid derived from the bark of the South American cinchona tree.

Hydroxychloroquine (HCQ) differs from chloroquine (CQ) only by the presence of a hydroxyl group in a B-position at the end of the ethyl side chain.

Indications

Approved
- Lupus erythematosus
- Malaria
- Rheumatoid arthritis

Unlicensed

Photosensitive disorders
- Polymorphous light eruption
- Porphyria cutanea tarda
- Solar urticaria
- Cutaneous manifestations of dermatomyositis

Granulomatous disorders
- Cutaneous sarcoidosis
- Generalized granuloma annulare

Benign disorders with lymphocytic infiltrates
- Lupus panniculitis
- Idiopathic panniculitis
- Jessner's lymphocytic infiltrate
- Lymphocytoma cutis
- Chronic erythema nodosum.

Miscellaneous
- Urticarial vasculitis
- Cutaneous or systemic vasculitis
- Oral lichen planus
- Chronic ulcerative stomatitis
- Morphea
- Graft versus host disease
- Follicular mucinosis

Mechanism of Action
- Not completely understood.
- Antimalarials inhibit toll-like receptors, mainly TLR9 & TLR7 and decrease levels of TNF-α and type I interferons.
- They also stabilize the lysosomes within injured cells and inhibit antigen presentation and synthesis of proinflammatory cytokines.
- Inhibit phospholipase A2 and the resultant effects on prostaglandin metabolism block UV light induced cutaneous effects.

Pharmacology
The antimalarials are well absorbed orally and bind particularly to pigmented tissues, including the retina. Metabolism mainly occur in liver and it is excreted renally with half-life of 40–50 days. Plasma level peaks at 4 hours for HCQ and 5 hours for CQ. Bioavailability of HCQ is 74% and CQ is 50%.

Hydroxychloroquine appears less toxic but also less effective than chloroquine.

Dosage
- Standard dosage range of HCQ-200–400 mg/day or 6.5 mg/kg/day.
- Dosage range of CQ-250–500 mg/day or 3 mg/kg/day.

Adverse Effects
Myelotoxicity—risk of agranulocytosis and aplastic anemia.

Cutaneous
- Blue-grey discoloration (shins, face and palate)
- Bleaching of hair roots.
- Hypersensitivity reactions: eczematous, lichenoid eruptions, urticaria, erythroderma.
- Induction or exacerbation of psoriasis
- Transverse pigmentary bands on nails.

Idiosyncratic

Oculotoxicity
- Antimalarial induced retinopathy ("Bull's eye maculopathy")
- Corneal deposits
- Loss of accommodation: chloroquine.

Neuromuscular toxicity
- Myalgia, fatigue and myopathy.
- Headache, dizziness, tinnitus, hearing loss, nightmares, irritability, seizures and psychosis.
- Cardiotoxicity—rarely cause QT prolongation.
- Gastrointestinal toxicity—nausea, vomiting, diarrhea, anorexia and heartburn.

Monitoring

Baseline

Ocular

Baseline slit-lamp, fundoscopic examination, visual field testing and assessment of visual acuity.

Laboratory

- Complete blood count
- Liver function tests
- Glucose-6-phosphate dehydrogenase (G6PD) screening (selected cases)
- Random or 24 hours urinary porphyrin screening.

Follow-up

Ocular—yearly slit lamp and fundoscopic test (after 5 years of therapy)

Laboratory

- Complete blood count (monthly for 3 months, then every 4-6 months)
- Chemistry profile (after 1 month, after 3 months then 4-6 months)

Drug Interactions

- Antacids impair absorption of antimalarials.
- Antimalarials may enhance the effects of hypoglycemic therapy.
- Macrolides (erythromycin, clarithromycin): QT prolongation with risk of torsades de pointes (with CQ)
- Dapsone: increased risk of hemolysis.
- Local anesthetics (benzocaine, prilocaine, tetracaine): increase risk of hemolysis, methemoglobinemia.
- Ionotropic agents (digoxin): decrease clearance of both HCQ and CQ with increased serum levels and adverse effects.
- Antiarrhythmics (propafenone): decrease clearance of both HCQ and CQ with increased serum levels and adverse effects.

Contraindication

- Hypersensitivity reaction to the drugs
- Documented retinopathy.

Pregnancy: safe in pregnancy.

Lactation: safe in nursing mothers.

Children: safe and effective in children.

SYSTEMIC RETINOIDS

Vitamin A (retinol) and related compounds with either structural (retinol derivative) or functional (vitamin A activity) similarities are known as retinoids. All-*trans*-retinoic acid (tretinoin), a naturally occurring metabolite, was the first retinoid to be synthesized with no significant advantages over vitamin A.

Mechanism of Action

1. Affect cellular growth, differentiation and morphogenesis;
2. Inhibit tumor promotion and malignant cell growth;
3. Exert immunomodulatory actions; and
4. Alter cellular cohesiveness

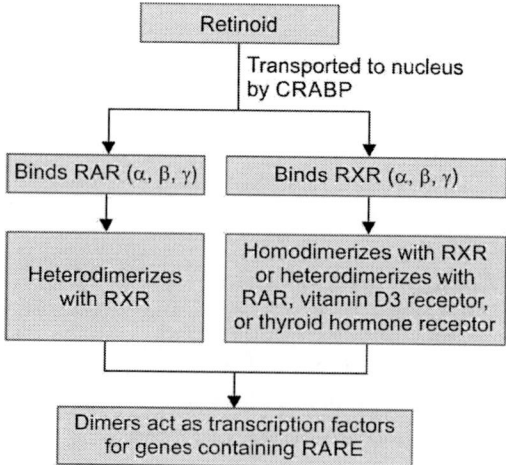

RAR = retinoic acid receptor, RXR = Retinoid X-receptor, CRABP = Cytosolic retinoic acid-binding protein

Classification

Synthetic Retinoids

1. **Isotretinoin:** Isotretinoin (13-cis-retinoic acid) is a naturally occurring retinoid resulting from the metabolism **of vitamin A**

Indication

Approved
Nodulocystic acne, Recalcitrant, especially if any scarring tendency.

Unlicensed
Follicular Disorders

Acne-related conditions
- Gram-negative folliculitis
- HIV-associated eosinophilic folliculitis
- Acne with solid facial edema

Rosacea
- Papulopustular (recalcitrant to other therapies)
- Granulomatous rosacea

Hidradenitis suppurativa

Dissecting cellulitis of scalp

Disorders of Keratinization
- Darier disease
- Pityriasis rubra pilaris
- Ichthyosis spectrum
- Keratodermas

Chemoprevention of Malignancies
- Organ transplantation patients
- Syndromes with increased risk of cutaneous malignancy
- Bazex syndrome
- Nevoid basal cell carcinoma syndrome
- Muir—Torre syndrome
- Xeroderma pigmentosa
- Frequent BCC or SCC (non-immuno-suppressed)
- Kaposi sarcoma

Other Inflammatory Dermatoses
- Lupus erythematosus (cutaneous features)
- Lichen planus—oral erosive, palmoplantar
- Lichen sclerosus et atrophicus

Miscellaneous
- Graft-versus-host disease
- Human papillomavirus infections

Mechanism of Action
Does not bind to RAR and RXR receptor

Pharmacology
- The oral bioavailability is 25% and is enhanced with food intake.
- There is very little lipid deposition in adipose tissue.
- The metabolism of retinoids is mainly via oxidation and chain shortening to biologically inactive, water-soluble products in the liver.
- In plasma, more than 99% of isotretinoin is protein-bound, mainly to albumin and elimination half-life is 20 hours.

Dosage
Isotretinoin 0.5–2 mg/kg/day

Adverse Effects

Acute
Mucocutaneous
- Xerosis with pruritus, Cheilitis, Dry mucosa: mouth, nose (epistaxis), eyes
- Skin fragility
- Retinoid dermatitis
- Palmoplantar peeling
- Photosensitivity
- Sticky sensation (palms, soles)
- Granulation tissue with pyogenic granuloma-like lesions (e.g., at sites of acne cysts, periungual)
- Intertriginous erosions with exuberant granulation tissue
- Nail fragility with softening, onycholysis, paronychia
- Facial swelling

- Staphylococcus aureus infection
- Telogen effluvium, hair thinning

Ocular

- Xerophthalmia
- Blepharoconjunctivitis
- Reduced night vision
- Blurred vision, photophobia, keratitis, corneal ulceration (rare)

Systemic

- Myalgias
- Arthralgias
- Anorexia, nausea, diarrhea, abdominal pain
- Headache, pseudotumor cerebri (rare)
- Fatigue, lethargy, irritability
- Depression, suicidal ideation (rare)
- Toxic hepatitis (rare)
- Pancreatitis secondary to hypertriglyceridemia (rare)

Metabolic

- Hyperuricemia
- Elevated liver function tests (usually transient, minor): AST, ALT, alkaline phosphatase, LDH, bilirubin.
- Hyperlipidemia: hypertriglyceridemia; increased cholesterol, VLDL and LDL; decreased HDL
- Elevated creatine kinase
- Hypercalcemia (rare)

Blood

- Leukopenia (with bexarotene)
- Agranulocytosis (with bexarotene)
- Thrombocytosis, thrombocytopenia

Chronic

Mucocutaneous

- Alopecia (rare)
- Dry eyes, corneal opacities (rare)

Systemic

- DISH syndrome-like bone changes
- Osteophyte and bony bridge formation, especially of vertebrae (rarely clinically significant at dosages for acne) Anterior > posterior spinal ligament calcification
- Extraspinal tendon and ligament calcification
- Osteoporotic changes in long bones (rare, with possible exception of long-term etretinate)
- Premature epiphyseal closure (rare)
- Periosteal thickening
- Myopathy (rare)

Contraindications

Pregnancy category X drug (avoid pregnancy and use two forms of effective contraception or abstinence continuously for 1 month before, during, and for 1 month after isotretinoin treatment)

Lactation: unsafe

Children: contraindicated in ≤ 12 years

Alitretinoin (9–cis-retinoic acid)

Alitretinoin is a naturally occurring pan-agonist retinoid.

Unlicensed indication

Refractory chronic hand eczema.

Mechanism of Action

Binds to both RARs and RXRs.

Pharmacology

- The absorption of oral alitretinoin from the gastrointestinal tract is variable; the absolute bioavailability of alitretinoin has not been determined.
- Alitretinoin is metabolized via oxidation by CYP3A4 enzymes of the liver into

4-oxo-alitretinoin, and both the parent drug and its metabolite also undergo isomerization into at-RA and 4-oxo-at-RA, respectively.
- Elimination is primarily renal, with the half-life of unchanged alitretinoin ranging between 2 and 10 hours.

Dosage

10–30 mg/day

Second-generation retinoids

Acitretin and Etretinate

Acitretin is the major metabolite and the pharmacologically active form of etretinate.

Indication

Approved

Psoriasis: Severe plaque-type psoriasis, Pustular psoriasis—generalized, pustular psoriasis—localized.

Unlicensed

Follicular Disorders

Acne-related conditions
- Gram-negative folliculitis
- HIV-associated eosinophilic folliculitis
- Acne with solid facial edema

Rosacea
- Papulopustular (recalcitrant to other therapies)
- Granulomatous rosacea
- Hidradenitis suppurativa
- Dissecting cellulitis of scalp

Disorders of Keratinization
- Darier disease
- Pityriasis rubra pilaris
- Ichthyosis spectrum
- Keratodermas

Chemoprevention of Malignancies
- Organ transplantation patients
- Syndromes with increased risk of cutaneous malignancy
- Bazex syndrome
- Nevoid basal cell carcinoma syndrome
- Muir–Torre syndrome
- Xeroderma pigmentosa
- Frequent BCC or SCC (nonimmunosuppressed)
- Kaposi sarcoma

Other Inflammatory Dermatoses
- Lupus erythematosus (cutaneous features)
- Lichen planus—oral erosive, palmoplantar
- Lichen sclerosus et atrophicus

Miscellaneous
- Graft-versus-host disease
- Human papillomavirus infections

Mechanism of Action

Only binds to RAR receptors

Pharmacology

- The oral bioavailability is 60% for acitretin and 44% for etretinate; and is enhanced with food intake.
- Etretinate is approximately 50 times more lipophilic than acitretin and binds strongly to plasma proteins, particularly lipoproteins and albumin. Etretinate is stored in adipose tissue (including subcutaneous fat), from which it is released slowly, with a long terminal half-life of up to 120 days.
- Acitretin metabolism does not accumulate in adipose tissue and is eliminated from the body more rapidly, with a half-life of 2 days.
- Hepatic metabolism, re-esterification to etretinate indirectly increased by alcohol consumption; main metabolite: *cis*-acitretin.

Dosage

Acitretin 25–50 mg/day

Contraindications

Pregnancy category X drug (it is 1 month before starting the drug and 3 years in USA and

2 years in Europe after discontinuation of the drug).)

Lactation: unsafe

Children: contraindicated in ≤ 12 years

Third-Generation Retinoids

Bexarotene

Bexarotene is an RXR-selective retinoid

Indications

Approved: Mycosis Fungoides: Resistant to at least one systemic therapy

Mechanism of Action

Binds to RXR

Pharmacology

- In plasma, bexarotene is highly bound (>99%) to various proteins.
- Bexarotene has a terminal half-life of between 7 and 9 hours.
- Bexarotene is metabolized by CYP3A4 and generates its own oxidative metabolites via hepatic CYP3A4 induction.
- Neither bexarotene nor its metabolites are excreted in the urine; their elimination is thought to occur primarily via the hepatobiliary system.

Dosage

300 mg/m^2/day

Adverse Effects

Other than side effects of systemic retinoids, bexarotene causes clinical signs of hypothyroidism with decreased free thyroxine (T4).

Contraindications

Pregnancy: Category X drug.

Lactation: unsafe

Children: contraindicated in ≤ 12 years

Monitoring for Isotretinoin and Acitretin

Baseline

Examination

- Careful history and physical examination
- Identify those patients at increased risk for toxicity or adverse effects
- Document concomitant medications that may interact with retinoids

Laboratory

- Serum or urine pregnancy test (in women of childbearing potential)
- Complete blood count (CBC) with platelets
- Liver function tests (AST, ALT, alkaline phosphatase, bilirubin)
- Lipid profile during fasting (triglycerides, total cholesterol, LDL and HDL cholesterol)
- Renal function tests (blood urea nitrogen, creatinine)
- Optional urinalysis (if patients have renal disease, proteinuria, diabetes or hypertension)

Special Tests

- Consider baseline X-rays of wrists, ankles or thoracic spine if plan long-term retinoid therapy
- Consider ophthalmologic examination if patients have a history of cataracts or retinopathy

Follow-up

Examination

- Clinical evaluation monthly for first 3–6 months, then every 3 months
- Assessment of patient response, improvement, and complaints of adverse effects
- Routine physical examination of lesional skin

- Additional/focused physical examination of any reported adverse effects

Laboratory
- Monthly for the first 3–6 months, then every 3 months
- Complete blood count (CBC) with platelet Liver function tests (AST, ALT)
- Fasting lipid (triglycerides, cholesterol- order LDL and HDL cholesterol periodically)
- Renal function tests (optional urinalysis)
- Serum or urine pregnancy test monthly for women of childbearing potential (and at end of therapy)

Special Tests
Periodically as indicated by symptoms
- Consider yearly X-rays of wrists, ankles or thoracic spine with long-term retinoid therapy
- Radiographic studies of significantly symptomatic joints with long-term therapy
- Complete ophthalmologic examination if patients report visual changes

Pregnancy Monitoring Guidelines

General Requirements
- Must have had two negative urine or serum pregnancy tests with a sensitivity of at least 25 mIU/mL before receiving the initial isotretinoin prescription.
- The second pregnancy test should be done during the first 5 days of the menstrual period immediately preceding the beginning of isotretinoin therapy.
- For patients with amenorrhea, the second test should be done at least 11 days after the last act of unprotected sexual intercourse (without using two effective forms of contraception).

Additional Guidelines
- Effective forms of contraception include both primary and secondary forms of contraception.
- Primary forms of contraception include: tubal ligation, partner's vasectomy, intrauterine devices, birth control pills, and injectable/implantable/insertable hormonal birth control products.
- Secondary forms of contraception include diaphragms, latex condoms, and cervical caps; each must be used with a spermicide.

Retinoic acid metabolism blocking agents
Retinoic acid metabolism blocking agents (RAMBAs) inhibit catabolism of at-RA by P450 enzymes in the CYP26 family, thereby raising the intracellular levels of endogenous at-RA in the skin and other targeted tissues. This limits systemic exposure and the potential for toxicity. Liarozole, an imidazole derivative without antifungal properties, is a RAMBA with low isoenzyme specificity that also inhibits P450-mediated pathways of steroid biosynthesis whereas talarozole, a triazole derivative, is a more selective and highly active CYP26 enzyme inhibitor.

Drug Interaction
1. Concomitant intake of tetracyclines group of drugs increases the risk of pseudotumor cerebri.
2. CYP3A4 inhibitors (Erythromycin >> clarithromycin > azithromycin) increase retinoids drug levels and resultant toxicity—lipids, liver toxicity, etc.
3. Combination with cyclosporine increases the level of cyclosporine.

Note
1. Renal toxicity is not characteristic of retinoid therapy. Isotretinoin has been safely administered to patients with end-stage kidney disease who were undergoing hemodialysis.
2. Patients with diabetes mellitus may have more difficult glucose control while taking a retinoid; however, the causal relationship remains uncertain. Acitretin has been shown to possibly reduce the efficacy of progestin-only contraceptives.

COLCHICINE

Colchicine is a naturally occurring alkaloid extracted from seeds and tubers of the plant *Colchicum autumnale*.

Indication

Approved

- Gout and pseudogout
- Familial Mediterranean fever

Unlicensed Dermatological Uses

- Neutrophilic dermatoses: Behcet disease, recurrent aphthous stomatitis, Sweet syndrome.
- Bullous dermatoses: dermatitis herpetiformis, linear IgA bullous dermatoses, IgA pemphigus, epidermolysis bullosa acquisita.
- Vasculitis: leukocytoclastic vasculitis, urticarial vasculitis.
- Papulosquamous dermatoses: psoriasis, palmoplantar pustulosis.
- Autoimmune connective tissue diseases: dermatomyositis, scleroderma, relapsing polychondritis.

Mechanism of Action

Colchicine has both antimitotic and anti-inflammatory properties.
- Antimitotic-binds to the dimers of tubulin, preventing their polymerization into microtubules, resulting in mitotic metaphase arrest and interference with cell motility.
- Anti-inflammatory—lysosomal degranulation, reduces adhesiveness of neutrophils to endothelial cells, inhibits macrophage activation and mast cell degranulation. It also inhibits cyclooxygenases COX-1 and COX-2.

Pharmacology

Colchicine is rapidly absorbed after oral administration reaching peak plasma levels in 30–120 minutes. Its terminal half-life is 20–40 hours. The drug I metabolized in the liver by CYP3A4 and P-glycoprotein and undergoes hepatobiliary excretion mainly in stool with 10–20% excreted unchanged in urine. The drug has a narrow therapeutic window with dose > 0.8 mg/kg being fatal.

Monitoring

Baseline

Laboratory

CBC, urea, creatinine, electrolytes and LFT.

Follow-up

- Complete blood count and differential white cell count every month.
- LFT, urea, creatinine, urinalysis every 3 months.

Dosage

Starting dose is 0.5 mg daily, increasing to 1–1.5 mg in divided doses. Maintenance dose is 0.5–2 mg.

Adverse Effects

- Neuromuscular toxicity and rhabdomyolysis.
- Hematological: Myelosuppression, leucopenia, pancytopenia, agranulocytosis, aplastic anemia.
- GI: Nausea, vomiting, watery diarrhea, abdominal cramps, paralytic ileus.
- Cutaneous: urticaria, SJS, TEN and alopecia universalis.

Drug Interactions

- Macrolide antibiotics, azole antifungals, calcium-channel blockers: increase colchicine levels with more adverse effects.
- Cyclosporin: concentrations increased resulting in increased risk of nephrotoxicity and neuromuscular adverse effects.

- Statins and fibrates (CYP3A4 substrates): increased risk of myopathy and rhabdomyolysis.
- Vitamin B12: absorption impaired resulting in megaloblastic anemia.

Contraindications

- Hypersensitivity to drug or its components
- Hematologic disorders
- Severe renal dysfunction.
- Coadministration of strong CYP3A4 and P-glycoprotein inhibitors.

Pregnancy: Category C

Lactation: Can be used in lactation.

Children: Safe to use in children.

BIOLOGICAL THERAPY/IMMUNOBIOLOGICS

Biologics are a class of drugs that are produced using a living system (microorganism, human, plant or animal cel). They are larger molecules and structurally more complex than traditional drugs. Biologics though more expensive than traditional drugs, target specific components of the immune system and have better safety profile.

Biosimilars: are biologic medications highly similar to the already approved biologic (reference) product with no clinically meaningful differences from the reference product. They are less expensive compared to the original biologic.

Immunobiologics consists of antibody based agents (mainly monoclonal antibodies), fusion proteins, recombinant cytokines and growth factors.

Classification According to Immunological Targets

- Cytokine/cytokine receptor blocking agents

Cytokine/cytokine receptor blocking agents	Drugs
TNF-α inhibitors	Etanercept, Infliximab, Adalimumab, Certolizumab pegol, Golimumab
IL-1 inhibitor	Anakinra, Canakinumab, Rilonacept
IL-17 inhibitor	Secukinumab, Brodalumab, Ixekizumab
IL-23 inhibitor	Guselkumab, Tildrakizumab, Risankizumab
IL-12/23 inhibitor	Ustekinumab
IL-4/13 inhibitor	Dupilumab
IL-13 inhibitor	Tralokinumab, Lebrikizumab
Il-31 receptor alpha inhibitor	Nemolizumab
IL-36 receptor antagonist	Spesolimab

- Anti-cell surface receptor antibodies

Cell surface receptor	Drugs
Anti CD4	Ibalizumab
Anti CD20	Rituximab
Anti CD6	Itolizumab

- Drugs inhibiting T lymphocyte costimulatory molecules
CTLA4–Ig—Abatacept
    CTLA4 Antibody—Ipilimumab
- Anti-IgE—Omalizumab, Ligelizumab
- B-lymphocyte stimulator (BLyS)-specific inhibitor—Belimumab

Nomenclature of monoclonal antibodies and fusion proteins explained by their source system
- Monoclonal antibodies have the suffix mab and fusion proteins have the suffix cept.

Antibody origin	Sub-stem B	Examples
Chimeric	-xi-	Rituximab, Infliximab
Humanized	-zu-	Omalizumab
Human	-u-	Secukinumab

Tumor necrosis factor (TNF) inhibitors: Classification

- Soluble TNF receptors: Etanercept
- Monoclonal antibodies: Infliximab, adalimumab, golimumab, certolizumab pegol

Mechanism of action

- Bind to both soluble and membrane bound TNF-α and prevent the cytokine from activating the receptors. Etanercept binds to TNF-β also.
- Induce apoptosis in T cells and monocytes by activating complement dependent cytotoxicity. (Adalimumab, Infliximab, Golimumab)

ETANERCEPT

It is a dimeric, fully human fusion protein consisting of two extracellular ligand binding domains of p75 TNFR (tumor necrosis factor receptor) linked to Fc domain of human immunoglobulin (Ig) G1.

Indications

Approved

- Ankylosing spondylitis
- Juvenile idiopathic arthritis (2 years or older)
- Plaque psoriasis (4 years or older)
- *Psoriatic arthritis*
- Rheumatoid arthritis

Unlicensed

- Neutrophilic dermatoses: Behcet disease, pyoderma gangrenosum, aphthous stomatitis, subcorneal pustular dermatoses, Sweet syndrome.
- Vasculitis: Giant cell arteritis, Takayasu arteritis, polyarteritis nodosa.
- Granulomatous dermatoses: generalized granuloma annulare, cutaneous sarcoidosis.
- Hidradenitis suppurativa
- Severe drug reactions: Stevens–Johnson syndrome, toxic epidermal necrolysis.
- Papulosquamous disorders: Pityriasis rubra pilaris, lichen planus
- Acute graft-versus-host disease.
- Autoimmune connective tissue disorders: Systemic sclerosis, Still disease, dermatomyositis, cutaneous lupus erythematosus, relapsing polychondritis
- Autoimmune bullous disorders: Mucous membrane pemphigoid
- Multicentric reticulohistiocytosis.

Pharmacology

Etanercept ha a half-life of 4.8 days. After subcutaneous injection peak level is reached in 2 days. Bioavailability is 58% with metabolism by proteolysis and metabolic byproducts eliminated in urine, bile or both.

Dosage

- 25 or 50 mg SC once or twice weekly accordingly.
- Children (2–17 years): 0.8 mg/kg/week in divided doses.

Monitoring

Baseline

History and physical examination

- To rule out tuberculosis, other acute and chronic infections
- To exclude malignancy, congestive heart failure, demyelinating diseases.

Laboratory

- Complete blood count
- Liver function test
- Blood urea, creatinine
- Serology: hepatitis B, C and HIV
- Urinalysis
- Pregnancy test
- Interferon-γ release assay (IGRA)

Chest X-ray

Follow-up monitoring

Annually: IGRA

CBC, LFT: clinician's decision

Drug Interactions

- Simultaneous use of IL-1 receptor antagonist (anakinra) or other DMARD increases risk of serious infection
- Live vaccines to be avoided

Pregnancy: Category B

Lactation

- Lactation: can be given during lactation, low risk

INFLIXIMAB

It is a chimeric IgG1human (75%)-mouse (25%) monoclonal antibody specific for TNF-α Infliximab is effective against both soluble and membrane bound TNF-α.

- Psoriatic arthritis (adults)
- Crohn disease (adults and children ≥ 6 years of age)
- Ulcerative colitis (adults and children ≥ 6 years of age)
- Rheumatoid arthritis
- Ankylosing spondylitis.

Unlicensed

- Severe acute generalized pustular psoriasis.

Neutrophilic dermatoses: Behcet disease, pyoderma gangrenosum, aphthous stomatitis.
- Granulomatous dermatoses: Cutaneous sarcoidosis
- Hidradenitis suppurativa
- GVHD
- Systemic vasculitis
- Granulomatous cheilitis
- Pityriasis rubra pilaris
- Reactive arthritis.
- Subcorneal pustular dermatosis
- Relapsing polychondritis
- Multicentric reticulohistiocytosis.
- Sjögren syndrome.

Pharmacology

It has a rapid onset of action with a half-life of 7–12 days in adults. Infliximab is metabolized by proteolysis into peptides or amino acids, which can be either recycled for protein synthesis or excreted by the kidneys.

Dosage

- 5 mg/kg/dose slow iv

Monitoring

Baseline

Similar to etanercept

Follow-up

Liver function tests: repeated at 3 months, then every 6–12 months.

Drug Interactions

- Simultaneous use of IL-1 receptor antagonist (anakinra), abatacept and tocilizumab increases risk of serious infection—not recommended as concurrent use
- Live vaccines to be avoided and to be administered 4 weeks before starting therapy.
- Concurrent administration of immuno-modulators like methotrexate may reduce the incidence of anti drug antibody to infliximab.

Pregnancy: Category B

Lactation: can be used.

ADALIMUMAB

Fully human IgG1 monoclonal antibody to TNF-α.

Indications

Approved

- Psoriatic arthritis
- Rheumatoid arthritis
- Juvenile idiopathic arthritis,
- Psoriasis (plaque type in adults)

- Ankylosing spondylitis.
- Crohn disease (adult and children)
- Ulcerative colitis
- Uveitis
- Hidradenitis suppurativa (≥ 12 years of age)

Unlicensed

- Neutrophilic dermatoses: Behcet disease, pyoderma gangrenosum, aphthous stomatitis.
- Granulomatous dermatoses; cutaneous sarcoidosis.
- Vasculitis: ANCA associated systemic vasculitis.
- Dermatomyositis.

Pharmacology

Bioavailability of adalimumab is 64% with half-life of 12 days. Peak concentration is reached in 131 hours and it is metabolized by proteolysis.

Dosage

- Loading dose of 80 mg/160 mg according to indications followed by 40 mg SC alternate weekly.

Monitoring

Similar to etanercept

Drug Interactions

- Simultaneous use of other targeted immunomodulators increases risk of serious infection—not recommended
- Avoid live vaccines.
- Methotrexate reduces the drug clearance.

Pregnancy: Category B

Lactation: can be used.

Children: recently approved in children ≥ 5 years of age for ulcerative colitis.

GOLIMUMAB

Human recombinant IgG1 monoclonal antibody specific for TNF-α.

Indications

Approved

- Rheumatoid arthritis (active Moderate-to-severe disease) in adults.
- Psoriatic arthritis (active disease) in adults.
- Ankylosing spondylitis (active disease) in adults.
- Ulcerative colitis (Moderate-to-severe disease) in adults.
- Polyarticular juvenile idiopathic arthritis and psoriatic arthritis in children aged 2 or older.

Pharmacology

Bioavailability of subcutaneous golimumab is 53%. Half-life is 2 weeks with exact metabolic pathway not clear.

Dosage

2 mg/kg iv infusion at weeks 0, 4, 8. Alternate 50 mg subcutaneous.

Monitoring

Similar to etanercept.

Drug Interactions

- Should not be administered simultaneously with other biologic DMARDs (infliximab, ustekinumab, rituximab) or JAK inhibitors due to increased risk of infection.
- Avoid live vaccines.
- Concurrent use of antivirals or antibiotics not recommended.
- Drugs metabolized by CYP450 enzymes (cyclosporine, warfarin) to be used with caution with monitoring for adverse effects.

Pregnancy: Category B.

Lactation: compatible.

CERTOLIZUMAB PEGOL

It is a humanized Fab' antibody fragment conjugated to polyethylene glycol that is an antagonist of both membrane bound and soluble TNF-α.

Indications

Approved
- Plaque psoriasis
- Psoriatic arthritis
- Rheumatoid arthritis
- Ankylosing spondylitis.
- Crohn disease.

Unlicensed
Neutrophilic dermatoses: Behcet disease, pyoderma gangrenosum.

Mechanism of Action

Certolizumab pegol does not have an Fc region compared to other TNF-α inhibitors and so has minimal Fc mediated effects like complement-dependent cytotoxicity or antibody dependent cytotoxicity. Absence of the Fc region also prevents its transport across placenta and so it is safe to use in pregnancy.

Pharmacology

Certolizumab being pegylated has better pharmacokinetics and bioavailability with increased half-life. Bioavailability is 80% with circulatory half-life of 14 days. It is degraded by the reticuloendothelial system to smaller peptides and amino acids and the elimination of the pegylated moiety is through kidneys.

Dosage

400 mg subcutaneous every 2 weeks.

Monitoring

Similar to etanercept.

Drug Interactions

- Coadministration with other biologic DMARDs (anakinra, TNF-α inhibitors, rituximab, abatacept) is contraindicated due to increased risk of infections.
- Live vaccines to be avoided.

Pregnancy: Category B.

Lactation: can be used.

Children: used in $\geq$ 2 years for juvenile polyarticular idiopathic arthritis.

Adverse Effects

Adverse effects of TNF-α inhibitors
- Common
  - Injection site reactions—redness, pain, itching, swelling, hemorrhage
  - Infusion reactions—with infliximab as it is administered iv, occur during or up to 3 hours following transfusion (20%)

Common symptoms—flushing, headache, pruritus, nausea, taste alterations, dyspnea

Severe hypotension, chest pain, dyspnea, anaphylaxis, convulsions
- Rare
  - Increased risk of infections—tuberculosis, bacterial infections, systemic fungal infections (histoplasmosis, aspergillosis, candidiasis) and other opportunistic infections. Upper respiratory tract infections are seen more with golimumab and certolizumab pegol.
  - Hepatotoxicity—transaminitis, cholestatic disease, hepatitis B, autoimmune hepatitis. Seen more with infliximab
  - Malignancy—risk of malignancies specially Hodgkin and cutaneous T cell lymphoma, non melanoma skin cancers and in children GI malignancies.

- Demyelinating disorders
- Congestive heart failure
- Cutaneous—paradoxical skin disorders; psoriasis, eczema, palmoplantar pustulosis, lichenoid dermatitis,
- Interstitial granulomatous dermatitis, cutaneous small vessel vasculitis, drug induced lupus erythematosus
- Hematological side effects—leucopenia, neutropenia, thrombocytopenia and pancytopenia

Contraindications

Absolute
- Hypersensitivity to component of formulation.
- Infliximab—allergy to murine proteins.

Relative
- Severe active infection—active tuberculosis including latent tuberculosis reactivation, invasive fungal, bacterial and viral (herpes zoster, hepatitis C) opportunistic infections
- Congestive heart failure (New York Heart association III or IV)
- Personal or family history of demyelinating disease or multiple sclerosis.
- History of lymphoreticular malignancy.

INTERLEUKIN 17 INHIBITORS

T-helper 17 cells produce interleukin 17 (IL17) which is made up of 6 cytokines (IL17A to IL17F) and 5 receptors subunits (IL17RA to IL17RE). These interleukins are essential in host defense against microbial infections and are implicated in the pathogenesis of various chronic inflammatory disorders.

IL17A inhibitors used in dermatology are of two groups:
- Monoclonal antibodies against IL17A: Secukinumab and ixekizumab.
- Monoclonal antibodies against IL17RA: Brodalumab.

Secukinumab

It is a human (Ig)G1 monoclonal antibody that binds to IL17A.

Indications

Approved
- Moderate-to-severe psoriasis (adults).
- Psoriatic arthritis.
- Ankylosing spondylitis.

Unlicensed
- Palmoplantar psoriasis
- Generalized pustular psoriasis.
- Hidradenitis suppurativa.

Mechanism of Action
Secukinumab on binding to IL-17A prevents its interaction with the IL-17 receptors.

Pharmacology
It has a bioavailability of 55–77% with peak levels reached in 6 days and a half-life of 22–31 days. Though the metabolism of Secukinumab is not clear, but being monoclonal antibodies it is expected to be proteolyzed to smaller peptides and amino acids. Mode of excretion is not clear.

Dosage
- 300 mg subcutaneous at weeks 0, 1, 2, 3 and 4 followed by 300 mg every 4 weeks.
- Pediatric: European medical agency has recommended a dose of 75 mg for children < 50 kg and 150 mg for children ≥ 50 kg aged ≥ 6 years.

Drug Interactions
- Coadministration of other immunosuppressives may increase the risk of infection by increasing the degree of immunosuppression.
- Live vaccines/live attenuated vaccines to be avoided within 2–3 half lives before

treatment, during and for 6 months after discontinuation.
- Patient with latex allergy/sensitivity-can develop reaction as both the removable cap to both prefilled syringe and autoinjector/pen contains natural rubber latex.

Pregnancy: Category B

Lactation: Use with caution as data limited.

Children: Safe for children aged 6 years and above.

IXEKIZUMAB

It is a humanized IgG4 monoclonal antibody that binds to IL-17A.

Indications

Approved
- Moderate-to-severe plaque psoriasis in adults.
- Psoriatic arthritis.
- Ankylosing spondylitis.
- Psoriasis in children ≥ 6 years.

Unlicensed
- Psoriatic erythroderma.
- Generalized pustular psoriasis.

Mechanism of Action

Ixekizumab binds to IL-17A and neutralizes it, thus preventing its interaction with IL-17 receptors.

Pharmacology

The bioavailability of ixekizumab is between 60–81% with peak levels reached in 4 days and half-life of 13 days.

Dosage

- 160 mg subcutaneous injection as loading dose followed by
- 80 mg every 2 weeks for 12 weeks and then every 4 weeks.
- Pediatric dosing: 160 mg loading and then 80 mg every 4 weeks if >50 kg
- 80 mg loading and then 40 mg every 4 weeks if 25–50 kg
- 40 mg loading and then 20 mg every 4 weeks if <25 kg.

Drug Interactions

- Coadministration of other immunosuppressives may increase the risk of infection by increasing the degree of immunosuppression.
- Live vaccines/live attenuated vaccines to be avoided within 2–3 half lives before treatment, during and for 6 months after discontinuation.

Pregnancy: Category not assigned due to insufficient data.

Lactation: Limited data, to be used with caution.

BRODALUMAB

It is a human monoclonal IgG2 antibody and a IL-17 receptor antagonist.

Indications

Approved
Moderate-to-severe plaque psoriasis in adults who have not responded to both topical and other systemic therapy.

Unlicensed
Psoriatic arthritis.

Mechanism of Action

It is a IL-17 receptor antagonist and thus inhibits interaction with cytokines IL-17A, AF,

C, E and F resulting in suppression of IL-17 related inflammatory responses.

Pharmacology

The bioavailability of brodalumab is 55% with peak levels reached in 3 days and a half-life of 10.9 days.

Dosage

210 mg subcutaneous injection every 2 weeks.

Drug Interactions

- Live vaccines to be avoided.
- Concurrent administration of drugs metabolized by hepatic CYP450 enzymes (cyclosporine, warfarin) may lead to their altered efficacy and dose adjustment may be needed.

Pregnancy: No data, so not assigned.

Lactation: Use with caution during breastfeeding till more data is available.

Children: Not used due to lack of data.

Monitoring of IL-17 Inhibitors

Baseline

- Personal and family history of GI symptoms especially for inflammatory bowel disease before starting them.

Laboratory

- Complete blood count.
- Liver function tests.
- Blood urea and creatinine.
- Serology for hepatitis B, C, HIV
- Urinalysis.
- Pregnancy test
- Tuberculosis screening: Chest X-Ray, IGRA

Follow-up

- Complete blood count every 6 months/if signs of infection.
- History and follow-up examination for GI symptoms (every 3–6 months)
- Annual tuberculosis screening to detect latent tuberculosis: IGRA, Chest X-ray for high-risk patients.

Adverse Effects Common to IL-17 Inhibitors

- Injection site reactions: erythema, induration, pain, bruising, hemorrhage (more with ixekizumab and brodalumab than secukinumab)
- Infections: upper respiratory infections, pharyngitis, nasopharyngitis, influenza, bronchitis, urinary tract infections, conjunctivitis, tinea, reactivation of latent tuberculosis (for high-risk patients)
    - Chronic mucocutaneous candidiasis. (secukinumab-1.7%, ixekizumab 3.3%, brodalumab 4%)
- Inflammatory bowel disease—new-onset and also exacerbation can occur.
- Hematological-neutropenia (mild, transient and self limited)
- Hypersensitivity reactions (e.g., angioedema, anaphylaxis) can develop.
- Suicidal ideation and behavior, including complete suicides (brodalumab)
- Cutaneous: lichenoid dermatitis, psoriasiform eruptions, hypertrichosis, new onset atopic dermatitis like eruption

Contraindications of IL-17 Inhibitors

Absolute

Hypersensitivity to the drug or components of formulation.

Relative

- Active inflammatory bowel disease
- History of suicidal ideas or recent suicidal behavior. (brodalumab)

Interleukin 12/23 Inhibitors

Ustekinumab

It is a fully human monoclonal IgG1κ antibody directed at the shared p40 subunit of IL-12 and IL-23.

Indications

Approved

- Moderate-to-severe plaque psoriasis in patients who are candidates for phototherapy or systemic therapy, aged 6 or older.
- Active psoriatic arthritis.
- Inflammatory bowel disease: severe active Crohn disease and ulcerative colitis.

Unlicensed

- Hidradenitis suppurativa,
- Systemic vasculitis: Takayasu arteritis, giant cell arteritis.
- Neutrophilic dermatoses: Behçet disease, pyoderma gangrenosum.
- Myelodysplastic syndrome.
- Papulosquamous disorders: pityriasis rubra pilaris, lichen planus.
- Synovitis, acne, pustulosis, hyperostosis, and osteitis (SAPHO) syndrome,
- Atopic dermatitis.
- Systemic lupus erythematosus.

Mechanism of Action

Ustekinumab blocks the p40 subunit (shared subunit of IL-12 and IL-23) and inhibits the interaction of these cytokines with the IL-12Rβ1 receptor resulting in inhibition of IL-12 and IL-23 signaling, activation, and cytokine production. This leads to downregulation of the immune system with anti-inflammatory effects.

Pharmacology

The bioavailability of Ustekinumab is 57% with a half-life of 3 weeks. Peak levels after subcutaneous injection is reached in 8.5 days. Details about metabolism and excretion are not known. Development of antidrug antibodies to Ustekinumab can lead to loss of efficacy.

Dosage

For dermatological indications: Weight ≤ 100 kg: 45 mg subcutaneously initially and after 4 weeks then every 12 weeks.
- Weight >100 kg: 90 mg subcutaneous initially and after 4 weeks then every 12 weeks.
- Pediatric: weight < 60 kg: 0.75 mg/kg subcutaneously and after 4 weeks then every 12 weeks.
- Weight 60–100 kg: 45 mg subcutaneously and after 4 weeks then every 12 weeks.
- Weight > 100 kg: 90 mg subcutaneously and after 4 weeks then every 12 weeks.

Monitoring

Baseline

- Complete blood count, liver function tests, electrolytes, urea, creatinine. CRP, ESR.
- Tuberculosis screening: Chest X-ray, IGRA
- Serology for hepatitis B, C, HIV.
- Varicella zoster virus serology-persons with a negative/uncertain history of varicella.
- Autoantibodies (ANA, dSDNA).
- Pregnancy test.
- Urinalysis.

Follow-up

- Complete blood count, liver function tests, electrolytes, urea, creatinine: at 3–4 months, then every 6 months.
- Regular clinical examination to detect infection, malignancies or other systemic disorders.

Adverse Effects

- Common: nasopharyngitis, headache, fatigue, upper respiratory tract infections, sinusitis, back pain, arthralgia, injection site erythema.

- Serious: Severe infections or exacerbation/reactivation of existing infection (bacterial, mycobacterial, fungal, viral)
- Malignancy (non-melanoma skin cancer)
- Hypersensitivity reactions/anaphylaxis
- Reversible posterior leukoencephalopathy syndrome
- Cryptogenic organizing pneumonia
- Interstitial or eosinophilic pneumonia

Drug Interactions

- None reported.
- Can be combined with methotrexate but not with other immunosuppressives.
- Live vaccines to be avoided.

Contraindications

Absolute

- Hypersensitivity to ustekinumab or any of the components.
- Severe active infections

Caution

- Latex hypersensitivity (with the pre-filled syringe dose)
- History of prior malignancy or present malignancy.
- Chroni/recurrent infections including latent tuberculosis.
- PUVA therapy.

Pregnancy: Category B.

Lactation: safe in nursing mothers.

Children: approved in children ≥ 6 years of age.

Interleukin 23 inhibitors

They are monoclonal antibodies that target the p19 subunit of IL-23. Guselkumab, tildrakizumab and risankizumab are the three drugs in this class.

Mechanism of Action

IL-23 inhibitors bind to the p19 subunit of IL-23 and prevents its interaction with IL-23 receptors on cell surface of various immune cells and release of proinflammatory cytokines. These inhibitors specifically inhibit the Th17 pathway.

Guselkumab also decreases mRNA expression of IL-17F and IL-22, and increases the level of IFN-γ produced by Th1 cells.

GUSELKUMAB

Guselkumab is a fully human, IgG1λ monoclonal antibody.

Indications

Approved

- Moderate-to-severe plaque psoriasis in adults.
- Active psoriatic arthritis.

Unlicensed

- Hidradenitis suppurativa.
- Palmoplantar pustulosis

Pharmacology

Guselkumab has a bioavailability of 49% following subcutaneous injection with peak levels reached in 5.5 days and half-life of 15–18 days. It is probably metabolized by proteolysis.

Dosage

100 mg subcutaneous injection on week 0, 4 and thereafter every 8 weeks.

Monitoring (Common to All IL-23 Inhibitors)

Baseline

- Complete blood count, liver function tests, electrolytes, urea, creatinine, CRP, ESR.
- Tuberculosis screening: Chest X-ray, IGRA
- Serology for hepatitis B, C, HIV.
- Varicella zoster virus serology-persons with a negative/uncertain history of varicella.
- Pregnancy test.
- Urinalysis.

Follow-up

- Complete blood count, liver function tests, electrolytes, urea, creatinine: at 3–4 months, then every 6 months.
- Regular screening and clinical examination to detect nonmelanoma skin cancers.
- Periodic screening to detect infections (tuberculosis, hepatitis B, C and HIV)

Adverse Effects

- Nasopharyngitis, upper respiratory infections.
- Injection-site erythema.
- Headache, arthralgia, back pain, pruritus.
- Increased risk of common infections like tinea, herpes simplex, gastrointestinal infections.

Drug Interaction

Live vaccines to be avoided.

Contraindications

Hypersensitivity to the drug or components of the formulation.

Pregnancy: no data.

Lactation: no data

Children: not evaluated.

TILDRAKIZUMAB

Tildrakizumab is a humanized monoclonal Ig-G1κ antibody that selectively inhibits IL-23p19.

Indications

Approved

- Moderate-to-severe plaque psoriasis in adults.

Pharmacology

Tildrakizumab has a bioavailability ranging between 73–80% with peak levels reached in 6 days with half-life of 23 days. Metabolism is probably by proteolysis with formation of smaller peptides and amino acids.

Dosage

100 mg subcutaneous injections at weeks 0, 4 and then every 12 weeks.

Adverse Effects

- Nasopharyngitis, headache, upper respiratory tract infections, bronchitis and gastroenteritis.
- Injection-site reaction: pain, erythema, hematoma.

Drug Interactions

Live vaccines to be avoided.

Contraindications

Hypersensitivity to the drug or components of the formulation.

Pregnancy: no data.

Lactation: no data

Children: insufficient data.

RISANKIZUMAB

It is a humanized IgG1 monoclonal antibody that binds to the p19 subunit of IL-23.

Indications

Approved

- Moderate-to-severe psoriasis in adults.
- Psoriatic arthritis.
- Crohn disease in adults.

Pharmacology

Risankizumab has a half-life of 20–28 days with bioavailability of 89% and peak levels of drug being reached in 4–10 days. Metabolism is by proteolysis into smaller peptides and amino acids.

Dosage

150 mg subcutaneous injection at weeks 0, 4, then every 12 weeks.

Adverse Effects

- Most common: nasopharyngitis, headache, gastroenteritis, and back pain.
- Others: upper respiratory tract infections, diarrhea, and arthralgia.

Drug Interactions

Live vaccines to be avoided.

Contraindications

Hypersensitivity to the drug or components of the formulation.

Pregnancy: no data.

Lactation: no data

Children: insufficient data.

RITUXIMAB

Rituximab is a chimeric murine human monoclonal IgG1κ antibody against CD20 antigen present on the surface of mature and pre-B-cells. It is made of two mouse variable regions, two human IgG1 heavy chains and two human κ light chains.

Indications

Approved

- Malignancies: Non-Hodgkin B cell lymphoma CD20+, chronic lymphocytic leukemia CD20+
- Vasculitis: Granulomatosis with polyangiitis, microscopic polyangiitis
- Rheumatoid arthritis
- Pemphigus vulgaris.

Unlicensed

- Autoimmune bullous dermatoses: pemphigus foliaceus, paraneoplastic pemphigus, epidermolysis bullosa acquisita, bullous pemphigoid, mucous membrane pemphigoid
- Autoimmune connective tissue disorders: Dermatomyositis, cutaneous lupus erythematosus
- Graft-versus-host disease.
- Vasculitis: Eosinophilic granulomatosis with polyangiitis.

Mechanism of Action

Rituximab kills CD20+ B cells by antibody mediated cellular damage, complement activated cytotoxicity and induction of CD20 signaling leading to cytolysis.

Pharmacology

Depends on the nature of the antibody isotype and the amount and location of CD20. IgG1 antibodies have a half-life of 21 days and are removed from circulation by phagocytosis.

Dosage

Rheumatoid arthritis protocol—1,000 mg iv infusion administered twice at 14 days gap with maintenance dose of 500 mg at 12 and 18 months (used for pemphigus vulgaris).

Alternate lymphoma protocol—375 mg/m^2 weekly for 4 weeks. (used for vasculitic disorders).

Monitoring

Baseline

- Screen for active infections and planned surgeries.
- History of prior or recent malignancy.
- History of cardiopulmonary disease.
- Vaccination history
- Pregnancy and lactation screening.

Laboratory

- Complete blood count with differentials.
- Liver function test.
- Urea, creatinine.

- Serum electrolytes: sodium, potassium, chloride, bicarbonate
- Serology for hepatitis B, C, HIV.
- Tuberculosis screening-IGRA.
- Flow cytometry for CD20 and CD3.
- Antidesmoglein 1, 3 titres.

Follow-up monitoring

Laboratory
- Complete blood count with differentials every 2–3 months.
- Periodic LFT, urea, creatinine, electrolytes.
- Periodic flow cytometry for CD20 and CD3.
- Periodic antidesmoglein 1, 3 titres.
- Annual tuberculosis screening.

Adverse Effects

Severe infusion reactions:
- 80% of fatal reactions occur with the first infusion, onset within half an hour to 2 hours.
- Headache, chills, nausea, pain, hypotension, urticaria, angoidema, bronchospasm, acute respiratory distress syndrome, myocardial infarction, ventricular fibrillation and even cardiogenic shock resulting in death.
- Mucocutaneous: Stevens–Johnson syndrome, toxic epidermal necrolysis, paraneoplastic pemphigus, lichenoid and vesiculobullous dermatitis.
- Neurological: Progressive multifocal leukoencephalopathy.
- Serious infections (bacterial, fungal, or viral) up to 1 year after completing therapy and reactivation of viral infections, especially hepatitis B, C, herpes simplex, varicella-zoster.
- Reactivation of tuberculosis, increased risk of *Pneumocystis jerovicci* pneumonia has also been seen.
- Cardiological: cardiac arrhythmia, myocardial infarction, cardiogenic shock.
- GI: bowel obstruction and perforation.
- Hematologic: Late-onset neutropenia (≥4 weeks after infusion) can develop, is self limiting.
  - Tumor lysis syndrome can develop in lymphoma patients, especially those with a high tumor burden resulting in acute renal failure.
- Decreased antibody responses to immunization, including COVID mRNA vaccines.
  - B cell lymphopenia can occur in infants exposed to rituximab in utero

Drug Interactions
- Coadministration with other myelosuppressive medications: increased risk of myelosuppression.
- Used together with other immunosuppressive drugs: increased immunosuppressive effects.
- Avoid live vaccines before and during treatment. All immunizations to be completed 4 weeks before treatment.
- Cisplatin: increased nephrotoxicity.

Contraindications
- Hypersensitivity (type I) to murine proteins.
- Hypersensitivity to Chinese hamster ovary cells or other components of the formulation.
- Active severe infections.
- Progressive multifocal leukoencephalopathy.
- Uncontrolled cardiac disease and heart failure.

Pregnancy: Category C

Lactation: avoid breast feeding during and for 6 months following stoppage of therapy.

Children: used off label following lymphoma protocol.

DUPILUMAB

Dupilumab is a recombinant, fully human IgG4 κ monoclonal antibody directed against α subunit of both type 1 and type 2 IL-4 receptors. It has been manufactured in Chicken Hamster Ovary cells by recombinant DNA technology.

Indications

Approved

- Moderate-to-severe, resistant, atopic dermatitis in adults and children ≥6 months not responding to conventional therapy.
- Asthma: as maintenance treatment in both children (≥ 6 years of age) and adults.
- Chronic rhinosinusitis with nasal polyposis in patients ≥12 years of age as maintenance treatment.
- Prurigo nodularis.
- Eosinophilic esophagitis in patients ≥12 years of age.

Unlicensed

- Dermatitis: allergic contact dermatitis, hand dermatitis.
- Chronic spontaneous urticaria.
- Alopecia areata.

Mechanism of Action

Dupilumab binds to the α subunit of both type 1 and type 2 IL-4 receptors, thus resulting in inhibition of downstream signaling of both IL-4 and IL-13 and reduction in Th2 mediated inflammation.

Pharmacology

Dupilumab shows non-linear pharmacokinetics with bioavailability of 64% after subcutaneous injection and peak levels reached after 1 week. It is metabolized by antibody-complex endocytosis into smaller peptides and amino acids. Antidrug antibodies are seen in 7% and is associated with decreased serum concentrations.

Dosage

- For dermatological indications-initial dose of 600 mg subcutaneous injection followed by 300 mg every other week.
- Dosage in pediatric patients: 6 months to 5 years age with body weight 5 kg to <15 kg—200 mg every 4 weeks
- 15 kg to < 30 kg: 300 mg every 4 weeks.
- Patients 6-17 years of age with body weight 15 kg to <30 kg: Initial loading dose 600 mg followed by 300 mg every 4 weeks.
- 30 kg to <60 kg: 400 mg initial dose followed by 200 mg every other week.
- ≥60 kg: 600 mg initial dose followed by 300 mg every other week.

Monitoring

No approved monitoring guidelines.

Baseline

Laboratory
- Complete blood count
- Urea and creatinine
- Liver function tests.
- Serology for hepatitis B, C, HIV.

Follow-up

- Complete blood count
- Urea and creatinine
- Liver function tests.

At 1 month, 4 months and then annually as per clinician's assessment.

Adverse Effects

- Injection site reactions: commonest.
- Ophthalmologic: conjunctivitis, keratitis, blepharitis, dry eye, eye pruritus.
- Infections: oral herpes, herpes zoster.

- Nasopharyngitis.
- Cutaneous: face and neck erythema, dermatitis, psoriasis/psoriasiform eruptions, lichen planus/lichenoid eruptions, and eosinophilic granulomatosis with polyangiitis, alopecia areata, vitiligo, detection of previously undetected cutaneous T cell lymphoma.
- Hypersensitivity reactions.

Drug Interactions

Dupilumab by inhibiting IL-4 and IL-13 can affect cytochrome enzyme formation and lead to change in various drug concentrations and their effects leading to close monitoring and dose adjustment.
- Anticonvulsants: phenytoin, carbamazepine, ethosuximide
- Anticoagulants: warfarin.
- Antiarrhythmics: procainamide, digoxin
- Immunosuppressives: cyclosporine, tacrolimus.
- Avoid live vaccines.

Contraindications

Hypersensitivity to dupilumab or components of the formulation.

Pregnancy: No data.

Lactation: acceptable during breast feeding.

Children: is approved in children ≥ 6 months of age.

IL-13 INHIBITORS

Il-13 inhibitors either bind to soluble IL-13 and prevents IL-4. Receptor α/L-13, Receptorα1 heterodimerization or blocks the binding of IL-13 to its receptors IL-13Rα1/IL-13Rα2 hampering endogenous regulation of IL-13. Lebrikizumab and tralokinumab are the two IL-13 inhibitors presently approved for dermatologic use.

LEBRIKIZUMAB

Lebrikizumab, a humanized IgG4κ monoclonal antibody with a high affinity for soluble IL-13.

Indications

Moderate-to-severe atopic dermatitis in adults and children ≥ 12 years of age with weight ≥ 40 kg. and older with disease not adequately controlled by topical therapies.

Mechanism of Action

It binds to soluble IL-13 preventing IL-4Rα/IL-13Rα1 heterodimerization and thus blocks downstream signaling. Lebrikizumab inhibits IL-13–induced responses including the release of proinflammatory cytokines, chemokines and IgE.

Pharmacology

Peak serum concentrations are achieved after 7–8 days of subcutaneous injection with a bioavailability of 86%. Its half-life is 24.5 days. The drug is broken down into smaller peptides and amino acids by catabolic pathways.

Monitoring

There are no approved monitoring guidelines.

Follow-up
- Complete blood count
- Urea and creatinine
- Liver function tests.

At 1 month, 4 months and then annually as per clinician's assessment.

Dosage

500 mg (two 250 mg injections) at week 0 and week 2, followed by 250 mg every 2 weeks until week 16.

Adverse Effects
- Ophthalmologic: conjunctivitis and keratitis-either new onset or worsening.

- Nasopharyngitis.
- Injection site reactions: pain, erythema.
- Hypersensitivity reactions-angioedema and urticaria.
- Infections: herpes zoster.
- Can affect immune responses to helminthic infections.

Drug Interactions

Avoid live vaccines while on Lebrikizumab therapy.

Contraindications

Hypersensitivity to the drug or formulation components.

Pregnancy: insufficient data

Lactation: no data to recommend usage.

Children: approved in children ≥ 12 years of age.

TRALOKINUMAB

Tralokinumab is a human IgG4λ anti-IL-13 monoclonal antibody antagonist.

Indications

Moderate-to-severe atopic dermatitis in patients ≥ 12 years of age not responding to topical therapy.

Mechanism of Action

Tralokinumab prevents IL-13 from binding to its receptors IL-13Rα1/IL-13Rα2, thus affects both downstream signaling heterodimerization (type 2 receptor) and endogenous regulation of IL-13.

Pharmacology

Bioavailability of tralokinumab after one subcutaneous injection is 76%. Its half-life is 22 days. Peak serum concentrations are reached after 5 days. Increased drug clearance occurs with increase in body weight.

Monitoring

No guidelines are approved. Clinicians may do a complete blood count, urea, creatinine and liver function tests at 1month, 4months and then annually.

Dosage

Initial dose of 600 mg followed by 300 mg as subcutaneous injection every other week.

Adverse Effects

- Infections: upper respiratory infections, eczema herpeticum.
- Ophthalmic: conjunctivitis, keratitis.
- Injection site reactions: pain, redness.
- Hematologic: eosinophilia.

Drug Interactions

Avoid live vaccines while on tralokinumab therapy.

Contraindications

Hypersensitivity to the drug or formulation components.

Pregnancy: insufficient data

Lactation: no data to recommend usage.

Children: can be used in children ≥ 12 years of age.

IL-31 RECEPTOR ANTAGONIST

Nemolizumab

It is a humanized IgG2 monoclonal antibody that acts as an IL-31 receptor antagonist.

Indications

Approved
Prurigo nodularis in adults.

Unlicensed
Itching associated with Moderate-to-severe atopic dermatitis in adults and children

> 13 years not controlled by existing therapy: approved in Japan.

Mechanism of Action

Nemolizumab inhibits IL-31 signalling by blocking IL-31 receptor activation by binding selectively to the alpha subunit of the receptor. Nemolizumab impedes IL-31–induced release of proinflammatory cytokines and chemokines.

Pharmacology

Peak concentrations were reached 6 days after subcutaneous injection. Mean half-life of nemolizumab is 16.7 days. Metabolic pathways are not clearly described but it is probably degraded to smaller peptides by catabolic pathways.

Monitoring

No monitoring guidelines are approved yet.

Dosage

- Adults < 90 kg weight-initial dose of 60 mg subcutaneous injection followed by 30 mg every 4 weeks.
- For adults weighing ≥ 90 kg-initial dose of 60 mg subcutaneous injection followed by 60 mg every 4 weeks.

Adverse Effects

- Headache-commonest.
- Atopic dermatitis exacerbation.
- Eczema.
- Nummular eczema.
- Hypersensitivity reactions facial angioedema.

Drug Interactions

- Avoid live vaccines while on nemolizumab therapy.
- CYP450 substrate drugs (warfarin, cyclosporin): dose needs to be modified and monitored for adverse effects.

Contraindications

Hypersensitivity to the drug or any component of the formulation.

Pregnancy: insufficient data

Lactation: no data to recommend usage.

Children: safety in children not yet proven.

IL-36 RECEPTOR ANTAGONIST

Spesolimab

It is a humanized monoclonal immunoglobulin G1 antibody produced by recombinant DNA technology in Chinese hamster ovary (CHO) cells.

Indications

Approved

Generalized pustular psoriasis (GPP) in adults and children ≥ 12 years with weight ≥40 kg for both rapid control of flares and prevention of long term recurrence.

Unlicensed

- Pyoderma gangrenosum
- Acrodermatitis continua of Hallopeau

Mechanism of Action

It binds to the IL-36 receptor thus preventing ligands (IL-36α, β and γ) from activating IL-36 receptor and stopping downstream activation of proinflammatory and profibrotic IL-36–mediated pathways.

Pharmacology

Spesolimab has a half-life of 25.5 days. Its metabolic pathway is not clearly defined but is likely to be broken down to smaller peptides by catabolic pathways.

Monitoring

Baseline
History, symptoms and signs of tuberculosis, other acute and chronic infections.

Laboratory
Chest X-ray, IGRA.

Follow-up
Annual IGRA.

Dosage
Single 900 mg IV infusion, if symptoms of flare persist repeat 900 mg after 1 week.

Adverse Effects

- Infections: increased risk of infections.
- Hypersensitivity reactions: immediate reactions (anaphylaxis) and delayed reactions such as drug reaction with eosinophilia and systemic symptoms (DRESS).
- Asthenia, fatigue, headache.
- Nausea and vomiting.
- Pruritus.
- Infusion site hematoma and bruising.

Drug Interactions

- No formal drug interactions studies have been conducted.
- Live vaccines to be avoided during use.

Contraindications

- Hypersensitivity to the drug or any component of the formulation.
- Avoid during active infections.

Pregnancy: insufficient data

Lactation: no data to recommend usage.

Children: safety and effectiveness in children < 12 years not yet proven.

IL-1 ANTAGONISTS

The three approved IL-1 antagonists are anakinra, canakinumab, and rilonacept.

Anakinra

Indications

Approved
- Cryopyrin-associated periodic syndrome (CAPS)
- Pustular eruptions and bone lesions of the autosomal recessive deficiency of the IL-1 receptor antagonist (DIRA).

Unlicensed
- Hidradenitis suppurativa.
- Pustular psoriasis.
- SAPHO syndrome, Schnitzler syndrome, PAPA syndrome.
- Pyoderma gangrenosum.

Mechanism of Action
Anakinra specifically targets IL-1 by competitively inhibiting both IL-1α and β at IL-1 receptor resulting in decrease in its inflammatory effects.

Pharmacokinetics
Bioavailability is 95%. It has a half-life of 4–6 hours and is rapidly eliminated through renal route. Due to its short half-life daily injections are needed.

Monitoring

Baseline
History and examination to rule out infection.

Laboratory
Complete blood counts should be performed monthly for 3 months and then quarterly

Tuberculosis screening: IGRA.

Follow-up
- Complete blood counts: monthly for 3 months, then quarterly.
- Annual tuberculosis screening.

Dosage
- Adults: 100 mg subcutaneous injection daily.
- Children: 1–2 mg/kg initial dose which can be increased to 8 mg/kg.

Adverse Effects
- Injection site reactions (most common)
- Hypersensitivity reactions (angioedema, anaphylaxis) can occur.
- Serious infections.
- Flu like symptoms.
- Hematological: neutropenia, thrombocytopenia.
- Increased liver enzymes.

Drug Interactions
Concurrent use with TNF-α inhibitors to be avoided.

Contraindications
- Hypersensitivity to the drug or components of the formulation.
- Active severe infections.
- Caution with dose adjustment (alternate day) in patients with renal impairment.

Pregnancy: insufficient data.

Lactation: safety not known.

Children: safety and efficacy established.

ANTI-IgE ANTIBODIES

Omalizumab
It is a recombinant monoclonal humanized (95%) murine monoclonal IgG1κ antibody against free human IgE.

Indications
Approved
- Moderate-to-severe persistent asthma in ≥ 6 years of age.
- Chronic idiopathic urticaria (CIU) non-responsive to H1 antihistamine treatment in ≥ 12 years of age.
- Nasal polyps in adults not responded adequately to nasal corticosteroids

Unlicensed
- Urticaria and angioedema: physical urticaria, cold urticaria, solar urticaria, bullous urticaria, severe delayed pressure angioedema, recurrent idiopathic angioedema.
- Autoimmune bullous disorders: bullous pemphigoid.
- Vasculitis: urticarial vasculitis.
- Mast cell disorders: mastocystosis.

Others
- Hyper-IgE syndrome.
- Allergy to peanut and latex.
- Systemic lupus erythematosus.
- Kimura disease.

Mechanism of Action
Omalizumab binds to the C-epsilon-3 domain, the same site where IgE binds to its receptor (FcεRI), preventing IgE from interacting with its receptor on eosinophils, basophils and mast cells. This results in lowered free IgE levels as also decrease in FcεRI on inflammatory cells and less release of mediators like histamine.

Pharmacology
The bioavailability is 62% after injection reaching peak serum concentrations after 7–8 days. Metabolism is by degradation in the reticuloendothelial system and endothelial cells with elimination by targeted binding (omalizumab–IgE complex formation). The mean half-life is 24 days.

Monitoring

Baseline

- Pretreatment total serum IgE levels if < 40 kU/L may lead to low response.
- Complete blood count to exclude thrombocytopenia (ROOK)
- No other laboratory investigations required both prior and during treatment.
- Postadministration monitoring for at least 1–2 hours for anaphylaxis is important.

Dosage

Chronic urticaria is 300 mg subcutaneously every 4 weeks.

Adverse Effects

- Common: nasopharyngitis, headache, sinusitis, joint pain, upper respiratory tract infection, nausea, cough.
- Injection site reactions.
- Type I (anaphylaxis) and type III (serum sickness) hypersensitivity reactions.
- Infections: increased risk of some helminthic infections.

Drug Interactions

- ACE inhibitors when used with omalizumab in chronic spontaneous urticaria can reduce its efficacy.
- Steroid to be gradually withdrawn following starting of omalizumab therapy.

Contraindications

Hypersensitivity to omalizumab or its excipient (polysorbate).

Pregnancy: Category B.

Lactation: Can be used in lactating mothers.

Children: Not licensed in children < 12 years of age.

B LYMPHOCYTE STIMULATOR (BLyS) SPECIFIC INHIBITOR

Belimumab

It s a fully human recombinant IgG1λ monoclonal antibody that inhibits soluble human B lymphocyte stimulator protein.

Indications

Approved

- Autoantibody-positive active systemic lupus erythematosus (SLE) in adults and pediatric patients ≥ 5 years of age who are on standard therapy.
- Active lupus nephritis in adults and pediatric patients ≥ 5 years of age as add on treatment.

Mechanism of Action

Belimumab blocks the binding of soluble BlyS to its receptors on B cells, thus inhibiting the survival of B cells, promoting apoptosis and impairing the differentiation of B cells into immunoglobulin-producing plasma cells.

Pharmacology

Bioavailability is 74–82% with terminal half-life of 19.4 days. It is probably degraded into smaller peptides and aminoacids by proteolytic enzymes.

Monitoring

Dosage

10 mg/kg iv at 2-week intervals for the first 3 doses and then at 4-week intervals.

Adverse Effects

- Infections: upper respiratory tract infection, urinary tract infection, nasopharyngitis, sinusitis, bronchitis, influenza, pneumonia.

- Infusion reactions: nausea, headache, skin rash, urticaria, myalgia, hypotension, anaphylaxis.
- GI: nausea, diarrhea.
- Neuropyschiatric: depression, suicidal tendencies, migraine, insomnia.
- Musculoskeletal: pain in extremities.

Drug Interactions

No formal drug interaction studies done.

Contraindications

- Hypersensitivity to belimumab.
- Live vaccines to be avoided.

Pregnancy: Category C.

Lactation: caution during breast feeding.

Children: can be used in children 5 years and above.

PDE4 INHIBITOR

Apremilast

It is a small molecule that works intracellularly to reduce the production of proinflammatory mediators and increase those that are anti-inflammatory.

Indications

Approved

- Psoriasis
- Psoriatic arthritis
- Oral ulcers associated with Behçet disease.

Unlicensed

Neutrophilic Dermatoses
- Behçet disease
- SAPHO syndrome

Autoimmune Connective Tissue Diseases
Discoid lupus erythematosus

Papulosquamous Dermatoses
- Lichen planus
- Pityriasis rubra pilaris

Pigmentary Disorders
Vitiligo

Dermatitis
Atopic dermatitis.

Others
- Hidradenitis suppurativa
- Alopecia areata

Mechanism of Action

- Apremilast inhibits phosphodiesterase 4, which is an intracellular enzyme that degrades cAMP.
- Increasing intracellular cAMP levels activates protein kinase A, leading to enhanced expression of several transcription factors including cAMP-response element binding protein (CREB), while inhibiting others such as nuclear factor kappa B (NF-κB).
- By inhibiting phosphodiesterase 4 and increasing intracellular cAMP levels, apremilast has multiple downstream effects: it decreases the production of inflammatory mediators such as TNF, IFN-γ, and interleukins (IL)-2,-12, and 23.
- It increases the production of anti-inflammatory mediators including IL-10; and it inhibits natural killer responses.

Pharmacology

- When administered orally, apremilast is 70–75% bioavailable.
- Nearly 70% of the drug is bound to plasma protein.
- It is metabolized by cytochrome P450 (CYP) enzymes, predominately CYP3A4 and also by CYP1A1 and CYP2A6.
- Apremilast has a terminal elimination half-life of 6–9 hours and is excreted in the urine and feces.

Dosage

- The recommended dosage for psoriatic arthritis and psoriasis is 30 mg twice daily. In order to reduce gastrointestinal symptoms, an upward titration of the dose by 10 mg/day is recommended, starting with an initial dose of 10 mg/day.

Dose Titration Schedule

Day 1	Day 2		Day 3		Day 4		Day 5		Day 6 and thereafter	
AM	AM	PM	AM	PM	AM	PM	AM	PM	AM	PM
10 mg	10 mg	10 mg	10 mg	20 mg	20 mg	20 mg	20 mg	30 mg	30 mg	30 mg

Monitoring

- Patients should be monitored for the development of adverse gastrointestinal manifestations (severe diarrhea, nausea, or vomiting). Dose reduction or treatment interruption should be prompted in these cases.
- Patients with an underlying psychiatric history managed with apremilast should be monitored closely and routinely, as treatment may increase the risk of depression and suicidal behaviors.
- Patients should also routinely have their weight monitored, as significant weight reductions may occur and require dose reduction or treatment interruption

Adverse Effects

Gastrointestinal

- Severe nausea, vomiting, diarrhea, especially first few weeks of therapy
- Weight loss

CNS

Headache

Respiratory

- Nasopharyngitis
- Upper respiratory tract infection

Psychiatric

- Depression
- Suicidal ideation/behavior

Drug Interaction

- CYP3A4 inducers like rifampicin, phenytoin, carbamazepine decrease the level of apremilast.
- CYP3A4 inhibitors like cyclosporine, itraconazole increase the level of apremilast.

Contraindication

- Apremilast is contraindicated in patients with known hypersensitivity to the drug or its components.
- Caution with creatinine clearance <30 mL/min

Pregnancy: Category C

Lactation: Not recommended

Children: Not recommended in patients under 18 years old.

JAK INHIBITORS

Janus kinase (JAK) is a family of cytoplasmic non-receptor tyrosine kinases that includes four members, namely JAK1, JAK2, JAK3, and TYK2. The JAKs transduce cytokine signaling through the JAK-STAT pathway, which regulates the transcription of several genes involved in inflammatory, immune, and cancer conditions.

Classification of JAK Inhibitors

- JAK inhibitors can be divided into two generations. The *first-generation* acts as non-selective inhibitors of JAKs. On the

other hand, *second-generation* drugs have selective inhibitory activity against JAKs. This difference in the selectivity of the two generations is associated with some differences in their safety and efficacy.
- JAK inhibitors may also be classified based on their binding mode and the type of interactions with the amino acids in JAKs into *reversible (competitive)* and irreversible (covalent) inhibitors.
- **Reversible inhibitor**:
  a. *ATP-Competitive Inhibitors:* The mechanism of action of these inhibitors depends on their competition with ATP for the catalytic ATP-binding site in JAKs. These inhibitors may also be classified based on the conformation of the kinase domain to which they bind.
     - **Type 1**: These inhibitors bind to the ATP-binding site of the JAKs under the active conformation of the kinase domain;
     - **Type 2:** Type II JAK Inhibitors also bind to the ATP-binding site of the kinase domain in the inactive conformation of JAKs
  b. *Allosteric JAK Inhibitors:* The allosteric JAK inhibitors include small molecule inhibitors that bind to a site other than the ATP-binding site in JAKs.
- **Irreversible inhibitor**: The mechanism of action of these inhibitors depends on the covalent interaction with the unique Cys909 residue in JAK3.

	Jak inhibitors	Target	Indications	FDA approval status
First generation	Baricitinib	JAK1/2	Rheumatoid arthritis, alopecia areata, COVID-19	Yes
	Tofacitinib	JAK1/3	Rheumatoid arthritis, psoriasis, psoriatic arthritis, inflammatory bowel disease	Yes
Second generation	Abrocitinib	JAK1	Moderate-to-severe atopic dermatitis (≥12 years)	Yes
	Upadacitinib	JAK1>2,3	Rheumatoid arthritis, psoriatic arthritis, atopic dermatitis	Yes
	Ritlecitinib	JAK3 and TEC kinase	Alopecia areata (≥12 years)	Yes
	Deucravacitinib	TYK2 inhibitor	Moderate-to-severe plaque psoriasis	Yes

ORAL JAK INHIBITORS

Tofacitinib

Indication

Approved

Rheumatoid arthritis, psoriasis, psoriatic arthritis, inflammatory bowel disease.

Unlicensed

Autoimmune Dermatoses
- Psoriasis
- Alopecia areata
- Vitiligo
- Dermatomyositis

Dermatitis
- Atopic dermatitis
- Photodermatoses
- Chronic actinic dermatitis

Other Dermatoses
- Erythema multiforme
- Hypereosinophilic syndrome

Pharmacology

- The absolute oral bioavailability is 74%.
- The protein binding of tofacitinib is approximately 40%. Tofacitinib binds predominantly to albumin and does not

appear to bind to α1-acid glycoprotein. Tofacitinib distributes equally between red blood cells and plasma.
- Clearance mechanisms for tofacitinib are approximately 70% hepatic metabolism and 30% renal excretion of the parent drug. The metabolism of tofacitinib is primarily mediated by CYP3A4 with minor contribution from CYP2C19.

Dosage
5 mg twice daily or 11 mg once a day.

Monitoring
Baseline
Clinical Evaluation
- History of malignancy and lymphoproliferative disorders
- History of herpes infections, interstitial lung disease, diverticulitis, renal dysfunction
- Perform thorough physical examination

Laboratory
- Complete blood count with leukocyte differential
- Liver enzyme panel
- Lipid panel
- Basic chemistry panel focusing on glomerular filtration rate
- Pregnancy test (for women of childbearing potential)
- Hepatitis B virus panel
- Hepatitis C virus panel
- Pretreatment evaluation for the presence of latent tuberculosis

Follow-up
Clinical Evaluation
- Annual thorough examination with special attention to possible nonmelanoma skin cancers and lymphoma
- Laboratory (4-8 Weeks After Therapy Initiation Then Every 3 Months Thereafter)
- Complete blood count
- Liver enzyme panel
- Lipid panel with focus on cholesterol levels

Adverse Effects
- ***Opportunistic infections***—fungal, TB, viral, bacterial EBV-associated posttransplant lymphomas, reactivation of latent TB and Herpes Zoster.
- ***Malignancy***: Lymphoma, lung, breast, gastric, colorectal, renal cell, prostrate, melanoma.
- ***Gastrointestinal***: Bowel perforations reported, especially with diverticulitis.
- ***Pulmonary***: Caution in patients with interstitial lung disease.
- ***Cardiovascular***: Decreased HR and prolonged PR interval.
- ***Hematologic***: Lymphocytopenia, neutropenia, anemia (Avoid if lymphocytes <500 cells/mm^3; ANC <500 cells/mm^3; Hb <9 g/dL).
- ***Metabolic***: Max lipid abnormalities 6–8 weeks [dose-dependent increases in total cholesterol, low-density lipoprotein (LDL) cholesterol, and high-density lipoprotein (HDL)]

Drug Interaction
- Fluconazole may increase serum concentrations of tofacitinib.
- Biologics, JAK inhibitors, traditional (azathioprine, cyclosporine, mycophenolates, etc.), chemotherapy, higher dose CS increase the risk of severe infections and/or myelosuppression.
- Methotrexate, leflunamide, hydroxychloroquine can be used simultaneously with tofacitinib at minimal risk if given at Rheumatology doses.
- Vaccines:
  – Live attenuated: Must wait at least 3 months after therapy to complete immunization.

- Killed, recombinant: Immunize at least 2 weeks prior starting tofacitinib; not adequate immune response, repeat in 3 months.

Contraindication

Hypersensitivity to the active substance/to any of the excipients of the formulation, active TB, serious infection like sepsis, severe hepatic impairment.

Pregnancy: Category C

Lactation: Contraindicated.

Children: Contraindicated below 2 years.

BARICITINIB

Indication

Approved

Rheumatoid arthritis, alopecia areata, COVID-19.

Pharmacology

- The absolute bioavailability of baricitinib is approximately 80%.
- Baricitinib is approximately 50% bound to plasma proteins.
- Baricitinib is a substrate of the Pgp, BCRP, OAT3 and MATE2-K transporters, which play roles in drug distribution.
- Elimination half-life is approximately 12–16 hours.
- Approximately 6% of the orally administered baricitinib dose is identified as metabolites (three from urine and one from feces), with CYP3A4 identified as the main metabolizing enzyme.

Dosage

- 2 mg once daily orally, with or without food. Increase to 4 mg once daily if the response to treatment is not adequate.
- For patients with nearly complete or complete scalp hair loss, with or without substantial eyelash or eyebrow hair loss, consider treating with 4 mg once daily, with or without food.

Drug Monitoring

Baseline

- Tuberculosis (TB) infection evaluation
- Viral hepatitis screening: HBsAg and Anti-HCV
- Complete blood count (CBC)-not recommended in patients with a platelet count <1,50,000/mm^3, absolute lymphocyte count <500/mm^3, absolute neutrophil count <1,000/mm^3, or Hb <8g/dL.
- Pregnancy test (for women of childbearing potential).

Follow-up

- CBC evaluations are recommended at baseline, 4 weeks after treatment initiation and 4 weeks after dose increase.
- Consider yearly screening for patients in highly endemic areas for TB. Monitor patients for the development of signs and symptoms of TB, including patients who were tested negative for latent TB infection prior to initiating therapy.
- Hepatitis B and C screening.
- Lipid parameters should be assessed approximately 4 weeks following initiation of therapy.

Adverse Effects

- ***Respiratory***: Upper respiratory tract infections, Lower respiratory tract infection
- Headache, fatigue.
- ***Skin***: Acne, Folliculitis of scalp, Herpes zoster, Genital Candida infections
- ***Metabolic***: Hyperlipidemia, Blood creatine phosphokinase increased, Liver enzyme elevations, Weight gain
- ***Urinary tract infections***

- **Blood**: Anemia, Neutropenia (Avoid if ANC less than 1,000 cells/mm^3, an absolute lymphocyte-count less than 500 cells/mm^3, Hemoglobin <8g/dL)
- **CVS**: Venous thromboembolic events (VTE), including deep venous thrombosis (DVT) and pulmonary embolism (PE).
- **GIT**: Nausea, Abdominal pain
- **Malignancy**: Non-melanoma skin cancer

Drug Interaction

- Baricitinib exposure is increased co-administered with strong OAT3 inhibitors (such as probenecid).

Contraindication

Hypersensitivity to the active substance/to any of the excipients of the formulation, active TB, serious infection like sepsis, severe hepatic impairment.

Pregnancy Category: Unknown

Lactation: Contraindicated

Children: Contraindicated below 2 years.

ABROCITINIB

Indication

Approved

Treatment of adults and paediatric patients 12 years of age and older with refractory, moderate-to-severe atopic dermatitis whose disease is not adequately controlled with other systemic drug products, including biologics, or when use of those therapies is inadvisable.

Pharmacology

- Oral bioavailability of abrocitinib is 60%, and food intake does not influence it.
- Elimination half-lives of abrocitinib and its two active metabolites, M1 and M2, range 3-5 hours.
- Abrocitinib is metabolized mainly by CYP2C19 and CYP2C9 and to a lesser extent by CYP3A4 and CYP2B6.
- The metabolites of abrocitinib are excreted predominantly in urine.

Dosage

- 100 mg orally once daily.
- 200 mg orally once daily is recommended for those patients who are not responding to 100 mg once daily.

Monitoring

Baseline

- Tuberculosis (TB) infection evaluation
- Viral hepatitis screening: HBsAg and Anti-HCV
- Complete blood count (CBC)-not recommended in patients with a platelet count <1,50,000/mm^3, absolute lymphocyte count<500/mm^3, absolute neutrophil count <1,000/mm^3, or Hb <8 g/dL.
- Pregnancy test (for women of childbearing potential).
- Liver enzyme panel
- Lipid panel

Follow-up

- CBC evaluations are recommended at baseline, 4 weeks after treatment initiation and 4 weeks after dose increase.
- Consider yearly screening for patients in highly endemic areas for TB. Monitor patients for the development of signs and symptoms of TB, including patients who were tested negative for latent TB infection prior to initiating therapy.
- Hepatitis B and C screening.
- Lipid parameters should be assessed approximately 4 weeks following initiation of therapy.

Adverse Effects

- **Skin**: Acne, Impetigo, contact dermatitis, herpes simplex, herpes zoster.

- **Upper respiratory tract infection**: Nasopharyngitis nausea, oropharyngeal pain.
- **GIT**: Upper abdominal pain, abdominal discomfort, vomiting, gastroenteritis.
- **CNS**: Headache, dizziness, fatigue
- **Metabolic**: Increased blood creatine phosphokinase, hyperlipidaemia.
- **Blood**: Lymphopenia, thrombocytopenia, thrombosis including DVT, PE, and arterial thrombosis.
- **Renal**: Urinary tract infection.
- **Hypertension**
- **Malignancy**: Non-melanoma skin cancer

Drug Interaction

- Coadministration of Abrocitinib with strong CYP2C19 inhibitors (e.g., Cimetidine, Omeprazole, Pantoprazole, lansoprazole, rabeprazole, Fluoxetine, indomethacin) increase the combined exposure of abrocitinib and its two active metabolites.
- Coadministration of Abrocitinib with drugs that are moderate to strong inhibitors of both CYP2C19 and CYP2C9 (Clopidogrel, fluconazole) increase the exposure of abrocitinib and its two active metabolites.
- Coadministration with antiplatelet therapy drugs may increase the risk of bleeding with thrombocytopenia.

Contraindication

- Concurrent Antiplatelet therapies except for low-dose aspirin (≤81 mg daily), during the first 3 months of treatment.
- Severe renal impairment or end-stage renal disease.
- Severe hepatic impairment.
- Active TB, active Hepatitis B or C infection.

Pregnancy: Category D

Lactation: Contraindicated

Children: Contraindicated below 12 years of age.

UPADACITINIB

Indication

Approved

- Rheumatoid arthritis
- Psoriatic arthritis
- Atopic dermatitis (Paediatric patients 12 years of age and older weighing at least 40 kg and adults)
- Inflammatory bowel disease

Pharmacology

- Upadacitinib is 52% bound to plasma proteins.
- Elimination Metabolism Upadacitinib metabolism is mediated by mainly CYP3A4 with a potential minor contribution from CYP2D6.
- Upadacitinib mean terminal elimination half-life ranged from 8 to 14 hours.

Dosage

Initiate treatment with 15 mg once daily. If an adequate response is not achieved, consider increasing the dosage to 30 mg once daily.

Monitoring

Baseline

- Tuberculosis (TB) infection evaluation
- Viral hepatitis screening: HBsAg and Anti-HCV
- Complete blood count (CBC)-not recommended in patients with a platelet count <1,50,000/mm^3, absolute lymphocyte count< 500/mm^3, absolute neutrophil count <1000/mm^3, or Hb <8 g/dL.
- Pregnancy test (for women of childbearing potential).

- Liver enzyme panel
- Lipid panel

Follow-up
- CBC evaluations are recommended at baseline, 4 weeks after treatment initiation and 4 weeks after dose increase.
- Consider yearly screening for patients in highly endemic areas for TB. Monitor patients for the development of signs and symptoms of TB, including patients who were tested negative for latent TB infection prior to initiating therapy.
- Hepatitis B and C screening.
- Lipid parameters should be assessed approximately 4 weeks following initiation of therapy.

Side Effects
- ***Respiratory***: Upper respiratory tract infections, Lower respiratory tract infection
- Headache, fatigue, pyrexia
- ***Skin***: Acne, Herpes zoster, Herpes simplex
- ***Metabolic***: Hyperlipidaemia, blood creatine phosphokinase increased, liver enzyme elevations
- ***Urinary tract infections***
- ***Blood***: Anaemia, Neutropenia, leukopenia (Avoid if ANC less than 1000 cells/mm^3, an absolute lymphocyte-count less than 500 cells/mm^3, Haemoglobin <8 g/dL)
- ***CVS***: Venous thromboembolic events (VTE), including deep venous thrombosis (DVT) and pulmonary embolism (PE).
- ***GIT***: Nausea, Abdominal pain, perforations.
- ***Malignancy***: Non-melanoma skin cancers

Drug Interaction
- Strong CYP3A4 Inhibitors like ketoconazole, clarithromycin, and grapefruit juice increases blood Upadacitinib level.
- Strong CYP3A4 inducer like rifampicin decreases blood Upadacitinib level.

Contraindication
- Hypersensitivity to the active substance/to any of the excipients of the formulation.
- Active TB, serious infection like sepsis.
- Severe hepatic impairment.

Pregnancy: Category D

Lactation: Contraindicated

Children: Contraindicated below 12 years of age.

RITLECITINIB

Indication
Approved

Treatment of severe alopecia areata in adults and adolescents 12 years and older.

Pharmacology
- Oral bioavailability is approximately 64%.
- Mean terminal half-life ranges from 1.3 to 2.3 hours.
- Metabolized by Glutathione S-transferase and CYP enzymes (CYP3A, CYP2C8, CYP1A2, and CYP2C9).

Dosage
- 50 mg orally once daily with or without food.
- If a dose is missed, administer the dose as soon as possible unless it is less than 8 hours before the next dose, in which case, skip the missed dose.

Monitoring
Baseline
- Tuberculosis (TB) infection evaluation
- Viral hepatitis screening: HBsAg and Anti-HCV
- Complete blood count (CBC)-not recommended in patients with a platelet

count <1,50,000/mm³, absolute lymphocyte count < 500/mm³, absolute neutrophil count <1000/mm³, or Hb <8 g/dL.
- Pregnancy test (for women of childbearing potential).
- Liver enzyme panel
- Lipid panel

Follow-up
- CBC evaluations are recommended at baseline, 4 weeks after treatment initiation and 4 weeks after dose increase.
- Consider yearly screening for patients in highly endemic areas for TB. Monitor patients for the development of signs and symptoms of TB, including patients who were tested negative for latent TB infection prior to initiating therapy.
- Hepatitis B and C screening.
- Lipid parameters should be assessed approximately 4 weeks following initiation of therapy.

Adverse Effects
- Headache, fatigue, pyrexia
- *Skin*: Acne, stomatitis, herpes zoster
- ***Hypersensitivity***: Serious reactions including anaphylactic reactions, urticaria and rash.
- *Metabolic*: Blood creatine phosphokinase increased, liver enzyme elevations
- *Blood*: Decreased RBC count, lymphopenia, thrombocytopenia (an absolute lymphocyte count <500/mm³ or, platelets <1,00,000/mm³)
- *CVS*: Venous thromboembolic events (VTE), including deep venous thrombosis (DVT) and pulmonary embolism (PE).
- *GIT*: Nausea, Abdominal pain.
- *Malignancy*: Non-melanoma skin cancers

Drug Interaction
- Strong CYP3A4 Inhibitors like ketoconazole, clarithromycin, and grapefruit juice increases blood Ritlecitinib level.
- Strong CYP3A4 inducer like rifampicin decreases blood ritlecitinib level.

Contraindication
- Patients with known hypersensitivity to ritlecitinib or any of its excipients
- Patients with Severe Hepatic Impairment

Pregnancy: Category D

Lactation: Contraindicated

Children: Contraindicated below 12 years of age.

DEUCRAVACITINIB

Indication

Approved
Treatment of adults with moderate-to-severe plaque psoriasis who are candidates for systemic therapy or phototherapy.

Unlicensed
- Generalized pustular psoriasis
- Erythrodermic psoriasis
- Psoriatic arthritis
- Moderate-to-severe scalp psoriasis
- Alopecia areata and alopecia universalis
- Nail psoriasis
- Systemic lupus erythematosus
- Discoid lupus erythematosus
- Subacute cutaneous lupus erythematosus
- Lupus nephritis
- Inflammatory bowel disease (Crohn disease and ulcerative colitis)
- Atopic dermatitis
- Erosive oral lichen planus

Pharmacology
- Oral bioavailability of deucravacitinib is 99%.
- The terminal half-life of deucravacitinib is 10 hours.

- Metabolism Deucravacitinib is metabolized by cytochrome P-450 (CYP) 1A2 to form major metabolite. It is also metabolized by CYP2B6, CYP2D6, carboxylesterase.

Dosage

6 mg taken orally once daily, with or without food.

Monitoring

Baseline

- Tuberculosis (TB) infection evaluation
- Viral hepatitis screening: HBsAg and Anti-HCV
- Complete blood count (CBC)—not recommended in patients with a platelet count <1,50,000/mm^3, absolute lymphocyte count <500/mm^3, absolute neutrophil count <1000/mm^3, or Hb<8 g/dL.
- Pregnancy test (for women of childbearing potential).
- Liver enzyme panel
- Lipid panel

Follow-up

- CBC evaluations are recommended at baseline, 4 weeks after treatment initiation and 4 weeks after dose increase.
- Consider yearly screening for patients in highly endemic areas for TB. Monitor patients for the development of signs and symptoms of TB, including patients who were tested negative for latent TB infection prior to initiating therapy.
- Hepatitis B and C screening.
- Lipid parameters should be assessed approximately 4 weeks following initiation of therapy.

Adverse Effects

- Upper respiratory infections: Common cold, sore throat, and sinus infection.
- Hypersensitivity including angioedema
- *Metabolic*: Elevated triglycerides, liver enzymes, blood creatine phosphokinase and rhabdomyolysis.
- Herpes simplex
- Mouth ulcers
- *Skin*: Folliculitis, Acne
- Malignancy including lymphomas.

Drug Interaction

No significant drug interaction

Contraindication

- Patients with known hypersensitivity to Deucravacitinib or any of its excipients
- Patients with Severe Hepatic Impairment.

Pregnancy: Not categorized, but should be avoided.

Lactation: Unknown

Children: Not established

ANTI-ANDROGEN

Finasteride

It is an androgen inhibitor.

Indication

Approved

Male pattern androgenetic alopecia

Unlicensed

- Female pattern androgenetic alopecia
- Hirsutism
- Acne vulgaris
- Hidradenitis suppurativa

Pharmacology

- Finasteride is well absorbed in the gastrointestinal tract, metabolized in the liver by CYP3A4, and excreted in urine and feces.
- The serum half-life is 5 to 6 hours.

Mechanism of Action

- It is a specific type II 5-α reductase inhibitor. This enzyme catalyzes conversion of testosterone to DHT. The type II isoenzyme is found in hair follicles on vertex and frontal scalp. Finasteride decreases both serum DHT and local scalp DHT in the hair follicle.
- The drug does not directly bind to the androgen receptor, and is not a traditional antiandrogen; however, DHT suppression secondarily reduces AR expression levels via feedback mechanisms.

Dosage

1 mg per day

Drug Monitoring

Prostate-specific antigen (PSA) value appropriate for men 50 years and older at baseline before treatment and again at 6 months.

Adverse Effects

Gynaecomastia, prostate cancer, severe myopathy, decreased libido, erectile and ejaculatory dysfunction, decreased ejaculate volume, and testicular pain.

Drug Interaction

It has a wide therapeutic index, and there are no important interactions as a result of this CYP metabolism.

Contraindication

- Hypersensitivity to finasteride or components formulation
- In women, pregnancy, lactation.
- Hepatic impairment

Pregnancy: Category X

Lactation: Contraindicated

Hildren: Contraindicated

Dutasteride: It is an androgen inhibitor.

Indication

Approved

Benign prostatic hypertrophy

Unlicensed

- Male pattern androgenetic alopecia
- Female pattern androgenetic alopecia
- Frontal fibrosing alopecia
- Hirsutism
- Acne vulgaris
- Hidradenitis suppurativa

Pharmacology

- Dutasteride is metabolized by CYP3A4.
- Dutasteride is approximately three times more potent than finasteride at inhibiting type II 5a-reductase and 100 times more potent at inhibiting type I 5a-reductase.129 Dutasteride can decrease serum DHT by more than 90% within 24 hours.
- It has a long half-life for terminal elimination of approximately 5 weeks.

Mechanism of Action

It inhibits dually and effectively both type I and type II 5-α reductase isoenzymes. Both isoenzyme types are located in the pilosebaceous unit.

Dosage

0.5 mg per day

Monitoring

Prostate-specific antigen (PSA) value is appropriate for men 50 years and older at baseline before treatment and again at 6 months.

Adverse Effects
- Reversible erectile dysfunction, decreased libido, ejaculation disorder.
- Gynecomastia
- Risk of prostate cancer.

Drug Interaction
- Drug that increases the serum level of dutasteride by inhibiting CYP3A4 include HIV drugs—protease inhibitors ritonavir, nelfinavir, tipranavir, fosamprenavir NNRTI – Delavirdine
- Hepatitis C virus protease inhibitors: Telaprevir, boceprevir
- Antifungal—azoles Ketoconazole > itraconazole
- Antidepressants—SSRI, Fluvoxamine, nefazodone
- Antibiotics—macrolides, fluoroquinolones, clarithromycin, ciprofloxacin
- Vasopressin receptor antagonist: Conivaptan
- Calcium channel blockers: Verapamil, diltiazem.

Contraindication
- Hypersensitivity to dutasteride or any component of product
- Use in children
- Use in women of childbearing potential

Pregnancy: Category X

Lactation: Contraindicated

Children: Contraindicated

SPIRONOLACTONE

It is a steroid molecule resembling mineralocorticoid. It is an aldosterone antagonist and a weak antiandrogen.

Indications
All indications of Spironolactone in dermatology are off-label

- Acne vulgaris
- Hirsutism
- Androgenic alopecia
- Hidradenitis suppurativa

Mechanism of Action
- Spironolactone competitively inhibits the binding of testosterone and dihydrotestosterone to the androgen receptor
- Inhibit androgen biosynthesis by direct inhibition of 17α-hydroxylase enzyme
- Inhibitory effect on 5-α reductase activity
- Variable progestational activity
- Reduces the response of LH to GnRH, thereby affecting the LH: FSH ratio

Pharmacology
Oral bioavailability of greater than 90% with 98% protein binding. Peak levels are reached 2-4 hours after oral administration. Half-life is 12.5 hours. It is rapidly metabolised in liver to primary metabolite Canrenone which is an aldosterone antagonist and is responsible for both diuretic and antiandrogen actions of the drug. Excretion is through urine and bile. Food increases absorption of spironolactone.

Dosage
Dosage for dermatological indications vary between 50–200 mg daily; may be divided into 2 times a day. Drug is started at a dose of 25–50 mg. Dose is slowly increased as tolerated. Menstrual abnormalities may occur at higher doses which may resolve after 2–3 months of therapy. If not improved, dose can be reduced to 50–75 mg daily or an oral contraceptive can be added or cyclic therapy of spironolactone can be given for 21 consecutive days, followed by 7 days drug holiday.

Adverse Effects
- Electrolyte abnormalities:
  - Hyperkalemia (serious)
  - Hyponatremia

- Hypocalcemia
- Hypomagnesemia
- Hypochloremic alkalosis
- Metabolic abnormalities
  - Hyperglycemia
  - Hyperuricemia (asymptomatic/gout)
- CVS
  - Hypotension
- Renal
  - Decreased renal function
- Reproductive
  - Menstrual abnormalities
    - Spotting
    - Breakthrough bleeding
    - Irregular menses
    - Oligomenorrhoea
    - Amenorrhoea
  - Teratogenicity-feminisation of developing male genitelia (to avoid, OCP+ spironolactone used)
- Cutaneous
  - Generalised pruritus
  - Alopecia
- Others
  - Gynaecomastia
  - Breast tenderness
  - Weight gain

Drug Interactions

- Drugs whose levels are increased with increased risk of side effects: Digoxin, lithium carbonate, ACE inhibitors, Angiotensin II receptor blockers, amiloride, low molecular weight heparin, drospirenone, cyclosporine, oral tacrolimus, SSRIs, Indomethacin
- Dietary and other supplements: Potassium salts, potassium rich foods (bananas, oranges, tomatoes)-risk of hyperkalemia

Monitoring

Baseline

Measurement of blood pressure and body weight

Laboratory

- Serum potassium, renal function test
- Circulating androgens (testosterone and DHEAS)

Follow-up

- Periodic measurement of blood pressure and body weight monthly
- Circulating androgens every 3-4 months

Contraindications

- Severe renal impairment
- Hyperkalemia
- Addison disease
- Hypersensitivity to spironolactone

Pregnancy: Category C

Lactation: Can be given to nursing mothers

Children: Unlicensed

Psychotropic Agents

Psychotropic drugs are medications that alter mood, perception, and behaviour. Most psychodermatologic patients fall primarily into one of the four underlying psychiatric diagnoses: (1) anxiety, (2) depression, (3) psychosis, and (4) obsessive-compulsive disorder.

Drugs Used for Anxiety

Acute Anxiety: Benzodiazepines

Benzodiazepines beneficial for acute anxiety include alprazolam, lorazepam and clonazepam.

Salient Features

a. Benzodiazepines are especially useful in the management of acute situational anxiety as the drug takes effect immediately and can almost always relieve anxiety if given in adequate doses.

b. Because of the potential risk of addiction with long-term use, the physician should try to limit the duration of the treatment to no more than 3 to 4 weeks.

c. Alprazolam differs from the older benzodiazepines, such as diazepam or chlordiazepoxide, because the half-life is short and predictable, and most of the previous dose is eliminated before the next dose.
d. Alprazolam may have a unique anti-depressant effect, whereas most other benzodiazepines generally have a depressant effect.
e. Tapering of alprazolam should be slow as rebound anxiety can develop following sudden stoppage.
f. **Adverse effect:** Sedation (on short-term use), physical dependency on long-term use

Dosage

- Alprazolam: 0.125–0.25 mg every 6–8 hours, as needed
- Lorazepam: 0.5–2 mg every 6–8 hours, as needed
- Clonazepam: 0.5–2 mg once or twice daily, as needed

Chronic Anxiety

Selective serotonin Reuptake Inhibitor (SSRI)

SSRI are the most widely prescribed class of antidepressants and are the first-line treatment for depression and chronic anxiety. The SSRI include fluoxetine, paroxetine, sertraline, escitalopram, and citalopram.

Salient Features

- They are potent and selective inhibitors of serotonin (5-HT) reuptake at the presynaptic terminal resulting in increase in 5-HT availability at serotonergic synapses.
- The onset of response to SSRI usually begins in about 1 to 2 weeks with 6 to 12 weeks required for full therapeutic effect. Fluoxetine has the longest half-life ranging from 1–6 days while paroxetine has the shortest half-life of 21 hours. Metabolism is mainly hepatic with excretion is via renal and fecal route.
- **Indications in dermatology:** Neurotic excoriations, body dysmorphic disorder, premature ejaculation

Dosage

Start with minimal effective dose and increase every week as tolerated
- Fluoxetine (10–20 mg/day, up to 40–60 mg/day)
- Paroxetine (10–20 mg/day, up to 50 mg/day)
- Sertraline (25–50 mg/day, up to 200 mg/day)
- Escitalopram (5–10 mg/day, up to 20 mg/day)
- Citalopram (10–20 mg/day, up to 40 mg/day)

Adverse Effects

- Gastrointestinal effects: Nausea, diarrhea, dyspepsia are the most common AE (more with sertraline)
- Suicidal thinking and behavior
- Discontinuation syndrome
- Hypomania and mania
- Anticholinergic Effects: Eyes—pupillary dilation and narrow angle glaucoma, excessive sedation
- Hypersensitivity reactions
- Cardiovascular: QTc prolongation (mainly with fluoxetine and citalopram)
- Metabolic: Altered appetite and weight Caution in patients with diabetes mellitus due to risk of hypoglycemia during treatment and hyperglycemia after treatment.
- Sexual dysfunction: Erectile dysfunction, less sexual desire, difficulty in having orgasm.
- Serotonin syndrome: Anxiety, being nervous or jittery, high fever, sweating, confusion, shaking, restlessness, lack of

coordination, major changes in blood pressure, tachycardia.
- Neurologic: Headache, dizziness, insomnia, movement disorders. Caution in patients with prior seizures.

Drug Interactions

- Tricyclic antidepressants (doxepin, amitriptyline): Levels increased by paroxetine, fluoxetine
- MAO inhibitors: CNS and CVS complications
- β blockers (propranolol, metoprolol): Increased risk of bradycardia and hypotension.
- Imidazole antifungals, calcium channel blockers, macrolides: Increase SSRI levels

Pregnancy: Category C.

Lactation: Safe

Selective Serotonin Norepinephrine Reuptake Inhibitor (SNRI)

Venlafaxine

Salient Features

- Inhibiting reuptake of both serotonin and norepinephrine. At low doses, venlafaxine functions like an SSRI, inhibiting serotonin, whereas at high doses (>225 mg/day) it inhibits both serotonin and norepinephrine.

Adverse effects nausea, insomnia, dizziness, drowsiness, dry mouth, sweating, weakness, and constipation. Others include sexual dysfunction, dose-related increase in blood pressure.

Dosage

75–150 mg/d extended release formulation.

Buspirone

It is a nonsedating anxiolytic medication that does not cause dependency.

Salient Features

- Buspirone is a partial agonist of the 5-HT (5-hydroxytryptamine) 1A receptor.
- Slow onset of action—2 to 4 weeks
- Dosage: The starting dose is 7.5 mg twice daily, subsequently increasing to 15 mg twice daily after 1 week, up to a maximum of 60 mg.
- **Adverse effects**: The most common AE are nausea, headache, dizziness, and fatigue,

Depression

SSRIs-discussed

Bupropion

Salient Features

- It is a norepinephrine-dopamine reuptake inhibitor, structurally related to amphetamine
- Full antidepressant effect—seen after at least 4 weeks of treatment or longer
- Adverse effects: Common-insomnia, agitation, headache, constipation, dry mouth, nausea, and tremor. Blood pressure should be checked at baseline and monitored during treatment, as bupropion may cause hypertension; seizure.

Mirtazapine

Salient Features

- Mirtazapine is an atypical antidepressant that may have a faster onset of action than SSRI antidepressants and lower risk for drug-drug interactions compared with many other antidepressants.
- Mechanism of action involves increased release of norepinephrine and serotonin. It has a high affinity for histamine H1 receptors, for which its sedative effects are attributed.
- **Dermatology indications**: Chronic pruritus due to renal, hepatic failure, inflammatory dermatoses, malignancy.

Dosage

Initially 15 mg before bedtime increase to 30 mg after 1 to 2 weeks.

Tricyclic Antidepressants (TCAs)

Doxepin

Salient Features

- In addition to its antidepressant effects, doxepin has strong antipruritic effects because it is a very powerful H1 antihistamine.
- Metabolism is by CYP 450 (CYP 2D6)
- Plasma protein binding is 80% with half-life 15 hours.

Dosage

- As antipruritic: 10–25 mg at bedtime
- As antidepressant: Start at 10–25 mg at bedtime and increase every 1–2 weeks to a therapeutic dose of 25–150 mg at bedtime or up to 300 mg in divided doses.

Pregnancy: Category C

Lactation: Not to be used

Amitriptyline: Tertiary amine TCA

Indications

- Vulvodynia
- Vestibulodynia (pain with sexual intercourse)
- Dysesthetic vulvodynia (neuropathic pain)
- Post-herpetic neuralgia (PHN)
- Trigeminal trophic syndrome
- Pain associated with chronic ulcers of pyoderma gangrenosum, polyarteritis nodosum, venous ulceration and epidermolysis bullosa.
- Neuropathic pruritus associated with notalgia paraesthetica, brachioradial pruritus, pruritus vulvae and male genital dysaesthesia

Mechanism of Action

Not fully known. Amitriptyline possibly inhibits the membrane pump mechanism responsible for the re-uptake of transmitter amines, such as norepinephrine and serotonin, thereby increasing their concentration at the synaptic clefts of the brain.

Dosage

- Start with 10 mg at night, 25–75 mg at night for PHN.
- Nortriptyline (another tertiary amine TCA): 10 mg

Drug Interactions

- Drugs increasing TCAs levels on coadministration: SSRI, SNRI, allylamine antifungals, H1 antihistamines.
- Anticholinergic drugs (glycopyrrolate): Increase anticholinergic side effects
- Sedative drugs: Increased sedation when combined
- MAO inhibitors: CNS and CVS complications
- Drugs decreasing TCA levels: Anticonvulsants, rifampicin

Adverse Effects

Doxepin: Sedation (commonest), prolongation of QTc interval, orthostatic hypotension, and anticholinergic side effects (dry mouth, constipation, urinary retention, narrow angle glaucoma, pupillary dilatation) discontinuation symptoms (dizziness, nausea, headache, insomnia, diaphoresis), suicidality

- **Amitriptyline and nortriptyline:** Sedation, drowsiness, dry mouth, blurred vision, constipation, hyperhidrosis, postural hypotension, nausea, confusion or a headache due to hyponatraemia, weight gain, heart rhythm disturbances

Contraindications

- Hypersensitivity to drug or components
- Acute recovery phase following myocardial infarction
- Glaucoma, urinary retention

Caution

- Elderly patients-risk of fall at night due to postural hypotension
- Cardiovascular disorders—pretreatment ECG for those with cardiac conduction disorders to rule out prolonged QTc interval and a repeat ECG for dysrhythmia following high dose usage.
- Patients with prior history of seizure disorders

Pregnancy: Category C.

Lactation: Safe

Psychosis

First-generation Antipsychotics

Pimozide

It is a centrally acting dopamine receptor D2 antagonist

Indication in Dermatology

- Delusion of parasitosis
- Trichotillomania
- Dermatitis artefacta

Dosage

- Start at 0.5-1.0 mg/day and increase by 0.5-1.0 mg every 2-4 weeks, as tolerated, to the lowest clinically effective dose—typically 2-6 mg/day
- Once adequate clinical response, maintain dose for at least three months, then gradually taper.

Adverse Effects

- Associated with QT prolongation, arrhythmias (doses ≥10 mg/day),
- Extrapyramidal symptoms (EPS): Akathisia, tardive dyskinesia (with long-term use)
- Drug interactions: Avoid if taking opiates, SSRIs macrolides, protease inhibitors, azole antifungals, grapefruit juice.
  - Baseline ECG often recommended when starting pimozide. Potassium and magnesium levels also to be monitored
  - Second-generation antipsychotics:
    - Risperidone, olanzapine and quetiapine are atypical antipsychotics and both dopamine (D2) and serotonin (5-HT2) receptor antagonists.

Risperidone

Dermatology indication: Delusion of parasitosis.

Dosage

- 0.5 mg/day, up to 4 mg/day
- Olanzapine (2.5 mg/day, up to 10-15 mg/day)

Adverse Effects

Risperidone: Sedation, QTc weight gain, hyperglycemia, galactorrhea, seizures, EPS, neuroleptic malignant syndrome, leucopenia
Olanzapine: Weight gain, diabetes, hyperlipidemia, hyperglycemia, galactorrhea, seizures, EPS, neuroleptic malignant syndrome, anemia.

Pregnancy: Category C.

Lactation: Can be given

Anticonvulsants in Psychodermatology

GABA agonists Gabapentin and Pregabalin

Indications in Dermatology

- All neuralgias mainly PHN
- Allodynia
- Dysesthesia
- Pruritus of unknown origin

Mechanism of Action

Centrally acting GABA agonist.

Dosage

- Gabapentin: Start at 300 mg/d up to 3600 mg/d given at night
- Pregabalin: 150 mg/d up to 600 mg/d

Adverse Effects

- Sedation, dizziness, ataxia
- Pancytopenia, Stevens-Johnson syndrome (rarely)

Pregnancy: Category C

HEDGEHOG PATHWAY INHIBITORS

Hedgehog signaling pathway plays a vital role in controlling cell proliferation, fetal development, hair follicle regulation, development of sebaceous glands, maintenance of stem cell populations and the etiology of various malignancies. Vismodegib and sonidegib are the two main hedgehog inhibitors used in dermatology.

Vismodegib

It is the first in the class of oral anti-cancer drugs that specifically inhibit the hedgehog (Hh) signaling pathway.

Indications

Approved

- Symptomatic metastatic basal cell carcinoma (BCC) in adults.
- Locally advanced BCC in adults where surgery and radiotherapy are not possible.

Unlicensed

- Malignancies: Nevoid basal cell carcinoma syndrome, melanoma, lymphoma.
- Genodermatoses: Neurofibromatosis 1.
- Autoimmune connective tissue disorders: Systemic sclerosis.
- Graft-versus-host disease.
- Photoaging.
- Trichoepithelioma.

Mechanism of Action

Vismodegib binds to smoothened transmembrane protein (SMO) and inhibits the induction of Hh target genes involved in cell proliferation and survival.

Pharmacology

It has a bioavailability of 32% after oral absorption and peak levels are reached in 2.4 days. More than 99% of vismodegib is bound to plasma proteins. It is metabolized by a combination of oxidation, glucuronidation and ring cleavage. It is a substrate for both CYP2C9 and CYP 3A4/5 and is excreted mainly in feces (82%). Half-life of vismodegib is 12 days after a single dose and 4 days following continuous dosing.

Monitoring

- Pregnancy test to be done 1 week before starting treatment. (STAT PEARLS)
- Women should employ effective contraceptive practices up to 7 months following treatment and men at least 3 months after last dose.
- CBC, LFT, urea, creatinine, serum electrolytes at baseline and periodic intervals.
- Creatine kinase levels to be done at baseline and at periodic intervals.

Dosage

150 mg od till disease progression or development of undesirable adverse effects.

Adverse Effects

- Teratogenicity: Craniofacial abnormalities, anorectal defects, fused or absent digits are the embryotoxicities seen.
- GI: Nausea, diarrhea, constipation, vomiting, decrease appetite.

- Musculoskeletal: Muscle spasms, arthralgia, premature epiphyseal fusion in children.
- Nervous system: Dysgeusia, ageusia.
- Cutaneous: Alopecia, pruritus.
- General: Fatigue, weight loss.
- Reproductive system: Amenorrhea.
- Malignancy: Keratoacanthoma and well differentiated squamous cell carcinoma.

Drug Interactions

- P-glycoprotein inhibitors (macrolides, cyclosporine, verapamil): Increase serum levels of vismodegib with increased risk of adverse effects.
- CYP450 inducers (rifampicin, anticonvulsants-phenytoin. Carbamazepine, phenobarbital): Decrease serum levels with reduced efficacy of vismodegib.
- CYP3A 4 inhibitors (antiretrovirals-ritonavir, indinavir, clarithromycin, triazole antifungals): Increase levels of vismodegib with more risk of adverse effects.
- Antacids (protein pump inhibitors, H2 antagonists, antacids containing calcium and magnesium): May decrease absorption and bioavailability of vismodegib.

Contraindications

- Hypersensitivity to drug or its components.
- Pregnancy and lactation.
- Avoid blood donation for at least 20 months and semen donation for at least 8 months after last dose.

Pregnancy: Category D, contraindicated.

Lactation: Avoid during breastfeeding and for 24 months after last dose.

Children: Not to be used below 18 years.

Sonidegib

It is a small molecule kinase inhibitor that inhibits the hedgehog signaling pathway.

Indications

Approved

- Locally advanced BCC in adults that recurs following surgery or radiotherapy.
- Locally advanced BCC in adult patients not suitable candidates for surgery or radiotherapy.

Unlicensed

Mechanism of Action

Sonidegib inhibits the transmembrane protein smoothened(SMO) and reduces Hh signaling genes that are associated with cell proliferation and survival.

Pharmacology

Less than 10% of the drug is absorbed after oral absorption, however fatty meals increase absorption. Sonidegib is ≥97% plasma protein bound and is metabolized by CYP3A with metabolites excreted by enterohepatic circulation. Elimination half-life is 28 days with 70% of drug excreted in feces and 30% in urine.

Monitoring

Baseline
Laboratory

- CBC, LFT, blood sugar, urea, creatinine
- Serum creatine kinase, amylase, lipase.
- Pregnancy test.

Follow up

Laboratory

CBC, LFT, urea, creatinine, serum creatine kinase at periodic intervals. Drug to be stopped if creatine kinase >2.5 times upper limit of normal with deteriorating renal function.

Dosage

200 mg orally once daily taken on an empty stomach till disease progression or undesirable adverse effect develop.

Adverse Effects

- Musculoskeletal: Muscle spasms, musculoskeletal pain, myalgia.
- Cutaneous: Alopecia, pruritus.
- Nervous system: Dysgeusia, headache.
- GI: Nausea, diarrhea, constipation, vomiting, decrease appetite.
- General: Fatigue, weight loss.
- Teratogenicity.

Drug Interactions

Similar to vismodegib but being a major substrate of CYP3A4 aas also being inhibitors of CYP2B6 and CYP2C9 it causes more interactions with drugs metabolized by these pathways with more adverse effects.

Contraindications

- Hypersensitivity to drug or its components.
- Pregnancy and lactation.
- Avoid blood and semen donation.

Pregnancy: Contraindicated.

Lactation: Avoid breastfeeding.

Children: Safety and efficacy not proven.

BETA-BLOCKERS

Beta-blockers are drugs that block norepinephrine and epinephrine (adrenaline) from binding to beta-adrenergic receptors.

Classification

Category	Properties	Drug
1st generation	Non-selective	Propranolol, timolol, pindolol, nadolol, sotalol
2nd generation	Beta-1 selective blocker	Atenolol, bisoprolol, metoprolol, esmolol
3rd generation	Non-selective	Carvedilol, labetalol
3rd generation	Beta-1 selective blocker	Betaxolol, nebivolol, celiprolol

Propranolol

It is a nonselective first generation beta-blocker

Mechanism of Action

- Immediate vasoconstrictive effects via β2–adrenergic receptors on haemangioma pericyte cells.
- Subsequent progressive reduction in volume and redness may be due to decreases in serum concentration of VEGF, b-FGF, and renin as well as induction of endothelial cell apoptosis.

Salient Features

- Oral β-blockers are effective in halting growth and expediting regression of cutaneous, ocular, airway and hepatic IHs as well as for complications, such as ulceration.
- Compared to systemic corticosteroids, propranolol has superior efficacy and a more favourable side-effect profile

Indications

Approved

Infantile hemangiomas.

Unlicensed

Wound healing, flushing, aquagenic urticaria, angiolymphoid hyperplasia with eosinophilia, erythromelalgia, hemohydrosis.

Dosage

- Initial: Usually ~1 mg/kg/day divided into 2 (or 3) doses
- Target: 2–3 mg/kg/day divided into 2 (or 3) doses‡; the target dose may be lower (~1 mg/kg/day) for ulcerated lesions, and the approved maximum is 3.4 mg/kg/day
- For a proliferating IH, treatment is typically continued for 6–12 months, depending on the clinical setting and course.

Adverse Effects

- Cutaneous: Triggering or aggravation of psoriasis, lichenoid reaction, Peyronie's disease, alopecia, erythema multiforme.
- Systemic: Cardiovascular—bradycardia, heart failure, postural hypotension, heart block.
  - Pulmonary: Worsening of chronic obstructive pulmonary disease and asthma.
  - Neurologic: Fatigue, insomnia, depression
  - Gastrointestinal: Nausea, vomiting, diarrhoea
  - Metabolic: Hypoglycaemia at risk patients

Contraindication

- Hypersensitivity to drug or components of formulation
- Variety of significant CV disorders—ischemic, valvular, arrhythmias, conduction abnormalities.

Pregnancy: Category C

Lactation: Safe

Children: Higher risk below 5 weeks of age

ORAL MINOXIDIL

Minoxidil

Originally developed as an antihypertensive agent, minoxidil has been known for decades to promote hair growth.

Mechanism of Action

- Minoxidil causes premature termination of the telogen phase, lengthens the anagen phase, and can increase follicle size, particularly of miniaturized follicles.
- Stimulation of vascular endothelial growth factor and prostaglandin synthesis may also play a role.
- Oral minoxidil relaxes vascular smooth muscle by opening ATP-dependent potassium channels. The increase in ATP results in a release of adenosine.
- Vascular endothelial growth factor (VEGF), a proposed promoter of hair growth, is stimulated by adenosine signalling pathways.
- Prostaglandins are stimulated by minoxidil in the dermal papillae.

Pharmacology

- Oral Minoxidil is at least 90% absorbed from the GI tract.
- The average plasma half-life in man is 4.2 hours.
- Minoxidil does not bind to plasma proteins and does not cross the blood brain barrier.

Indications

Unlicensed

In androgenetic alopecia.

Dosage

0.25 to 1.25 mg daily are usually used for FPHL and doses ranging from 2.5 to 5 mg/day for MPHL.

Adverse Effects

Hypotension, headache.

Contraindication

- Hypersensitivity to the product.
- It is not recommended for pregnant or nursing women.

Pregnancy: Category C

Lactation: Not recommended

Children: Not recommended in patients under 18 years old.

ORAL VITAMINS

Niacinamide

Nicotinic acid (niacin, vitamin B_3) is an essential dietary constituent, the deficiency of which leads to pellagra. In the body, nicotinic acid (niacin) is converted to niacinamide (nicotinamide), which functions as a crucial coenzyme.

MOA: It inhibits PARP-1 [poly-(adenosine) diphosphate-ribose polymerase-1] which is involved in NFκB (Nuclear factor-kB)-mediated transcription. This leads to dysregulation of adhesion factors (such as intracellular adhesion molecule-1), thereby altering leucocyte chemotaxis.

- It also reduces interleukin 1 (IL-1), interleukin 12 (IL-12), tumor necrosis factor-alpha (TNF-α), major histocompatibility complex II (MHC-II) and macrophage migration inhibitor factor-1 and is anti-inflammatory.

Indications

Unlicensed

- Bullous pemphigoid
- Prophylaxis and treatment of pellagra caused by poor nutrition, Hartnup disease, or carcinoid tumors.
- Photodermatoses.

Side Effects

- **GIT:** Nausea, vomiting, hepatotoxicity
- **CNS:** Headache, Schizophrenia
- **Myopathy**

Contraindication

- Hypersensitivity to niacinamide or components of formulation.

- In patients of jaundice/liver disease, diabetes, gout, or peptic ulcer.

Pregnancy: Newer rating—compatible.

Zinc

Zinc is a trace element involved in many cellular processes. The recommended doses for elemental zinc are 0.5–1 mg/kg/day in divided doses in children and 15–30 mg/day in adults.

Mechanism of Action

- Modulates the actions on macrophage and neutrophil functions, natural killer cell/phagocytic activity, and various inflammatory cytokines.
- Zinc stabilizes cell membranes, acts as a cofactor for various metalloenzymes (like MMPs), is involved in superoxide dismutase and metallothionein functions, and participates in basal cell mitosis and differentiation

Indications

Infection
- Verruca vulgaris
- Cutaneous leishmaniasis
- Leprosy

Inflammatory disorders
- Acne vulgaris
- Rosacea
- Hidradenitis suppurativa
- Psoriasis
- Behcet's disease
- Vitiligo
- Alopecia areata.

THALIDOMIDE

Thalidomide is an *N*-phthalimidoglutarimide. It was initially used as a nonbarbiturate sedative-hypnotic, but subsequently withdrawn several years later due to its potent teratogenic effects. The drug has an orphan drug status and has been used since 1998 for erythema nodosum leprosum and other indications in dermatology.

Indications

Approved
- Erythema nodosum leprosum
- Unlicensed
- Neutrophilic dermatoses
  - Behcet disease
  - Severe aphthous stomatitis
  - Pyoderma gangrenosum
- HIV-associated dermatoses
  - AIDS-associated oral stomatitis
  - AIDS-associated Kaposi sarcoma
- Lymphocytic infiltrates
  - Cutaneous lupus erythematosus
  - Jessner lymphocytic infiltrate
  - Cutaneous lymphoid hyperplasia
- Papulosquamous disorders
  - Lichen planus—oral and refractory generalized lichen planus
  - Lichen planopilaris–recalcitrant form
- Vesiculobullous disorders
  - Bullous pemphigoid
  - Mucous membrane pemphigoid
  - Recurrent erythema multiforme

Others
- Chronic graft-versus-host disease
- Cutaneous sarcoidosis
- Nodular prurigo/actinic prurigo
- Cutaneous lesions of adult Langerhans cell histiocytosis
- Uremic pruritus
- Weber-Christian disease
- Postherpetic neuralgia.

Mechanism of Action

Not clear, exhibits multiple effects
- Hypnosedative effect: Due to glutarimide ring and it easily penetration into central nervous system.
- Immunomodulatory and anti-inflammatory effects:
  - Inhibits TNF-α, IL-6, IL-12, IL-8 and matrix metalloproteinase 2 thus affecting cellular immune response.
  - Humoral immunity is affected by suppression of IFN-γ and increased production of IL-4 and IL-5.
  - It suppresses both phagocytosis and chemotaxis of neutrophils and also monocyte phagocytosis.
  - Inhibits mediators of inflammation like histamine, serotonin, prostaglandins and acetylcholine.
- Neural and angiogenic effects: Has direct effects on neural tissue and inhibits angiogenesis.

Pharmacology

Absorbed slowly from GI tract after oral administration with peak plasma levels reached within 2–6 hours after administration. It undergoes hydrolytic degradation into 12 cleavage products. The half-life of thalidomide is 5–7 hours with excretion being mainly nonrenal. The drug actively crosses placenta due to its lipid solubility. Thalidomide is poorly water soluble.

Dosage

100–300 mg/day starting dose to be taken at bedtime or 1 hour after evening meal with a glassful of water. Following improvement tapering to be done by 50 mg every 2–4 weeks. Tapering attempts of patients on maintenance therapy should be done every 3–6 months. **(FitzPatrick)**

Monitoring

System for Thalidomide Education and Prescribing Safety (STEPS) requires monitoring of patients during treatment.

Baseline

Complete history to assess risk of thrombotic, cardiac and neurological disorders along with physical examination.

Laboratory

- Pregnancy test in females of childbearing age group within 24 hours before 1st dose.
- Complete blood count including platelet count.
- Urea, creatinine, electrolytes
- Liver function tests
- Thyroid function tests
- Coagulation profile (INR, APPT and derived fibrinogen)
- Nerve conduction studies (sensory nerve action potential measurement-SNAP).
- HIV patients—viral load

Follow Up

Physical examination including neurological examination monthly for first 3 months, then every 1–6 months.

Laboratory

- Pregnancy tests: Weekly for the 1st month, then monthly for females of childbearing age with regular menstrual periods and every 2 weeks for those with irregular menstrual periods.
- Complete blood counts with platelet counts: Monthly till dose stability, then every 2–3 months.
- Nerve conduction study every 6 months.

Focus on contraception and pregnancy prevention programme is of paramount importance.

Adverse Effect

- Psychiatric: Headache, mood changes, dizziness.
- Neurologic: Sedation (most common), peripheral neuropathy: Axonal neuropathy, mild proximal muscle weakness with symmetric painful paresthesia of hands and feet along with sensory loss of lower limbs is most common.
- Thromboembolic events: Risk is higher in smokers, history of hypercholesterolemia and arterial thrombosis.
- GI: Nausea, constipation, appetite increase.
- Mucocutaneous: Xerostomia, xerosis, itching, red palms, brittle fingernails, exfoliative dermatitis.
- Endocrinal: Both hypothyroidism, and hyperthyroidism, hypoglycemia.
- Reproductive: Teratogenicity—100% chance of birth defects if prescribed between 21 and 36 weeks of gestation. Phocomelia and ear malformations common, menstrual irregularities, decreased libido.
- Hematologic: Leucopenia
- Cardiac: Bradycardia, peripheral edema.

Drug Interactions

- Increased sedation: With hypnotics, antipsychotics, sedative H_1 antihistamines, barbiturates, alcohol and opioid derivatives
- Peripheral neuropathy: Metronidazole, vincristine, isoniazid.
- Teratogenicity: CYP 3A4 inducers like griseofulvin, rifamycin, anticonvulsants impair hormonal contraceptives.
- Increased risk of bradycardia: Beta blockers, neostigmine:
- Increased risk of thromboembolic disorders: Bisphosphonates, erythropoiesis-stimulating agents, corticosteroids (though hormonal contraceptives also increase the risk of thromboembolic events but benefit outweighs risk.
- Increase risk of myelosuppression and infections: Immunosuppressives (biologics, JAK inhibitors and conventional immunosuppressants.)
- Vaccines: Live vaccines to be administered 3 months after completion of treatment.

Contraindications

Absolute

- Hypersensitivity to the drug
- Pregnancy
- Women of childbearing age/potential
- Men in sexual contact with women of childbearing age/potential
- Pre-existing peripheral neuropathy.

Relative

- History of neuritis or neurological disorder
- Hypothyroidism
- Constipation, congestive heart failure
- Hypertension
- History and presence of risk factors for thromboembolism.
- Renal dysfunction
- Hepatic dysfunction.

Pregnancy: Category X.

Lactation: Not recommended

Children: Can be used in children when absolutely necessary.

LENALIDOMIDE

Second generation thalidomide analogue.

Mechanism of Action

Same as thalidomide but effect on T cells, IL-2 and IFN-γ more than thalidomide.

Pharmacology

Rapidly and highly absorbed in fasting conditions. It has a short half-life of 3-4 hours. 82% of oral dose is excreted in urine within 24 hours.

Indications

Approved

- Follicular or mantle cell lymphoma, multiple myeloma and deletion 5q myelodysplastic syndrome.
- Unlicensed in dermatology
- Severe refractory cutaneous lupus erythematosus
- Prurigo nodularis
- Chronic actinic dermatitis
- Scleromyxedema.

Adverse Effects

- Neutropenia and thrombocytopenia more with lenalidomide
- Peripheral neuropathy, sedation and constipation
- Less with lenalidomide
- Thromboembolic events in the form of deep vein thrombosis and pulmonary embolus more compared to thalidomide specially in predisposed patients.

Drug Interaction

- Increases level of digoxin
- Increased risk of thromboembolism in patients on prothrombotic agents
- Monitoring
- Similar to thalidomide
- Contraindication
- Same as thalidomide

SYSTEMIC PSORALEN PLUS ULTRAVIOLET A PHOTOCHEMOTHERAPY (PUVA)

- Psoralens are naturally occurring linear furocoumarins that are found in a large number of plants (*Ammi majus, Psoralea corylifolia*). There are several synthetic psoralen compounds too.
- For oral mainly 8-MOP (methoxsalen) is used. The synthetic compound, 4,5',8-trimethylpsoralen (TMP, trioxsalen), is less phototoxic than 8-MOP after oral administration, but more phototoxic when delivered via bathwater.

Indications

Approved

- Psoriasis
- Mycosis fungoides/Sézary syndrome
- Vitiligo

Unlicensed

- **Neoplastic:** Histiocytosis X (Langerhans' cell histiocytosis)
- **Papulosquamous/Dermatitis**
  - Atopic dermatitis
  - Seborrheic dermatitis
  - Chronic hand dermatitis
  - Palmoplantar pustulosis
  - Lichen planus
  - Parapsoriasis
  - Pityriasis lichenoides
  - Lymphomatoid papulosis
- **Photosensitivity dermatoses**
  - Polymorphous light eruption
  - Erythropoietic protoporphyria
  - Solar urticaria
  - Chronic actinic dermatitis
- **Other pruritic dermatoses**
  - Dermographism
  - Aquagenic urticaria/pruritus
  - Chronic urticaria
  - Polycythemia vera
  - Idiopathic pruritus
  - Urticaria pigmentosa
  - Prurigo nodularis
- **Other immunologic**
  - Dermatoses
  - Alopecia areata
  - Graft-versus-host disease
  - Morphea
  - Systemic sclerosis
- **Miscellaneous dermatoses**
  - Transient acantholytic dermatosis (Grover disease)
  - Pigmented purpuric dermatoses
  - Ichthyosis linearis circumflexa
  - Scleromyxedema
  - Generalized granuloma annulare.

Mechanism of Action

Ground state psoralen molecules are activated to the excited singlet state by absorption of photons in the UVA waveband, with peak absorption between 320 and 330 nm. The singlet state undergoes decay to the triplet state and is responsible for most photochemical effects.

Two types of photochemical reaction occur:

- Type I (direct) photochemical reactions result in photoaddition of the compound to pyrimidines in deoxyribonucleic acid (DNA), forming monofunctional adducts, cross-linking of adjacent strands of DNA (bifunctional adducts) and conjugation of proteins.
- Type II (indirect) photochemical reactions produce of reactive oxygen species and free radicals damaging cell membranes and cytoplasmic constituents.

Pharmacology

- Intake of food before taking psoralens slows absorption and reduces the peak serum levels. So, it is better to take a light meal before ingesting psoralens.
- Intake of food before taking psoralens slows absorption and reduces the peak serum levels. Thus, the medication should be taken 30 minutes after a light meal, which decreases nausea associated with 8-MOP.
- With oral therapy, 75 to 80% of 8 MOP, and 98 to 99% of 5-MOP, respectively.
- It undergoes first-pass metabolism.

Dosage

A dosage of 8-MOP of 0.6 to 0.8 mg/kg body weight is administered orally 2 hours before sun exposure.

Treatment Protocols

Oral PUVA/PUVASOL: A dosage of 8-MOP of 0.6 to 0.8 mg/kg body weight is administered orally 2 hours before sun exposure; treatments are usually given two or three times weekly at least 48 hours apart to permit evaluation of any erythema resulting from the preceding treatment. Eye protection with UVA-blocking glasses is required when the patient is exposed to sunlight on the day of treatment, from time of psoralen ingestion until sunset that day. On the day of treatment, after ingestion of psoralens, photoprotection should be practiced, including application of broad-spectrum sunscreen with sun protection factor (SPF) of 30 on exposed areas, taking care that sunscreen is not on the skin when UVA exposure is administered.

Adverse Effects

Short-Term

Phototoxic Reactions
- Symptomatic erythema
- Pruritus
- Subacute phototoxicity
- Photo onycholysis
- Koebner phenomenon
- Friction blisters on hands and feet
- Ankle edema

Due to Methoxsalen
- Gastrointestinal disturbance
- Central nervous system disturbance
- Bronchoconstriction
- Hepatic toxicity
- Drug fever
- Exanthems

Others
- Cardiovascular stress
- Herpes simplex recurrences
- Photosensitive eruptions

Long-term
- Nonmelanoma skin cancer
- Melanoma

Contraindication

Absolute
- Pemphigus and pemphigoid
- Lupus erythematosus with photosensitivity
- Xeroderma pigmentosum
- Pregnancy
- Lactation
- History of idiosyncratic reaction to psoralen compound.

Relative
- Photosensitivity/photosensitizing medications
- Prior exposure to ionizing radiation or arsenic
- History or family history of melanoma
- History of skin cancer or chronic photodamage
- Severe cardiac, liver or renal disease
- Very young age

Pregnancy category: C

Lactation: Contraindicated

Children: Not recommended below 12 years.

BOTULINUM TOXIN

Botulinum toxin (BoNT) is a neurotoxin product from the cultures of *Clostridium botulinum*. *Clostridium botulinum* produces seven known serologically distinct and immunologically independent neurotoxins, serotyped A, B, C, D, E, F, and G.

Pharmacology

- All BoNT serotypes have a generally conserved small core neurotoxin protein (150 kDa).

- Serotype A (BoNTA) is the most potent and longest lasting.
- Serotype E appears to have a rapid onset of approximately 24 hours, and a short duration of approximately 30 days. This has advantages for those who want to try neurotoxin but are afraid they may not like it.
- There may also be a role for serotype E in the reduction of postoperative pain and prevention of postoperative scarring.

MOA

- **Inhibition of neuromuscular function**: Any process that significantly interferes with even one component of vesicle exocytosis will impair neuromuscular function. SNARE proteins are the target of the BoNT light chain, resulting in postsynaptic cellular dysfunction and ultimate paralysis if enough cells are unable to contract.
- **Recovery of neuromuscular function**: Once the vesicular-transport machinery is damaged, the acute effects are irreversible. Muscle weakness is seen in 2 to 4 days, with peak paralysis in 7 to 10 days. Within 1 month the peripheral nerves begin to sprout new, smaller, unmyelinated nerve endings. After about 3 months a functional connection is re-established in the original nerve terminal.

Formulation

- Onabotulinum toxin A
- Abobotulinum toxin A
- Incobotulinum toxin A
- Rimabotulinum toxin B

Indications

Cosmetic

Upper Face
- Glabellar complex and vertical frown lines
- Horizontal forehead lines
- Crow's feet

Mid Face
- Bunny lines
- Infraorbital wrinkles
- Nasal tip elevation
- Gummy smile

Lower Face
- Perioral lines
- Marionette lines
- Popply chin
- Masseter

Neck
- Platysmal bands
- Horizontal necklines
- Nefertiti lift

Noncosmetic

Hyperhidrosis

Complications

- Pain, swelling, erythema, bruising
- Ptosis (eyelid, brow, lip)
- Hand weakness (hyperhidrosis treatment)
- Dysphagia
- Headache
- Distant inflammation, anaphylaxis, flu-like symptoms, metallic taste
- Xerophthalmia
- Ectropion
- Diplopia
- Hypertension, arrhythmia, myocardial infarction

Contraindication

Hypersensitivity to toxin/components formulation (including cow's milk protein).

Pregnancy category: C

VACCINES IN DERMATOLOGY

HPV vaccine: A vaccine is an antigenic substance prepared from the causative agent of a disease or a synthetic substitute, used to provide immunity against disease.

Mechanism of Action

- Virus-like particles (VLPs) resemble native virions morphologically and immunologically, and they carry neutralization epitopes on their surface.
- Systemic immunizations with VLPs induce high-titer, long-lasting, and type restricted neutralizing antibodies.
- Chimeric VLPs have been engineered to incorporate an early protein such as E7 into an L1 or L1/L2 capsid. The induction of cytotoxic T-lymphocyte responses to the E7 oncoprotein, in addition to antibodies directed against the L1 capsid protein, provides both therapeutic and prophylactic benefit.

Types

1. Quadrivalent vaccine of HPV-6,-11,-16,-18 VLPs (Gardasil)
2. Bivalent vaccine of HPV-16,-18 VLPs (Cervarix)
3. 9 valent vaccine (Gardasil-9): VLPs for HPV-6 and -11 as well as high-risk HPV types 16, 18, 31, 33, 45, 52, and 58.

Indications

- Advisory Committee on Immunization Practices (ACIP) recommends (all females and males in the following age ranges):
  - Routine HPV vaccination is recommended at 11 to 12 years. It can be administered starting at 9 years of age.
  - For adolescents and adults aged 13 to 26 years who have not been previously vaccinated or who have not completed the vaccine series, catch-up vaccination is recommended.
  - For adults 27 years and older, catch-up vaccination is not routinely recommended.
- The 9-valent vaccine is FDA-approved for females and males ages 9 to 45 years to prevent anogenital warts as well as cervical, vulvar and vaginal cancers, anal cancer, and HPV-related head and neck cancers.

Schedule

- **Individuals initiating the vaccine series at 9 to 14 years of age:** Two doses of HPV vaccine should be given at 0 and at 6 to 12 months. If the second dose was administered <5 months after the first, the dose should be repeated a minimum of 12 weeks after the second dose and a minimum of 5 months after the initial vaccine dose.
- **Individuals initiating the vaccine series at 15 years of age or older:** Three doses of HPV vaccine should be given at 0, 1 to 2 (typically 2), and 6 months.
- The minimum intervals between the first two doses is 4 weeks, between the second and third doses is 12 weeks, and between the first and third dose is 5 months. If a dose was administered at a shorter interval, it should be repeated once the minimum recommended interval since the most recent dose has passed.
- **Immunocompromised patients:** Three doses of HPV vaccine should be given at 0, 1 to 2, and 6 months regardless of age.

Safety

- HPV vaccination during pregnancy is not recommended.
- Lactating females can receive the immunization series since subunit vaccines do not affect the safety of infant breastfeeding.

Vaccination for the Prevention of Shingles (Herpes Zoster)(Shingrix)

Shingrix is a recombinant zoster vaccine.

Indication

SHINGRIX is a vaccine indicated for prevention of herpes zoster (HZ) (shingles):
- In adults aged 50 years and older.
- In adults aged 18 years and older who are or will be at increased risk of HZ due to immunodeficiency or immunosuppression caused by known disease or therapy.

[Limitations: SHINGRIX is not indicated for prevention of primary varicella infection (chickenpox)]

Schedule

Two doses (0.5 mL each) administered intramuscularly according to the following schedules:
- A first dose at Month 0 followed by a second dose administered 2-6 months later.
- For individuals who are or will be immunodeficient or immunosuppressed and who would benefit from a shorter vaccination schedule: A first dose at Month 0 followed by a second dose administered 1 to 2 months later.

Adverse Reactions

- Local: Pain, redness, and swelling.
- Systemic: Myalgia, fatigue, headache, shivering, fever, and gastrointestinal symptoms.

Contraindication

- History of severe allergic reaction (e.g., anaphylaxis) to any component of the vaccine or after a previous dose of SHINGRIX.
- **Use in pregnancy and lactation**: There is currently no recommendation for SHINGRIX use in pregnancy; therefore, delaying SHINGRIX until after pregnancy may be considered.

CHAPTER 3

Topical Drugs

TOPICAL DRUGS

Topical Antibacterials

Topical antibacterials are usually used in the prevention and treatment of cutaneous infections. They are also an integral part of the therapeutic armamentarium of acne.

Two broad categories of topical antibacterial agents:
- Drugs used primarily for wound care and minor topical bacterial infections.
- Drugs used primarily for acne and rosacea.
- Drugs used for wound care and minor topical bacterial infections.
- Mupirocin:
  - Mupirocin is naturally derived from *Pseudomonas fluorescens* and is chemically unrelated to other antibiotics.
  - Mechanism of action: It reversibly binds to bacterial isoleucyl t-RNA synthetase thus inhibiting bacterial RNA, protein and cell wall synthesis. Mupirocin is bactericidal and effective against both penicillinase-producing and methicillin-resistant *S. aureus*, *S. pyogenes*, some Gram-negative organisms. It is ineffective against anaerobes.

Indications

- Cutaneous bacterial infections caused by *Staphylococcus* and *Streptococcus* like impetigo, folliculitis, lacerations, burns, secondarily infected eczema and leg ulcers.
- Nasal decolonization of methicillin-resistant *S. aureus* (MRSA) in both patients and healthcare workers. Intranasal application of Mupirocin twice daily for 5 days is usually effective.

Salient Features

- Topical absorption is minimal and cutaneous metabolism is <3%, leaving most of the drug on the skin for antibacterial activity. (Inkelman W, Gratton D. Topical antibacterials. Clin Dermatol. 1989;7:156-162.)
- Mupirocin may be less effective on weeping wounds because 95% of the drug is protein-bound. (Leyden JJ. Review of mupirocin ointment in the treatment of impetigo. Clin Pediatr. 1992;31:49-53)

Dosage

2% ointment or cream applied twice daily.

Adverse Effects

Skin irritation: Burning, stinging or pain and pruritus.

Pregnancy: Category B.

Lactation: Probably compatible

Children: Safe.

FUSIDIC ACID

Fusidic acid is an antibiotic with a steroidal structure derived from the fungus *Fusidium coccineum*. Its active ingredient is sodium fusidate.

Mechanism of Action

It acts by interfering with bacterial protein synthesis, by preventing the translocation of the elongation factor-G (EF-G) from the ribosome. It is effective against Gram-positive bacteria like *S. aureus*, *Corynebacterium* species and some Gram-positive anaerobes.

Indications

- Staphylococcal primary skin infections like impetigo.
- For elimination of nasal carriage of *S. aureus* (2nd choice to mupirocin)
- Erythrasma and pitted keratolysis

- In combination with topical steroids for treating infected eczemas.

Salient Features

Fusidic acid can penetrate normal, damaged as well as avascular skin.

Dosage

2% cream or ointment used twice/thrice daily for 14 days.

Adverse Effects

Sensitization (occasional).

Pregnancy: Category B

Lactation: Probably compatible

Children: Safe to use

RETAPAMULIN

Retapamulin is a semisynthetic pleuromutilin class of topical antibacterial derived from an edible mushroom *Citophilus scyphoides*.

Mechanism of Action

It is bacteriostatic and acts by binding to a unique site protein L3 on the 50S ribosomal subunit thus inhibiting peptidyl transferase and preventing translation.

Indication

- Primary impetigo due to MSSA (Methicillin sensitive *S. aureus*) or *S. pyogenes* in adults and children more than 9-months-old.
- Staphylococcal folliculitis
- Secondarily infected wounds and dermatitis.

Salient Feature

Retapamulin is active against multiple gram-positive aerobic cocci including MSSA, MRSA and mupirocin resistant *S. aureus*, *S. pyogenes*.

Dosage

1% ointment twice daily for 5 days.

Adverse Effects

Local reactions—pruritus, paresthesia, pain irritation at application site, allergic contact dermatitis.

Pregnancy: Category B

Lactation: Probably compatible.

Children: Not to be used in infants <9 months of age.

OZENOXACIN

It is a nonfluorinated quinolone bactericidal antibiotic.

Mechanism of Action

Ozenoxacin acts by inhibiting bacterial DNA synthesis by inhibiting DNA gyrase A and topoisomerase IV.
- It has bactericidal action against both Gram-positive and Gram-negative bacteria including MRSA, mupirocin, fusidic acid, ciprofloxacin resistant strains of *S. aureus*, *S. pyogenes*, *Cutibacterium acne*.

Indication

- Impetigo caused by *S. aureus* and *S. pyogenes* in adults and children aged 2 months and older.

Dosage

It is used as 1% cream twice daily for 5 days.

Adverse Effects

Development of rosacea and seborrheic dermatitis.

Pregnancy: category: Unknown

Lactation: Unknown

Children: Not below 2 months.

NEOMYCIN

Neomycin is a bactericidal aminoglycoside antibacterial agent produced by *Streptomyces fradiae*. It is made of three major chemically related compounds, neomycin A neomycin B (framycetin) and neomycin C.

Mechanism of Action

- It acts by binding to the 30S subunit of bacterial ribosome to inhibit protein synthesis.
- Neomycin kills Gram-negative organisms like *Proteus* sp, *E. coli*, *Serratia* sp, *H. influenzae*. Among Gram-positive bacteria it is active against *Staphylococcus*.

Indication

- Neomycin is combined with Bacitracin to increase Gram-positive coverage against *S. aureus* and *S. pyogenes* and with Polymyxin B to increase coverage against *Pseudomomas aeruginosa*.
- Triple combination of Neomycin, Bacitracin and Polymyxin B is used in the treatment of superficial pyodermas, prophylaxis against infection in minor wounds, burns and secondarily infected dermatitis.

Dosage

0.5% cream 2-3 times a day for 7 days.

Adverse Effects

- Neomycin is the most common cause of postoperative allergic contact dermatitis in dermatologic surgery and in leg ulcers.
- Cross reactivity with other aminoglycosides like gentamycin.

Pregnancy: Category D

Lactation: Probably compatible

Children: Neomycin in combination with Polymyxin B can be safely used in children ≥2 years of age.

Gentamycin

Gentamycin is an aminoglycoside antibiotic derived from *Micromonospora purpurea*.

Mechanism of Action

It inhibits bacterial protein synthesis by irreversibly binding to 30S ribosomal subunit and is bactericidal against *S. aureus* and Gram-negative organisms like *P. aeruginosa*, *E. coli*, *Proteus sp*. Gentamycin is ineffective against anaerobic bacteria.

Indications

- Treatment of burns, bedsores, impetigo and other pyogenic skin infections.
- Used as Gentamycin collagen sponges to reduce postoperative complications following surgical excision in hidradenitis suppurativa.

Dosage

Adults and children ≥1 year of age— 1% cream applied three or four times daily.

Adverse effects

Allergic contact dermatitis and cross sensitivity with other aminoglycosides.

Pregnancy: Category C

Lactation: Safe

Children: To be used in children ≥ 1 year of age.

NADIFLOXACIN

Nadifloxacin is a potent broad-spectrum fluorinated quinolone with bactericidal properties.

Mechanism of Action

- It inhibits DNA gyrase thus preventing bacterial DNA synthesis and replication.
- Nadifloxacin has antibacterial action against Gram-positive bacteria including MRSA and MSSA, *Strepto pyogenes, S. epidermidis*, Gram-negative bacteria and anaerobes including *C. acnes*.

Indication

- Superficial bacterial infections like impetigo, sycosis barbae.
- Acne vulgaris.

Dosage

1% cream twice daily.

Side effects: Minimal—burning, itching, erythema at local site.

Pregnancy: Limited data in pregnancy.

Lactation: Limited data.

Children: Safety not established.

SILVER SULFADIAZINE

Silver sulfadiazine (SSD) is an inexpensive, widely used topical anti-infective agent in the prevention and treatment of infected wounds caused by second- and third-degree burns.

Mechanism of Action

The exact mode of action is not clear, however in wounds, SSD acts by delivering continuous low concentrations of silver ions interfering with DNA transcription, bacterial respiration and uncoupling ATP synthesis.

Indication

- Second and third degree burn wound.
- Treatment of venous leg ulcers, pressure ulcers, neuropathic diabetic foot ulcers.
- Treatment of mild infections like *Pseudomonas cellulitis*, toe-web infections, ecthyma gangrenosum.

Dosage

1% cream applied once or twice daily.

Adverse Effects

- Pruritus, burning sensation, brownish-grey discoloration of skin, Stevens-Johnson syndrome and photosensitivity.
- Caution while application to large burn areas due to significant absorption and renal insufficiency.

Contraindication

In patients with hypersensitivity to sulfonamides.

Pregnancy: Category B

Lactation: No data in lactation

Children: Avoid in neonates.

ANTISEPTICS

Gentian Violet

Gentian violet is a triphenylmethane dye having anti-infective action against bacteria, fungus, helminths and trypanosoma.

Mechanism of Action

Its exact mechanism of action is not known, but it has multiple modes of action which includes alteration of redox potential, inhibition of reduced nicotinamide adenine dinucleotide phosphate oxidases, uncoupling of oxidative phosphorylation and bacterial cell wall formation inhibition.

Indications

- Treatment of MRSA-colonized ulcers and pyodermas. Its low cost, ease of application and stability makes it a good option, treatment of nasal carriage of MRSA.
- In infected eczemas.

Adverse Effects

Staining of sites of application.

HYDROGEN PEROXIDE

It is a potent broad spectrum antimicrobial effective against bacteria, viruses, yeast and protozoa.

Mechanism of Action

It produces free hydroxyl radicals that damage cellular lipids, proteins and DNA.

Indication

- As skin antiseptic at 3–6% concentrations (vol/vol)
- Acne—both inflammatory and non-inflammatory lesions.

Alcohol

Alcohol based antiseptics are widely used as surface disinfectants and skin antiseptic agents.

Mechanism of Action

Alcohol based antiseptics act by protein denaturation or by inhibition of mRNA and protein synthesis and thus microbial membrane damage.

Salient Features

- They act against vegetative bacteria, viruses and fungi but not against bacterial spores.
- Alcohols are combined with other antiseptics like chlorhexidine for residual activity as their effect is short lasting.
- Concentrations ranging between 60–90% are bactericidal.

CHLORHEXIDINE

It is a divalent cationic biguanide antiseptic used extensively in healthcare setup to prevent infections.

Mechanism of Action

Chlorhexidine is a broad-spectrum antimicrobial which inhibits bacterial spore outgrowth and as a membrane active agent causes protoplast lysis. It is active against both Gram-positive and Gram-negative bacteria, some enveloped viruses and fungi. It has long term residual action compared to other antiseptics.

Indications

- In immunocompetent patients it decreases the recurrence rate of *S. aureus* pyoderma and furunculosis.
- Preoperative cleansing with Chlorhexidine prevents both superficial and deep incisional infections postsurgery.

Adverse Effects

Mild skin irritation.

POVIDONE-IODINE

It is a complex of triiodide and polyvinylpyrrolidone.

Mechanism of Action

Though not clearly understood, but free iodine inhibits electron transport and cellular respiration, destabilizes membrane integrity, denatures nucleic acids and inhibits protein synthesis. Povidone-iodine kills both Gram-positive and Gram-negative bacteria, viruses, fungi and protozoa.

Indication

- Presurgical skin disinfectant (10% concentration).
- Reducing bacterial colonization in chronic nonhealing wounds.

Adverse Effects

Irritant contact dermatitis with tissue necrosis following long term contact.

Triclosan

It is a chlorinated bisphenol antiseptic used in many hygiene and personal care products like mouthwashes, deodorants, handwashes in concentrations up to 2%.

Mechanism of Action

Triclosan inhibits bacterial fatty acid biosynthesis and is effective against Gram-positive and most Gram-negative bacteria except *Pseudomonas* spp.

TOPICAL ANTIACNE DRUGS

Benzoyl Peroxide

Benzoyl peroxide (BPO) is an organic peroxide originally derived from chlorhydroxyquinoline, a byproduct of coal tar.

Mechanism of Action

- Bactericidal against *Cutibacterium acnes* mainly acting by its powerful oxidizing action. It is converted to benzoic acid after cutaneous absorption. Benzoic acid is metabolized by cysteine releasing free radical oxygen species which oxidizes bacterial proteins.
- Keratolytic and anti-inflammatory effects.

Indications

- As monotherapy or combination with topical antibiotic (Clindamycin) or topical retinoid (Tretinoin and Adapalene) as first line treatment of mild to moderate acne vulgaris. Combination therapy is more efficacious with acceptable safety profile than monotherapy.
- Combination of BPO with Clindamycin is effective in reducing the papular and pustular lesions of rosacea.

Dosage

Adults and children ≥12 years of age—use on the affected area(s) of the skin 1 or 2 times a day.

Adverse Effects

- Irritant dermatitis—main adverse effect
- True contact allergy—0.2%-1%
- Can bleach fabric, hair and other colored materials.

Pregnancy: Category C

Lactation: Probably compatible

Children: Used in children ≥12 years of age.

CLINDAMYCIN

Synthetic derivative of lincomycin.

Mechanism of Action

Inhibits bacterial protein synthesis by irreversibly binding to 50s subunit of bacterial ribosome. Effective against most aerobic Gram-positive cocci (except *Enterococcus* species), community acquired MRSA, Gram-positive and Gram-negative anaerobes.

Indications

- Mild to moderate Acne vulgaris in combination with BPO and topical Tretinoin (no longer recommended as monotherapy

due to increased resistance of *C. acnes* to Clindamycin).
- Treatment of erythrasma, folliculitis, pitted keratolysis, rosacea, Fox-Fordyce disease and periorificial facial dermatitis.

Dosage

Adults and children ≥12 years of age—two daily application.

Adverse Effects

- Mild local reactions—burning, itching, dryness and erythema.
- Contact allergy—very rare
- Gram-negative folliculitis—rarely associated
- *Pseudomembranous colitis*—extremely rare.

Pregnancy: Category B

Lactation: Safe

Children: Used in children ≥12 years of age.

AZELAIC ACID

Azelaic acid is a naturally occurring 9-carbon dicarboxylic acid produced as a by-product of metabolism of the yeast *Malassezia furfur*. It has antibacterial, anti-inflammatory and comedolytic properties.

Mechanism of Action

- Exact mechanism of antibacterial action is not clear. It inhibits bacterial protein synthesis and is bacteriostatic against Staphylococcus, *Cutibacterium acnes* and some Gram-negative organisms like *E. coli, P. aeruginosa, P. mirabilis*
- Competitive inhibitor of tyrosinase – can be used in treatment of hypermelanosis
- Keratolytic and comedolytic – it inhibits the growth and differentiation of keratinocytes
- Interacts with peroxisome proliferators activated receptor Y (PPAR-γ) thus suppresses UV-B light induced expression of IL-1β, IL-6 and TNF-α-this action is responsible for its effectiveness in rosacea.

Indications

- Mild to moderate acne vulgaris – improvement in acne is seen after 1 to 2 months and is maximal after 4 to 6 months of continuous use. However, it does not decrease the rate of sebum production. Azelaic acid is applied initially once daily for 1–2 weeks and if tolerated increased to twice daily application.
- Rosacea – twice daily application of azelaic acid for up to 12 weeks has been effective in improving erythema and inflammatory lesions of moderate rosacea.
- Perioral dermatitis
- Post inflammatory hyperpigmentation following acne vulgaris specially in darker skinned patients.

Dosage

Adults and children ≥ 12 years of age – 15–20% cream or gel applied twice daily

Adverse Effects

- Mild-dryness, itching, scaling or burning sensation can be seen in 10%

Pregnancy: Category B

Lactation: Compatible

Children: Used in children ≥ 12 years of age

Erythromycin

Erythromycin is a macrolide antibacterial isolated from *Streptomyces erythraceus*.

Mechanism of action

Erythromycin is bactericidal and inhibits bacterial protein synthesis by irreversibly binding to the 50s subunit of bacterial ribosome. It is bactericidal against Gram-positive cocci, *Cutibacterium acnes* and several

Gram-negative bacteria like *H. influenzae, Chlamydia sp, T. pallidum, Ureaplasma urealyticum, Mycoplasma pneumoniae.*

Indications

- Mild to moderate acne vulgaris – erythromycin is used in combination with BPO or Zinc 1.2% as incidence of erythromycin resistance when used as monotherapy is very high in the range of 50-100% depending of geographical regions.
- Combination of erythromycin and BPO can be an alternative treatment in rosacea
- Topical erythromycin is a first line treatment for erythrasma and pitted keratolysis

Dosage

Adults and children ≥ 12 years of age – 2-4% gel, lotion applied once or twice daily

Adverse Effects

- Mild – erythema, scaling, itching, burning, dryness
- Allergic contact dermatitis – rare

Pregnancy: Category B

Lactation: Safe

Children: Used in children ≥ 12 years of age

METRONIDAZOLE

It is a synthetic nitroimidazole antibacterial and antiprotozoal.

Mechanism of Action

The nitro group of metronidazole is reduced by mitochondrial ferredoxin in bacteria and the reduced metabolite inhibits bacterial nucleic acid synthesis by DNA strand breaking.

Indication

- Rosacea –0.75% gel as initial treatment of inflammatory lesions or for maintenance.
- Cutaneous ulcer – treatment of both benign and malignant malodorous ulcers and anaerobe infected decubitus ulcers

Adverse effects

Rare – dryness, burning, itching and stinging.

Pregnancy: Category B

Lactation: Better to avoid use in nursing mothers.

Children: Safety in children not established.

DAPSONE

Dapsone (4,4'-diaminodiphenyl sulfone) as a topical formulation is effective in the treatment of inflammatory lesions of moderately severe acne vulgaris.

Mechanism of Action

The exact mechanism of action of topical dapsone in acne is not clear, but its anti-inflammatory and anti-neutrophilic actions may be the cause of its beneficial effects. The action of dapsone on *C. acnes* remains poorly understood.

Indication

- Moderate acne

Dosage

Twice daily application of 5% topical dapsone, 7.5% gel once daily.

Adverse Effects

- Transient dryness, erythema, scaling, local burning sensation and sunburn. Treatment with topical dapsone does not require pretreatment G6PD screening or laboratory monitoring for hemolytic anemia.
- Dapsone when mixed with BPO can cause orange brown discolouration of clothing

Pregnancy: Category C

Lactation: Moderately high risk so to be avoided in nursing mothers

Children: Used in children ≥ 9 years of age.

Sodium Sulfacetamide

Sodium sulfacetamide has both antibacterial and anti-inflammatory properties.

Mechanism of Action

It inhibits *C. acnes* by inhibiting bacterial dihydropteroate synthetase thus prevents conversion of p-aminobenzoic acid to folic acid.

Indications

- Acne vulgaris
- Rosacea
- Seborrheic dermatitis and perioral dermatitis

Dosage

Sulfacetamide 10%—sulfur 5%, applied twice a day.

Adverse Effects

- Dryness, transient pruritus
- Combination with BPO preparations can cause orange brown staining of clothes
- Avoid in patients with known hypersensitivity to sulfonamides.

Pregnancy: Category C

Lactation: Moderate-high risk.

Children: Used in children ≥ 12 years of age.

TOPICAL ANTIFUNGAL AGENTS

Topical antifungals are generally considered first-line therapy for uncomplicated, superficial dermatomycoses owing to their high efficacy and low potential for systemic adverse effects.

Classification

Polyenes	Nystatin, Amphotericin B, Hamycin
Imidazoles	Miconazole, Clotrimazole, Ketoconazole, Oxiconazole, Econazole, Sulconazole, Sertaconazole, Luliconazole, Efinaconazole, Bifonazole, Tioconazole.
Allylamines	Terbinafine, Naftifine
Benzylamines	Butenafine
Benzoxaborole	Tavaborole
Hydroxypyridone	Ciclopirox
Whitfield ointment	3% salicylic acid, 6% benzoic acid in petrolatum
Other antifungals	Selenium sulphide
Thiocarbamates	Tolciclate, Tolnaftate
Morpholine derivatives	Amorolfine

Mechanism of Action

Mechanism of Action	Antifungal agents
Bind to fungal cell membrane ergosterol and form pores	Amphoteric B, Nystatin, Hamycin
Inhibition of ergosterol and lanosterol synthesis	Allylamines, benzylamines, tolnaftate
Inhibition of ergosterol synthesis	Azoles
Ciclopirox olamine	Chelates polyvalent cations (e.g. Fe3+) that have important functions in fungal cytochromes, catalases, and peroxidases; it thereby inhibits respiration, blocks transport of amino acids and alters cell membrane permeability
Selenium sulfide	Antimitotic properties; reduces cellular adhesion in the stratum corneum, facilitating shedding of fungi
Tavaborole	Blocks fungal protein synthesis via inhibition of the fungal leucyl-transfer ribonucleic acid (tRNA) synthetase

Polyenes

- First agents to have specific antifungal properties.
- Includes nystatin, amphotericin B, hamycin

Nystatin

Salient Features

- Produced by *Streptomyces noursei* and *Streptomyces albidus*. It has a structure and mode of action similar to that of amphotericin B but associated systemic toxicity has limited nystatin's use to topical applications.
- Has both fungistatic and fungicidal activity.
- Not active against dermatophyte infections

Indication

Cutaneous or mucocutaneous candidiasis

Dosage

- Cutaneous application-twice daily to affected areas.
- Oral candidiasis: Suspension – 4 to 5 times daily.

Vaginal cream-One 100,000–unit applicatorful inserted into the vagina one or two times a day for two weeks.

Adverse Effects

- Burning, pruritus, rash, eczema, and pain on application.
- Hypersensitivity(rare)

Pregnancy category: C

Lactation: Compatible

Children: Safe

AZOLES

Miconazole

Miconazole is a synthetic-substituted 1-phenethyl imidazole derivative.

Salient Features

- Miconazole penetrates the stratum corneum well, and is can be detected there even 4 days after a single application. Systemic absorption is minimal.
- It is effective in the treatment of tinea pedis, tinea corporis, tinea cruris, pityriasis (tinea) versicolor, and cutaneous candidiasis.
- Miconazole also demonstrates activity against some Gram-positive bacteria
- Effective in the treatment of erythrasma, impetigo, and ecthyma caused by group A β-hemolytic streptococci or pathogenic staphy lococci.
- Twice-daily application is recommended in all clinical situations except pityriasis versicolor, in which once-daily application is sufficient.

Adverse Effects

Irritation, burning, maceration, and allergic dermatitis at application sites

Pregnancy category: C

Lactation: Probably Compatible

Children: Safe

Clotrimazole

Salient Features

- Broad spectrum of activity against most strains of *Trichophyton, Epidermophyton,* and *Microsporum* species, also active against Gram-positive bacteria.
- It is also used in the treatment of oropharyngeal (troches) and vaginal (intravaginal tablet, cream) candidiasis.
- Twice daily application is effective for cutaneous lesions.
- Oral troches slowly dissolve in the mouth and should be administered four to five times daily for 2 weeks.
- Intravaginal clotrimazole may be effective following once daily tablet insertion for 1 to 2 days

Adverse Effects

Erythema, burning, irritation, stinging, peeling, blistering edema, pruritus, and urticaria at the site of application

Pregnancy: Category B

Lactation: Compatible

Children: Safe

Ketoconazole

Salient Features

- Ketoconazole is a synthetic antimycotic with a broad spectrum of activity against dermatophytes and yeasts.
- It is used in treatment of dermatophytosis (tinea corporis, cruris, pedis), cutaneous candidiasis and pityriasis versicolor.
- Shampoo formulation is also used in treatment of serborrhoeic dermatitis.

Adverse Effects

Irritation, pruritus, and stinging, contact dermatitis

Pregnancy: CategoryC

Lactation: Probably compatible

Children: Safe

Oxiconazole

Oxiconazole nitrate is an acetophenone-oxime derivative of imidazole.

Salient Features

- First topical antifungal agent to be approved for once daily application.
- Topical oxiconazole is rapidly absorbed into the stratum corneum. Fungicidal concentrations of oxiconazole are found in the epidermis within 5 hours of topical application with maximum concentrations achieved as early as 100 minutes following application.
- It is present in the epidermis at therapeutic levels for 7days, permiting once-daily dosing.

Adverse Effects

Pruritus, burning, irritation, erythema, maceration, and fissuring

Pregnancy: Category B

Lactation: Probably compatible

Children: Safe

Econazole

It is deschloro derivative of miconazole.

Salient Features

- Econazole inhibits most strains of *Trichophyton, Microsporum,* and *Epidermophyton, C. albicans,* and *M. furfur.*
- Econazole has also shown activity against some Gram-positive and Gram-negative bacterial organisms.
- Econazole foam relives pruritus

Dosage

- Cutaneous candidiasis-twice daily for 2 weeks
- For dermatophytosis and pityriasis versicolor – once daily for 2–4 weeks.

Adverse Effects

Erythema, burning, stinging, and pruritus.

Pregnancy: Category C

Lactation: Probably compatible

Children: Safety and efficacy have not been established in children younger than 12 years of age.

Sulconazole

Sulconazole has a sulfide bond between constituent azole heterocyclic rings.

Salient Features

- Percutaneous absorption of sulconazole exceeds that of other azole compounds.
- It is used in the treatment of dermatophytosis, pityriasis versicolor, and cutaneous candidiasis.
- Antibacterial activity against Gram-positive bacteria.
- Effective therapy for impetigo and ecthyma caused by group A β-hemolytic streptococci and staphylococci.

Dosage

- For of dermatophytosis, pityriasis versicolor, and cutaneous candidiasis – 1% cream and solution applied 1–2 daily for 2–4 weeks.
- For impetigo and ecthyma-twice daily for 14 days.

Adverse Effects

Allergic contact dermatitis

Pregnancy: Category C

Lactation: Probably compatible

Children: No study data in children.

Sertaconazole

Salient Features

- It is relatively lipophilic compared with other azoles, leading to a greater reservoir effect in the stratum corneum
- It has dual mechanism of action and depending on the exact organism and drug concentration, Sertaconazole can be either fungistatic or fungicidal. It inhibits lanosterol 14α-demethylase and also binds to nonsterol cell membrane lipids, leading to altered membrane permeability resulting in leakage of intracellular contents in susceptible microbes.
- It has modest activity against Gram-positive bacteria
- Approved for tinea pedis, use in other dermatophytosis is unlicensed.

Dosage

Tinea pedis-2% cream applied twice daily for 4 weeks

Adverse Effects

Allergic contact dermatitis

Pregnancy: Category C

Lactation: Unknown

Children: Safe in children ≥ 12 years of age.

Luliconazole

- Luliconazole has a unique chemical structure with the imidazole moiety incorporated into the ketene dithioacetate structure. This increases its potency against filamentous fungi along with broad spectrum antifungal action.
- Indicated for the topical treatment of interdigital tinea pedis, tinea cruris, and tinea corporis caused by the organisms *Trichophyton rubrum* and *Epidermophyton floccosum*

Dosage

- Tinea pedis – once daily for 2 weeks.
- Tinea corporis and cruris: Once daily for 1 week.

Adverse Effects

Contact dermatitis and cellulitis

Pregnancy: Category C

Lactation: Compatible

Children: Not to be used below 2 years in tinea corporis and below 12 years in tinea cruris and pedis.

Efinaconazole

First topical triazole approved for the treatment of onychomycosis of the toenails.

Salient Features

- Its binding to keratin is not strong, and low keratin affinity results in increased availability of free drug to the nail infection site.
- Antifungal activity seen against dermatophytes, *Candida* sp and nondermatophyte molds.
- Approved for mild to moderate tinea unguium without lunula involvement caused by *T. rubrum* and *T. mentagrophytes* in immunocompetent adults.

Dosage

Once daily to toenails for 48 weeks.

Adverse Effects

Mild-to-moderate application site reactions (in the form of irritation, itching, burning, redness).

Pregnancy: Category C

Lactation: Probably compatible

Children: Not below 6 years

Allylamines and Benzylamines

Naftifine: Naftifine is a synthetic allylamine antifungal.

Salient Features

- It is highly lipophilic and so penetrates and achieves high concentrations in the stratum corneum and hair follicles.
- Both fungicidal and fungistatic.
- Naftifine's spectrum activity includes a broad range of dermatophytes, yeasts, and saprophytes.
- Effective in treatment of tinea corporis, tinea cruris and candidiasis.
- Naftifine cream is also an effective monotherapy for moccasin tinea pedis.

Dosage

1% or 2% cream or gel applied once daily for 2 weeks.

Adverse Effects

Mild burning, stinging, itching, erythema, irritation, and rarely, allergic reactions.

Pregnancy: Category B

Lactation: Probably compatible

Children: Not below 2 years

Terbinafine

Terbinafine is a broad-spectrum synthetic antifungal of allylamine family, with both fungistatic and fungicidal properties.

Salient Features

- Terbinafine is highly lipophilic, resulting in high concentration in and efficient binding to the stratum corneum, sebum, and hair follicles, so chance of reinfection is less.
- Persistent concentrations well above the MIC for the common dermatophytes 7 days after topical application.

Dosage

1% cream to be applied once or twice daily till clinical improvement.

Adverse Effects

Pruritus, acute irritant contact dermatitis, irritation, burning/tingling sensation and dryness at the site of application.

Pregnancy: Category B

Lactation: Probably compatible

Children: Not below 12 years

Butenafine

Butenafine is the first and only in the benzylamine class of antifungals.

Salient Features

Fungicidal concentrations in the skin, particularly the stratum corneum, for at least 72 hours after application; this effect may be as a result of interaction with or fixation to cutaneous lipids, leading to a depot effect.

Dosage

1% cream once daily for 2 weeks.

Adverse Effects

Burning, itching, and redness at application sites

Pregnancy: Category C

Lactation: Probably compatible

Children: Not below 12 years

Ciclopirox Olamine

It is a hydroxypyridone antifungal with both an unique structure and mode of action unrelated to the other available antifungals.

Salient Features

- Approved for the treatment of tinea pedis, tinea corporis, tinea versicolor, and cutaneous candidiasis; the lacquer is approved for onychomycosis.
- Shampoo is used for seborrheic dermatitis of scalp.
- Ciclopirox has also demonstrated anti-inflammatory activity. It inhibits prostaglandin and leukotriene synthesis in human polymorphonuclear (PMN) leukocytes.

Dosage

- For cutaneous infections-cream is applied twice daily for 4 weeks.
- For seborrheic dermatitis scalp-apply 1 teaspoon of 1% shampoo (or up to 2 teaspoons for long hair) two times a week for four weeks with at least three days between each application.
- For nail fungal infection – 8% nail lacquer on affected nail and surrounding 5mm skin once daily for 48 weeks.

Adverse Effects

- Burning sensation or pruritus upon application
- Allergic hypersensitivity

Pregnancy: Category B

Lactation: Probably compatible

Children: Safety and effectiveness in children below the age of 10 years have not been established.

Selenium Sulfide

Salient Features

- Selenium sulfide is currently indicated for the treatment of pityriasis versicolor and seborrheic dermatitis of the scalp.
- It is also effective in the treatment of confluent and reticulated papillomatosis of Gougerot and Carteaud.
- It appears to have a cytostatic effect on cells of the epidermis and follicular epithelium. This property allows for the shedding of fungi in the stratum corneum via a reduction in corneocyte adhesion.

Dosage

For seborrheic dermatitis scalp-2.5% lotion on the scalp two times a week for two weeks, then use one time a week or less often. 1% lotion to be used on the scalp two times a week.

For tinea versicolor-2.5% lotion on the body one time a day for seven days.

Adverse Effects

Itching, redness.

Pregnancy: Category C

Lactation: Not established

Children: Not established

Tavaborole

It is an oxaborole antifungal used for the treatment of onychomycosis caused by both *Trichophyton rubrum* and *trichophyton mentagrophytes*.

Salient Features

- Tavaborole can penetrate the nail plate due to its small size, hydrophilicity, and antifungal activity.
- Nail concentrations of tavaborole were found to be 20 times higher than the minimum fungicidal concentration against the dermatophytes after 3 months treatment.
- Tavaborole undergoes extensive metabolism with renal excretion.

Dosage

Once daily application of 5% solution for 48 weeks.

Adverse Effects

Application site erythema, dermatitis, exfoliation and ingrown toenail.

Pregnancy: Category C

Lactation: Probably compatible

Children: Not below 6 years

AMOROLFINE

Amorolfine is a phenylpropyl morpholine derivative topical antifungal.

Mechanism of Action

It exerts both fungistatic and fungicidal action. It acts at two steps in the biosynthesis pathway of ergosterol by inhibition of $\delta 14$ sterol reductase and cholestenol δ-isomerase. This results in the accumulation of $\delta 14$ sterol ignosterol and depletion of ergosterol in the fungal cell membranes, which leads to increased permeability of the membrane and disruption of fungal metabolism.

Indication

- Onychomycosis (used as nail laquer)
- Superficial dermatophytosis like tinea corporis, tinea cruris.

Dosage

- As 0.25% cream once daily for 2-3 weeks (up to 6 weeks) for superficial dermatophytosis.
- 5% nail lacquer 1-2 times/week for 6-12 months for finger and toenil onychomycoses respectively.

Adverse Effects

Pain, erythema, itching, discoloration, irritation, and rarely, allergic contact dermatitis at the site of application.

Pregnancy category: B

Lactation: Probably compatible

Children: Not below 12 years

TOPICAL ANTIVIRALS

Topical and intralesional (IL) antiviral agents can be broadly classified under three categories:

Viricidal drugs	Immune-enhancing drugs	Cytodestructive drug
Acyclovir Pencyclovir Cidofovir Foscarnate Idoxuridine	Imiquimod Interferon HPV vaccine	Bleomycin Podophyllin/podophyllotoxin Trichloroacetic acid (TCA) Cantharidin Salicylic acid 5-Fluorouracil Potassium hydroxide (KOH) Hydrogen peroxide (HP)

Viricidal Drugs

Acyclovir

Acyclovir is an acyclic analogue of the nucleoside guanosine

Mechanism of Action

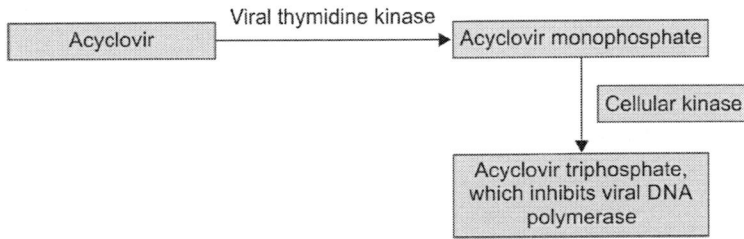

Salient Feature

Effective against HSV-1, HSV-2 and less effective against VZV.

Indications

Approved
- Initial genital herpes simplex
- Limited nonlife-threatening mucocutaneous HSV in immunocompetent patients.

Dosage

Application of acyclovir 5% ointment for initial genital HSV is recommended every 3 hours, 6 times daily for 7 days.

Side Effects Application site reactions include mild pain and burning.

Contraindication

Hypersensitivity to the drug or any of the components of the formulation.

Pregnancy: Category B drug

Lactation: Safe in lactation

Children: Safe

Penciclovir Penciclovir is an acyclic purine nucleoside analogue of guanine and is structurally related to ganciclovir

Mechanism of Action

- Penciclovir exhibits more efficient phosphorylation, a higher affinity of viral DNA polymerases for the triphosphate form, and increased stability of the triphosphate form, leading to a longer duration of activity compared to acyclovir.
- It exhibits inhibitory activity against Herpes simplex virus 1(HSV-1), HSV-2, Varicella-Zoster virus, and Epstein-Barr virus.

Indication

Approved

Recurrent herpes labialis in immunocompetent patients.

Dosage

1% penciclovir cream is to be applied at the earliest sign or symptom to all lesions every 2 hours (or at least 6 times daily) for 4 days.

Side Effects

Application site reactions include mild pain and burning.

Contraindication

Hypersensitivity to the drug or any of the components of the formulation.

Pregnancy: Category B drug

Lactation: Safe in lactation

Children: Safe (12 years of age or older)

CIDOFOVIR

Cidofovir is an acyclic nucleotide that exhibits antiviral activity against a broad range of DNA viruses

Mechanism of Action

- On entry into virally infected cells, cidofovir undergoes two stages of phosphorylation to form the active metabolite cidofovir diphosphate which acts as a competitive inhibitor of deoxycytosine-5-triphosphate for incorporation into viral DNA by viral DNA polymerases.
- Active against HPV, human herpes viruses, and Molluscum contagiosum.
- Cidofovir does not depend on viral thymidine kinase for its phosphorylation

Indication

Unlicensed

- Molluscum contagiosum
- Verruca vulgaris
- Condyloma acuminata
- Herpes simplex
- Basal cell carcinoma
- High-grade intraepithelial neoplasia in HIV-infected patients
- Human polyomavirus-7 related rash and pruritus in a lung transplant patient.

Dosage

1% or 3% cream used twice daily for variable duration depending on the indication of usage.

Adverse Effects

Application site reactions include mild pain and burning.

Contraindication

Hypersensitivity to the drug or any of the components of the formulation.

Pregnancy: Category C drug

Lactation: Safe in lactation

Children: Safe

IMMUNE-ENHANCING DRUGS

Imiquimod

It is a nonnucleoside heterocyclic amine which activates Toll-like receptor 7, thus inducing potent antiviral and antitumor effect.

Indication

Approved

- External genital and perianal HPV infections
- Actinic keratosis and superficial BCC in immunocompetent adults.

Unlicensed

- Verruca plana
- Bowen's disease

- Molluscum contagiosum
- Refractory genital herpes simplex virus infection
- Melanoma-in-situ
- Nodular BCC
- Melanoma metastases
- T cell lymphoma
- Paget disease
- Leishmaniasis

Dosage

Anogenital warts: Imiquimod 5% cream should be applied thrice weekly upto 16 weeks to the affected area at bedtime and left in place for 6 to 10 hours before being washed off.
- In Basal cell carcinoma, 5% cream to be applied for five consecutive days in a week for 6 weeks
- Actinic keratosis: Twice weekly for 16 weeks.

Side Effects

- Local: Pruritus, erythema, edema, irritation, ulceration at application site
- Systemic: Flu-like systemic symptoms- fever, headache, fatigue, diarrhea, and myalgias

Contraindication

- Hypersensitivity to the drug or any of the components of the formulation.
- Ulceration of genitalia
- Sunburn

Pregnancy: Category C drug

Lactation: Safe in lactation

Children: Safe (age 12 years and over)

Interferon α

- Topical and intralesional preparations have been used in the treatment of condyloma acuminata for their immunomodulatory, antiproliferative, and antiviral properties.
- It is not very cost effective for treatment of condyloma.

Intralesional Immunotherapy

- These include Candida albicans, MMR vaccine, or Trichophyton skin test antigens to treat benign genital and non-genital warts.

Candidal Antigen

- It stimulates the production of T-helper cytokines that activate cytotoxic and natural killer cells to eradicate HPV infection.
- It has been used in treatment of verruca vulgaris (sessions ranging from every 2 to every 4 weeks with IL injection of 0.1 to 0.3 mL), anogenital wart and molluscum contagiosum.

MMR Vaccine

- Measles, mumps, rubella (MMR) viral vaccine accelerates the clearance of virus and viral infected cells by stimulation of cell-mediated and humoral immunity.
- It has been used in a dose of 0.5 mL injected into each cutaneous wart once in two weeks for up to 5 sittings

Trichophyton Skin Antigen

- Trichophyton antigen has been prepared as an allergic extract from Trichophyton species by adding extracting solution.
- 0.3 mL injected every 3 weeks, maximum of 5 sittings

Cytodestructive drugs

Drugs	Mechanism of action	Salient features
Podophyllin and podofilox Crude extract of cytotoxic material from the roots of May apple plant (*Podophyllum peltatum* or *podophyllum emodi*)	Podophyllotoxin, the active ingredient, is an antimitotic agent that arrests cells in metaphase by binding reversibly to tubulin.	• **Approved**: Patient-applied podofilox 0.5% solution or gel and 0.15% cream was found to have better clearance rates than office-applied podophyllin 20% and 25% in the treatment of anogenital warts. • Podofilox is applied by the patient twice daily for 3 consecutive days followed by a 4-day rest period for up to 4 weeks • Podophyllin (25% podophyllin in compound tincture benzoin) is applied once weekly over lesions and washed off after 4 hours till resolution. • Adverse effects: Inflammation, burning, erythema, erosions. • Contraindicated in cervical wart. • Podofilox is pregnancy category C and podophyllin is category X.
Cantharidin	Acts by interfering with mitochondria leading to epidermal cell death, acantholysis, and clinical blister formation. (It has no direct antiviral effect.)	1. Approved: Molluscum contagiosum for adults and paediatric patients 2 years of age or older. (Cantharidin 0.7% solution) 2. Also has been used in verruca vulgaris (to be applied for 4 to 24 hours with adhesive tape) 3. Inadequate application may result in annular wart with central flattening known as doughnut wart.
Trichloroacetic acid (TCA)	It causes hydrolysis of cellular proteins, leading to inflammation and cell death	1. TCA may be formulated in different strengths (typically 60%–90%). A thin amount is applied to each wart and allowed to turn white or 'frost,' indicating precipitation of denatured proteins. 2. TCA is applied in the office with repeated applications up to three times weekly until resolution. 3. Has been used in anogenital warts including cervical warts and mucosal wart, non-genital wart. 4. Adverse effects: Local pain and ulceration.
Potassium hydroxide	It penetrates and destroys the skin by dissolving the keratin	1. 5–10% solution has been used once daily nighttime application for verruca vulgaris and molluscum contagiosum (even twice daily application is effective for MC) 2. Adverse effects: Transient burning, stinging, pain and pigment disturbances.
5–Fluorouracil	5–FU is a cytotoxic fluorinated pyrimidine analogue that penetrates abnormal skin to a greater extent than normal skin.	1. Topical 5% 5-FU was safe, effective, and well tolerated (once daily). 2. Approved in multiple actinic keratosis and superficial basal cell carcinoma 3. Unlicensed use in verruca vulgaris, verruca plana and resistant condyloma of genitalia 4. Adverse effects-erythema, edema, mucositis and erosive dermatitis. 5. Pregnancy category X 6. Contraindicated in lactation

Continued...

Continued...

Drugs	Mechanism of action	Salient features
Sinecathechin	It contains epigallocatechin gallate, which protects cells from oxidative damage, induces apoptosis, and inhibits telomerase activity.	1. Sinecathechin (15% ointment) is a topical high-grade green tea polyphenol extract approved for treatment of external genital and perianal warts. 2. Unlicensed use: Recalcitrant molluscum contagiosum 3. The ointment is applied three times daily for up to 4 months. 4. Adverse effects: Erythema, ulceration, pruritus and pain 5. Contraindicated in pregnancy
Salicylic acid and lactic acid	Keratolytic agent – reduces corneocyte adhesion	1. Once daily application 16–60% cream, lotion, plaster, collodion 16%. 2. Used in verruca vulgaris, corns, calluses 3. Pregnancy category C.
Hydrogen peroxide	It is a powerful oxidizing agent with strong biocidal activity.	1% cream and 3%, 6% solution have been used twice daily in molluscum contagiosum.
Berdazimer sodium	It exerts antiviral effect by releasing nitric oxide that causes nitrosylation and NF-κB modulation	1. It has been approved for treatment of molluscum contagiosum in patients aged 6 months or older. 2. 10.3% gel is applied once daily for 12 weeks

TOPICAL ANTIPARASITIC AGENTS

Permethrin

Permethrin is a synthetic pyrethroid derived from the pyrethrum flower *Chrysanthemum cinerariaefolium*.

Mechanism of Action

- Permethrin acts on the arthropod cell membrane. It inhibits closure of voltage-gated sodium channels, thereby inhibiting nerve repolarization. The constant influx of sodium leads to repetitive firing of the nerves resulting in the insect reaching a state of knockdown followed by paralysis and death.
- It is weakly ovicidal, since ova do not have fully developed central nervous system.

Indication

Approved

Scabies

Unlicensed

Pediculosis capitis and pubis Demodex folliculitis

Dosage

5% cream for scabies treatment and 1% cream rinse for head lice. 5% cream is used for pubic lice and also for head lice in those resistant to 1% cream rinse.

Scabies

Adult and infants (2 months and above): Apply from neck to toe for 8 hours overnight. Repeat in 1 week.

Pediculosis Capitis

Overnight application to scalp and neck with rinsing in the morning. Repeat in 1 week.

Adverse Effect

- Stinging, irritation, and tingling.
- Rarely, hypersensitivity reactions.

Contraindication

- Known hypersensitivity

- Persons with sensitivity to *Compositae* should not use permethrin as there is chance of cross-reactions.

Pregnancy: Category B

Lactation: Safe

Children: Safe in patients 2 months of age and older.

Ivermectin

Ivermectin is synthetically derived from avermectin, a naturally occurring compound produced from *Streptomyces*.

Mechanism of Action

It works by binding to ligand-gated (glutamate and γ-aminobutyric acid)chloride channels, increasing their permeability with subsequent influx of chloride into the cells. The resulting hyperpolarization leads to paralysis and death.

Indication

Approved
- Pediculosis capitis, inflammatory rosacea

Unlicensed
- Scabies, larva migrans

Dosage

- **Pediculosis capitis:** Apply 0.5% lotion to dry scalp and hair. Leave on for 10 minutes and then rinse thoroughly with warm water.
- **Rosacea:** Apply 1% cream once daily over affected areas.

Adverse Effects

Irritation and localized burning.

Pregnancy: Category C

Lactation: Safe, but direct application to nipple and areola is to be avoided.

Children: Approved in children older than 6 months.

Malathion

Malathion is a weak organophosphate that is converted to malaoxon.

Mechanism of Action

It irreversibly inhibits acetylcholinesterase, resulting in neuromuscular paralysis in arthropods.

Indication

Approved
Pediculosis capitis.

Unlicensed
Scabies

Dosage

Apply 0.5% lotion to scalp and neck overnight and rinse in the morning. Repeat in 7–9 days.

Adverse effect

- Potentially flammable, skin and scalp irritation, contact hypersensitivity reaction.

Pregnancy: Category B

Lactation: Safe

Children: Not approved for children < 6 years of age.

Crotamiton

Crotamiton has weak scabicidal activity along with an antipruritic effect. It is colorless or pale-yellow oil used in the treatment of scabies.

Mechanism of Action

Crotamiton inhibits TRPV4 (transient receptor potential vanilloid 4) channel that is expressed in the skin and primary sensory neuron.

Indication Scabies (approved)

Dosage

A total dose of 30g of 10% cream/lotion should be applied from the neck down for 2 consecutive days.

Adverse Effect

Irritation, redness and swelling

Pregnancy Category: C

Lactation: No data

Children: Safe

Lindane

Lindane also known as gamma-benzene hexachloride, is an organochlorine insecticide.

Mechanism of Action

Lindane inhibits inositol in insect tissue. This affects neurotransmission thereby producing respiratory and muscle paralysis and ultimate death of the parasite.

Indication

- Scabies
- Pediculosis capitis and pubis

Adverse Effects

- CNS: Seizures, excitability, agitation, delirium, tremors, dizziness
- Systemic absorption may lead to aplastic anaemia
- Cutaneous: Burning, pruritus

Contraindication

GBH is to be avoided in:
- Patients with seizure disorders
- Patients with acutely inflamed raw skin
- Hypersensitivity to drug

Pregnancy and lactation: Contraindicated

Children: Children weighing less than 50 kg to avoid.

Spinosad

Spinosad is a 5:1 mixture of spinosyn A and spinosyn D, macrolactones obtained from soil actinomycete *Saccharopolyspora spinosa*.

Topical pediculicide acts by interfering wirh nicotinic acetylcholine and GABA receptors, causing louse paralysis and death. It is ovicidal

Dosage

0.9% suspension approved for patients 4 years and older applied from neck to foot and left for 6 hours (single application).

Indication: Approved: Scabies
Head lice infestation

Adverse Effects

Dryness, irritation and redness of skin

Scalp application
- Can cause eye redness
- Rarely hypersensitivity reactions

Contraindication

Hypersensitivity to drug or excipients

Pregnancy: Category B

Lactation: No data

Children: Safe in children 4 years and above

TOPICAL GLUCOCORTICOIDS

Topical corticosteroids (TCS) are the gold standard of the dermatological therapy.

Salient Features

Hydrocortisone is the backbone of most TCS molecules.

- The Stoughton Vasoconstriction assay is the most commonly used test for TCS 'potency' as it corresponds well with clinical efficacy and is reproducible.
- The pharmacokinetics and subsequently the potency depends on the structure of TCS molecule, the vehicle, its concentration in the vehicle and the characteristics of the skin on which TCS is to be applied.

Classification of topical steroids

WHO potency group	Class	Topical glucocorticoid agent and formulation
Ultrahigh (superpotent)	1	• Betamethasone dipropionate ointment and gel 0.05% • Clobetasol propionate ointment, cream, gel, lotion, foam, solution ("scalp application"), spray, and shampoo 0.05% • Desoximetasone spray 0.25% • Diflorasone diacetate ointment 0.05% • Fluocinonide cream 0.1% • Flurandrenolide tape 4 mcg/cm^2 • Halobetasol propionate ointment, cream, lotion, and foam 0.05%
High	2	• Betamethasone dipropionate ointment, cream, and lotion 0.05% • Clobetasol propionate cream 0.025% • Desoximetasone cream, ointment 0.25% or gel 0.05% • Diflorasone diacetate cream and ointment 0.05% • Fluocinonide cream, ointment, gel, and solution 0.05% • Halcinonide cream, ointment, and solution 0.1% • Halobetasol propionate lotion 0.01% • Mometasone furoate ointment 0.1% • Triamcinolone acetonide ointment 0.5%
	3	• Amcinonide cream and lotion 0.1% • Betamethasone dipropionate cream, lotion, and spray 0.05% • Betamethasone valerate ointment 0.1% and foam 0.12% • Diflorasone diacetate cream 0.05% • Fluticasone propionate ointment 0.005% • Triamcinolone acetonide ointment 0.1% or cream 0.5%
Moderate (medium)	4	• Betamethasone valerate foam 0.12% • Desoximetasone cream 0.05% • Fluocinolone acetonide ointment 0.025% • Flurandrenolide ointment 0.05% • Hydrocortisone valerate ointment 0.2% • Mometasone furoate cream and lotion 0.1% • Triamcinolone acetonide cream and ointment 0.1% or spray 0.2%
	5	• Betamethasone dipropionate lotion 0.05% • Betamethasone valerate cream and lotion 0.1% • Clocortolone pivalate cream 0.1% • Fluocinolone acetonide cream 0.025% or oil and shampoo 0.01% • Fluticasone propionate cream and lotion 0.05% • Flurandrenolide cream and lotion 0.05% • Hydrocortisone butyrate cream, ointment, lotion, and solution 0.1% • Hydrocortisone probutate cream 0.1% • Hydrocortisone valerate cream 0.2% • Prednicarbate cream and ointment 0.1% • Triamcinolone acetonide ointment 0.025% or lotion 0.1%

Continued...

Continued...

WHO potency group	Class	Topical glucocorticoid agent and formulation
Low	6	• Alclometasone dipropionate cream and ointment 0.05% • Betamethasone valerate lotion 0.05% • Desonide cream, gel, ointment, lotion, and foam 0.05% • Fluocinolone acetonide cream and solution 0.01% • Triamcinolone acetonide cream and lotion 0.025%
	7	• Dexamethasone sodium phosphate cream 0.1% • Hydrocortisone (acetate) cream, ointment, gel, lotion, and solution 0.5%–2.5% • Methylprednisolone acetate cream 0.25%

Indication

- **Dermatitis**
  - Atopic dermatitis
  - Dyshidrotic eczema
  - Nummular eczema
  - Lichen simplex chronicus
  - Diaper dermatitis
  - Seborrheic dermatitis
- **Papulosquamous disease**
  - Lichen planus
  - Lichen planopilaris
  - Pityriasis rosea
  - Psoriasis—intertriginous
  - Psoriasis—plaque or palmoplantar
- **Autoimmune Bullous Dermatoses**
  - Bullous pemphigoid
  - Cicatricial pemphigoid
  - Pemphigoid gestationis
  - Pemphigus foliaceus
  - Pemphigus vulgaris
  - Epidermolysis bullosa acquisita
- **Autoimmune Connective Tissue Diseases**
  - Dermatomyositis
  - Lupus erythematosus
  - Morphea
- **Neutrophilic Dermatoses**
  - Behçet disease
  - Pyoderma gangrenosum
- **Others:**
  - Alopecia areata
  - Acne keloidalis nuchae
  - Chondrodermatitis nodularis helicis
  - Cutaneous T-cell lymphoma, patch-stage
  - Granuloma annulare
  - Jessner lymphocytic infiltrate
  - Lichen sclerosis et atrophicus
  - Pruritic urticarial papules and plaques of pregnancy
  - Pruritus— scrotal, vulvar and perianal
  - Sarcoidosis
  - Vitiligo
- **Mechanism of Action**

Anti-inflammatory Effect

a. **Direct/immediate effects**: Stabilizes lysosomal membrane, potentiate vascular response to catecholamines, inhibit mast cell sensitization and resultant release of histamines.

b. **Glucocorticoid receptor (GCR)-mediated/delayed effects**: Induction of anti-inflammatory proteins e.g. lipocortin (inhibits phospholipase A2), vasocortin and vasoregulin.

c. **Miscellaneous**: Decreased chemotaxis of proinflammatory cells at the sites of inflammation and subsequent reduced cytokines production.

Anti-proliferative effects: Inhibits mitoses of keratinocytes, fibroblast proliferation inhibition with resultant decreased collagen, elastin fibers and glycosaminoglycans.

Immunosuppressive effects: Depletion of Langerhans cell in epidermis and dermis, induction of lymphocytes and eosinophils apoptosis.

Adverse Effects

a. Systemic
- Hypothalamic-pituitary-adrenal axis suppression
- Iatrogenic Cushing syndrome
- Growth retardation in both infants and children

b. Local
- Epidermal atrophy—shiny, wrinkled, fragile skin with hypopigmentation, striae, telangiectasia, purpura, stellate pseudoscars.
- Glaucoma/cataracts
- Allergic or irritant contact dermatitis. Allergic contact dermatitis is suspected when a steroid responsive dermatoses being treated with TCS either fails to respond or worsens on therapy. Allergy can be due to excipients (penetration enhancers, preservatives), packging allergens (nickel in tube) or the active ingredient itself. It is diagnosed by patch testing and occasionally by prick or intradermal tests. Positive patch test reactions to budesonide and tixocortol-21-pivalate are considered as good indicators of corticosteroid allergy.
- Facial hypertrichosis
  - Tachyphylaxis
- Perioral dermatitis, rosacea, acne
  - TSDF (topical steroid dependant facies)
- Folliculitis, miliaria
- Genital ulceration
- Increased risk of bacterial, fungal, and viral infections
- Delayed wound healing
  - CS are currently divided into **five groups based on cross-reactivity** defined by patch testing: (A) hydrocortisone type, (B) triamcinolone acetonide type, (C) betamethasone type, (D1) betamethasone dipropionate type, and (D2) methylprednisolone aceponate type. TCS can cross react within each group, but only rarely between groups.
  - **The vehicle of a TCS preparation** can increase the side effects of the TCS or cause local adverse effects itself. Components of the vehicle can cause itching, burning, stinging, urticaria, irritant and allergic contact dermatitis. Propylene glycol and sorbitan sesquioleate are the two most common allergens present in TCS vehicles.

Dosage and Application

- Applied once or twice daily
- Selecting the correct vehicle and the potency of TCS is important
  - Ointments: For thick hyperkeratotic lesions
  - Creams: For acute exudative lesions and in intertriginous areas.
  - Lotions and gels: For hair bearing areas.
  - Foams: For scalp
- A **fingertip unit (FTU)** is the amount of ointment expressed from a tube with a 5 mm diameter nozzle, applied from the distal skin crease to the tip of the palmar aspect of the index finger. One FTU weighs 0.49 g and covers 312 cm^2 in adult men, and in adult women weighs 0.43 g and covers 257 cm^2 on average. There are specific guidelines regarding the amount of FTUs to be used in specific body areas for both adults and children.

Monitoring

- Not to be used unsupervised.
- High potency steroids not to be used for more than 2 weeks specially on face, genitals and intertriginous areas to avoid adverse effects.

Contraindications

Absolute

- Known hypersensitivity to the topical corticosteroid
- Known hypersensitivity to a component of the vehicle

Relative

- Bacterial, mycobacterial, fungal, viral infection
- Scabies infestation
- Ulceration

Pregnancy: Only when potential benefits justify possible risk to the fetus

Lactation: Used with caution at sites other than the breast or nipple

Children: Safely used in children

TOPICAL RETINOIDS

- Topical formulations of vitamins are increasingly used in dermatologic conditions and for cosmetic indications, their anti-inflammatory, anti-oxidant modulation of proliferation and differentiation of cells, wound healing, moisturizing effect, and photo-protective properties.

Vitamin A

- Vitamin A or retinol is a fat-soluble vitamin. Retinoids are natural and synthetic analogues of retinol that contain different polar end groups and are defined as molecules that bind to and activate specific nuclear receptors (retinoic acid receptors and retinoid X receptors).

Classification

Generation	Structure	Examples	Receptor binding affinity
First generation	Naturally occurring Non-aromatic	All trans retinol Tretinoin Isotretinoin (13 cis retinoic acid) Alitretinoin (9–cis retinoic acid, Panretin)	Nil RAR-α, β, γ RAR-α, β, γ RAR-α, β, γ RXR-α, β, γ
Second generation	Monoaromatic	No topical retinoid Systemic retinoids: Acitretin, etretinate, (withdrawn)	RAR-α, β, γ RXR-α, β, γ
Third generation	Polyaromatic	Adapalene Tazarotene Bexarotene, (Rexinoid)	RAR-α (weak), β, γ RAR-α (weak), β, γ RXR-α, β, γ
Fourth generation	Pyranones	Trifarotene Seletinoid G	RAR-γ PPAR α/γ

Mechanism of Action

Name of the Retinoid	Mechanism of Action
All-trans retinol	Gene transcription after transformation to all-trans retinoic acid
Tretinoin	Gene transcription influencing cellular growth and differentiation Normalizes follicular epithelial keratinization and differentiation Inhibits matrix metalloproteinase production by down-regulation of transcription factors Stimulates synthesis of collagens and fibrillin

Continued...

Continued...

Name of the Retinoid	Mechanism of Action
Adapalene	Normalizes follicular epithelial differentiation Inhibits polymorphonuclear leucocyte chemotaxis Decreases leukotriene and prostaglandin production by downregulation of 5 and 15 lipoxygenase Reduces Toll-like receptor-2 expression by keratinocytes Regulates epidermal immune system by increasing CD1d and decreasing IL10 expression by keratinocytes
Tazarotene	Blocks initiation of ornithine decarboxylase activity leading to reduced cell proliferation & hyperplasia Reduces migration inhibitory factor-related protein (MRP-8), downregulates the expression of involucrin, keratinocyte transglutaminase1, elafin, keratin 6 and 16 Induces tazarotene inducible genes (TIG)1, 2 and 3 resulting in decreased keratinocyte proliferation
Alitretinoin	Modulates gene expression resulting in pro-apoptotic and anti-proliferative action Downregulates IL-6 Alters viral encoded oncogenes expression
Bexarotene	Increases apoptosis by decreasing antiapoptotic protein and via caspase-3 activation.
Trifarotene	Downregulates dystonin-affects cell adhesion by weakening hemidesmosomes Induces aquaporin-3 and peptidyl arginine deiminase 1 resulting in improved cutaneous hydration Downregulates membrane metallo-endopeptidase resulting in improvement in skin texture.

Adverse Effects

- The most typical adverse effect of topical retinoids is irritant contact dermatitis, often known as retinoid dermatitis. It is characterized by variable erythema, scaling, itching, burning, stinging, and dryness.
- Retinoid dermatitis usually occurs within the first month of therapy and subsequently subsides. Reducing the frequency, contact time or amount of topical retinoid application temporarily is effective in preventing and treating the condition.
- Tretinoin can cause photosensitivity.
- Tazarotene can cause koebnerization of psoriasis.

Tretinoin

- Tretinoin represents an oxidized form of all-*trans* retinol. It is endogenously synthesized in the skin from all-*trans* retinol after delivery of this compound to basal keratinocytes via the bloodstream.

Mechanism of Action

Discussed earlier

Pharmacology

- Systemic absorption < 2% in normal skin. Normally present in the skin.
- Isomerization to 13–*cis*-Retinoic acid in epidermis.
- Excretion by desquamation and by biliary route.

Indication

Approved
- Acne vulgaris
- Photoaging, e.g. fine facial wrinkling, mottled pigmentation, facial roughness.

Unlicensed

- Rosacea
- Disorders of cornification: Ichthyoses, Darier disease, primary inherited and acquired palmoplantar keratodermas, keratosis pilaris, acanthosis nigricans, Kyrle disease, disseminated superficial actinic porokeratosis (DSAP).
- Oral Lichen planus.
- Post-inflammatory hyperpigmentation, melasma, and photoaging-related hyperpigmentation
- Actinic keratosis, Lentigens
- Pre-malignant, malignant disorders and cutaneous chemoprophylaxis
- Androgenetic alopecia
- Striae distensae
- Milia-en-plaque
- Infections: Verruca plana, molluscum contagiosum

Contraindication

- Pregnancy
- Lactation
- Hypersensitivity to the vehicle
- Caution for eczematous skin, sunburn, permanent wave solutions, electrolysis, hair depilatories or waxes

Pregnancy Category: C

Alitretinoin

Alitretinoin is a naturally occurring pan-agonist retinoid that binds to both RARs and RXRs.

Mechanism of Action

Discussed earlier.

Salient Feature

- Systemic absorption is minimal. Normally present in the plasma.
- Onset of action is seen in 2 weeks with clinical improvement seen in 4–8 weeks.

Indications

Approved

AIDS related cutaneous lesions of Kaposi sarcoma (0.1% gel)

Unlicensed

- Non AIDS related Kaposi sarcoma
- Hand dermatitis
- Photoaging

Contraindication

- Pregnancy
- Breast feeding
- Hypersensitivity to vehicle

Pregnancy Category: D

Adapalene

Adapalene is a photostable, rigid, and highly lipophilic synthetic retinoid with higher affinity for RAR-β/γ than for RAR-α.

Mechanism of Action

Discussed earlier.

Salient Features

- Its lipophilic properties may contribute to better pilosebaceous uptake and anti-acne activity.
- Given its negligible transdermal absorption, the teratogenic risks of topical adapalene appear to be minimal.
- Minimal biotransformation due to chemical rigidity.
- Excretion by desquamation and by biliary route.

Indications

Approved

Acne vulgaris

Unlicensed

- Darier disease
- Acanthosis nigricans

- Photoaging
- Rosacea
- Post-inflammatory hyperpigmentation, melasma, and photoaging-related hyperpigmentation
- Actinic keratosis.

Contraindication

- Pregnancy (relative)
- Hypersensitivity to adapalene or the vehicle

Pregnancy Category: C

Tazarotene

Tazarotene is a prodrug that is rapidly converted by cutaneous esterase to its free carboxylic acid (tazarotenic acid), which is the active metabolite.

Mechanism of Action

Discussed earlier

Salient Features

- It has a higher affinity for RAR-β/γ than RAR-α and no affinity for RXR.
- Systemic absorption of the prodrug is practically non-existent because of its rapid skin metabolism to tazarotenic acid.
- Total systemic absorption is up to 5% of the drug applied in normal skin and 15% of the amount applied in psoriatic skin.
- The half-life of tazarotene is less than 20 minutes.
- The terminal half-life of tazarotenic acid is approximately 18 hours.
- Onset of action is 2 weeks with 8–12 weeks time required for clinical improvement.

Indications

Approved

- Acne vulgaris
- Psoriasis involving < 20% body surface area.

Unlicensed

- Papulosquamous disorder: Pityriasis Rubra Pilaris.
- Disorders of keratinization: Darier disease, lamellar ichthyosis, keratosis pilaris.
- Cutaneous T-cell lymphoma.
- Chemoprophylaxis for non-melanoma skin cancer.
- Nail disorders: Nail dystrophy, brittle nail, onychomycosis

Contraindication

- Pregnancy.
- Hypersensitivity to tazarotene or the vehicle
- Eczematous skin, sunburn, exposure to weather extremes.

Pregnancy category: X

BEXAROTENE

Bexarotene is a synthetic retinoid that binds selectively to the RXR ligand. Many authors use the term 'rexinoid' (given the RXR binding) to categorize bexarotene.

Indication

Approved

CTCL (early stage IA and IB)

Unlicensed

- Lymphomatoid papulosis
- Hand dermatitis
- Psoriasis
- Alopecia areata

Adverse Effects

Rash, pruritus, pain, contact dermatitis at application site

Contraindication

- Pregnancy

- Breast feeding
- Hypersensitivity to vehicle

Pregnancy category: X

TRIFAROTENE

Trifarotene, a fourth-generation retinoid with 20-fold higher affinity for RAR-γ than RAR-α/β.

Mechanism of Action

Discussed earlier

Indication

Approved

Acne vulgaris on face and trunk (≥9 years of age)

Unlicensed

Lamellar ichthyosis

Pharmacology

- Rapidly metabolized in hepatic microsomes, thereby minimizing systemic drug levels.
- Plasma protein binding is approximately 99.9%.
- Elimination-The terminal half-life ranges from 2 to 9 hours.
- Trifarotene is primarily metabolized by CYP2C9, CYP3A4, CYP2C8, and to a lesser extent by CYP2B6.

Dosage

0.005% cream once daily in the evening.

Adverse Effects

- Local irritation-erythema, dryness, scaling, burning, pruritus and sunburn. Tolerability on the trunk is better than on the face.
- Acne exacerbation, allergic contact dermatitis, discoloration, erosion, pain on the skin, rash and swelling – less common.

Contraindication

- Pregnancy
- Active eczema
- Hypersensitivity to trifarotene

TOPICAL IMMUNOMODULATORS

Immunomodulators

Classification

Class	Drugs
Macrolactams	• Tacrolimus • Pimecrolimus • Sirolimus • Cyclosporine
Contact sensitizers	• Diphenylcyclopropenone • Dinitrochlorobenzenes • Squaric acid dibutyl ester
Immuno-stimulators	• Imiquimod • Resiquimod
Miscellaneous	• Vitamin D analouges • Anthralin • Zinc • Interferon

Topical Calcineurin Inihibitors

They are the macrolactams.

Mechanism of Action

- Both tacrolimus and pimecrolimus binds to intracellular FK 506–binding protein and this complex blocks enzyme calcineurin. This results in inhibition of transcription of genes coding IL2 which hampers T cell activation and proliferation.
- Inhibits inflammatory mediator release from neutrophils, basophils and mast cells
- Downregulates expression of both IL-8 receptors on keratinocytes and FcεRI on Langerhans' cells.

Tacrolimus

Tacrolimus is a macrolide produced by the soil bacterium *Streptomyces tsukubaensis*.

Indications

Approved

Contact dermatitis

Unlicensed

- Seborrheic dermatitis
- Dyshydrosiform hand eczema
- Juvenile plantar dermatosis
- Papulosquamous disorders
    - Psoriasis
    - Cutaneous, oral and genital Lichen planus
    - Lichen planus pigmentosus
    - Lichen striatus
    - Pityriasis lichenoides
- Pigmentary disorders
    - Vitiligo
- Autoimmune connective tissue disorders
    - Cutaneous lupus erythematosus
    - Cutaneous lesions of dermatomyositis
    - Morphea
- Inflammatory disorders
    - Pyoderma grangrenosum
    - Lichen sclerosus mainly anogenital lesions
    - Cutaneous Crohn disease
- Disorder of pilosebaceous unit
    - Rosacea
- Vesiculobullous disorders
    - Pemphigus vulgaris
    - Bullous pemphigoid
    - Hailey-Hailey disease
    - Paraneoplastic pemphigus
- Miscellaneous
    - Zoons balanitis
    - Plasma cell vulvitis
    - Granuloma annulare
    - Necrobiosis lipoidica
    - Granuloma faciale
    - Chronic actinic dermatitis
    - Graft-versus-host disease

Dosage

Apply locally twice daily (0.03% ointment for 2-15 years, 0.1% for 16 years and above).

Adverse Effects

- Burning sensation at application site
- Itching
- Erythema
- Facial flushing following alcohol ingestion
- Rosacea like dermatitis
- Skin infections like herpes simplex, warts
- Flulike symptoms, fever, headache following excessive systemic absorption

Drug Interactions

- Proper drug interaction studies have not been done
- Simultaneous use of topical tacrolimus with CYP3A4 inhibitors like itraconazole, fluconazole, ketoconazole, erythromycin, calcium channel blockers and cimetidine in patients with extensive or erythrodermic disease should be done with caution

Contraindication

- **Absolute**
  Hypersensitivity to tacrolimus or any components of the ointment
- **Relative**
  Children less than 2 years of age
  Active skin infection (at site to be treated)

Pregnancy Category: C

Lactation Category: Can be applied to nipples after nursing but nipplesare to be cleaned before next feeding.

Low risk to nursing infant

Pimecrolimus

Semisynthetic derivative of ascomycin, a macrolide obtained from *Streptomyces hydroscepicus var ascomyceticus.*

Indications

- Dermatitis
    - Atopic dermatitis (approved)
    - Contact dermatitis

- Seborrheic dermatitis
- Dyshidrotic eczema
- Papulosquamous disorders
  - Psoriasis
  - Lichen planus
  - Lichen striatus
- Pigmentary disorders
  - Vitiligo
- Autoimmune connective tissue disorders
  - Cutaneous lupus erythematosus
- Disorder of pilosebaceous unit
  - Rosacea
- Miscellaneous
  - Perioral dermatitis
  - Behcet disease
  - Zoon balanitis
  - Vulval lichen sclerosus
  - Chronic actinic dermatitis
  - Granuloma faciale
  - Lymphocytic infiltrate of Jessner
  - Darier disease
  - Cutaneous mastocytosis

Dosage

Apply 1% cream locally twice daily accordingly (2 years and above age group)

Adverse Effect

- Burning sensation
- Itching
- Irritation
- Erythema
- Facial Acne
- Folliculitis
- Molluscum contagiosum

Drug Interaction

- None

Contraindications

Absolute
- Hypersensitivity to pimecrolimus or any components of the cream

Relative
- Children less than 2 years of age
- Active skin infection (at site to be treated
- Pregnancy Category: C
- Lactation Category: Can be applied to nipples after nursing but nipplesare to be cleaned before next feeding.
- Low risk to nursing infant

Sirolimus

Sirolimus, also known as rapamycin is a macrolide compound.

Indications

Approved

Genodermatoses
- Facial angiofibromas associated with Tuberous sclerosis complex in patients ≥ 6 years age

Unlicensed

Vascular Anomalies
- Port wine stain
- Microcystic lymphatic malformation
- Neviform/multi-segmental angiokeratoma

Papulosquamous Disorders
- Oral lichen planus

Benign hair Follicle Tumours
- Trichoepithelioma
- Adenoma sebaceum

Mechanism of Action

Mammalian(mechanistic) target of rapamycin inhibitor(mTOR) inhibitor having immunosuppressive, anti-proliferative and antiangiogenic effects.

Dosage

- Complete all age-appropriate vaccinations as recommended by current immunization guidelines prior to application.

- Apply 0.2% gel to the skin of the face affected with angiofibroma twice daily.

Adverse Effects
- Dry skin
- Skin irritation
- Acne
- Pruritus
- Eye irritation
- Erythema
- Acneiform dermatitis
- Contact dermatitis
- Ocular hyperaemia
- Skin hemorrhage
- Solar dermatitis
- Photosensitivity

Drug Interactions
CYP3A4 Inhibitors: During concomitant use of sirolimus with CYP3A4 inhibitors, monitor for adverse reactions.

Pregnancy: Insufficient data, pregnancy category not assigned

Lactation: Not recommended

Children: Not below 6 years

Vitamin D Analogues
Vitamin D (calcitriol) is a fat-soluble vitamin available in 2 forms: Ergocalciferol (D2) and cholecalciferol (D3). Currently available topical vitamin D analogues include:
- Calcitriol (naturally occurring bioactive form, 0.0003%)
- Calcipotriene (also known as calcipotriol, 0.005%)
- Maxacalcitol
- Tacalcitol (0.0002%)

Mechanism of Action
Vitamin D receptors (VDR) are found in keratinocytes, melanocytes, Langerhans cells, endothelial cells, and fibroblasts. VDR is activated by its ligands, calcitriol, or synthetic analogues to form a drug-receptor complex. This complex, in association with retinoic acid receptor X (RXR-α), binds to vitamin D response elements, leading to further activation or suppression of genes containing these elements.
- Effect on keratinocytes: Decreases proliferation, modulates differentiation, increases ceramide synthesis and helps in cornified envelope formation.
- Effect on immune cells: Inhibits IL-2, IL-6, and IFNγ production by Th1 cells, inhibits IL-17 production by Th17 cells, inhibits cytotoxic T cells and natural killer cells, increases Reg T cell activity and IL-4 production by Th2 cells.
- Effects on melanocytes: Increases activity of tyrosinase and melanogenesis, strengthens melanocyte stability by regulating activation, proliferation, migration, and pigmentation pathways.
- Effect on dendritic cells: Decreases MHC class II, CD40, CD80, and CD86 expression

CALCIPOTRIENE
Calcipotriene (calcipotriol) is a synthetic analogue of calcitriol.

Indication
Approved
- Psoriasis

Unlicensed
- Disorders of keratinization: X-linked ichthyosis, Lamellar ichthyosis, Epidermolytic hyperkeratosis, Sjögren–Larsson syndrome
- Autoimmune dermatoses: Morphea, Vitiligo,
- Neoplastic diseases: Cutaneous T-cell lymphoma

Miscellaneous Dermatoses

- Acanthosis nigricans
- Confluent and reticulated papillomatosis
- Disseminated superficial actinic porokeratosis
- Erythema annulare centrifugum
- Grover disease
- Inflammatory linear verrucous epidermal nevus (ILVEN)
- Lichen amyloidosis
- Pityriasis rubra pilaris
- Prurigo nodularis
- Verruca vulgaris

Salient Features

- It binds to the VDR with the same affinity as calcitriol, but is less likely to cause hypercalcemia, owing to its rapid local metabolism when applied topically.
- Maximum weekly dose 100g.

Adverse Effects

- Local: Irritation, burning, and stinging at the application site. Allergic contact dermatitis.
- Systemic:
- Use of excessive amounts of topical vitamin D analogues can lead to hypercalcemia and hypercalciuria.
- Patients with renal disease and those receiving medications that can increase the serum calcium level (e.g. thiazide diuretics, high doses of oral vitamin D) may be at increased risk of developing hypercalcemia.

Contraindication

Absolute

None

Relative

- Conditions causing hypercalcemia
- Treatment of >30% of the body surface area is not recommended.

Pregnancy Prescribing—category C

CONTACT SENSITIZER

Topical contact allergens' consist of a class of compounds that treat various dermatoses by inducing an allergic contact dermatitis in a previously unsensitized host, and maintaining the dermatitis at the site of the skin disease being treated.

Diphenylcyclopropenone (DCP)

Indications

- Viral warts
- Alopecia areata
- Melanoma

Mechanism of Action

- Alteration in cytokine parameter with nonspecific inflammation
- It inhibits progression of immune response to another unrelated antigen—in alopecia areata
- Viral loaded cell lysis and death due to non-specific CMI response—in viral wart.

Dosage

2% on a small area (2-4 cm^2) as starting sensitiz-ing dose. Later on 0.001 to 0.1% weekly on larger area.

Adverse Effect

- Itching
- Irritation
- Burning
- Erythema
- Blister
- Contact dermatitis
- Spread of contact dermatitis
- Urticaria
- Dyscromia in confetti
- Vitiligo
- Leukoderma
- Erythema multiforme or like reaction
- Regional adenopathy

- Sleep impairment
- Flu-like syndrome

Drug Interaction

- Cross-sensitivity to other chemicals.

Contraindication

- Hypersensitivity.

Pregnancy Category

- Not categorized.

Lactation Category

- Not known.

Children Avoid in children younger than 12 years age.

SQUARIC ACID DIBUTYL ESTER (SADBE)

Indications

- Viral warts
- Alopecia areata

Mechanism of Action

- Non-specific cell-mediated immune response, triggering virus-infected cell lysis and death.
- 'Antigenic competition' theory proposes that an immunoreaction to one antigen may inhibit the development of the immune response to another unrelated antigen

Dosage

2% SADBE in acetone, once weekly or accordingly.

Monitoring

- None.

Adverse Effect

- Itching
- Irritation
- Burning
- Erythema
- Contact dermatitis
- Spread of contact dermatitis
- Urticaria
- Dyscromia in confetti
- Vitiligo
- Leukoderma
- Erythema multiforme or like reaction
- Regional adenopathy
- Sleep impairment
- Flu-like syndrome
- Benign lymphoplasia.

Requirement

- Refrigeration to maintain potency of the drug.

Contraindication

- Hypersensitivity.

Pregnancy Category

- Not categorized.

Lactation Category

- Not known.

Children: Not recommended

Imiquimod/Resquimod

It is a nonnucleoside heterocyclic amine which activates Toll-like receptor 7, thus inducing potent antiviral and antitumor effect.

Resiquimod

Resiquimod is second generation imidalazoquinoline.

Indications

Unlicensed
- Actinic keratosis

- Recurrent genital HSV-2 infection
- Cutaneous T cell lymphoma
- Vaccine adjuvant

Mechanism of Action

- **Resiquimod** is an agonist of toll-like receptors (TLR) 7 and 8 on dendritic cells, macrophages, and B-lymphocytes resulting in immune response.
- Also, it appears to activate Langerhans' cells, leading to an enhanced activation of T-lymphocyte.

Side Effects

Erythema, irritation, tenderness, erosion, pruritus

Pregnancy category: Not established

Lactation: Not established

Children: Unknown

Anthralin

Anthralin is the synthetic form of the chrysarobin found in the bark of the South American araroba tree.

Indications

Approved

Chronic plaque psoriasis

Unlicensed

- Alopecia areata (Short contact therapy):
  - Anthralin 0.5% cream is applied to affected areas of the scalp daily for 10 minutes, followed by washing with shampoo/soap and water.
  - 10-minute increments done every 4–5 days until slight irritation (e.g. erythema, scaling, pruritus) occurs
  - If excessive irritation develops, treatment is withheld for several days and resumed at the last tolerated application time.
  - If there is no irritation with a 60-minute contact time, 1% anthralin is applied for 10 minutes and application times increased as mentioned earlier.
  - If there is no irritation with 1% anthralin applied for 60 minutes, overnight application is considered.

Mechanism of Action

- Anthralin induces an inflammatory response at sites of application, which may result from generation of extracellular oxygen free radicals.
- Inhibition of mitochondrial respiration and cell growth are thought to reduce keratinocyte proliferation and lead to antipsoriatic effects.
- Anthralin also has anti-Langerhans cell effects.

Adverse Effects

- Irritation at application sites (depending on the concentration and contact time).
- Staining of skin, clothing.
- Nephrotoxicity-extensive application causes systemic absorption and causes toxicity.

Pregnancy category: C

Lactation: No recommended

Children: Not recommended

TOPICAL PHOSPHODIASTERASE-4 INHIBITORS

Crisaborole

Crisaborole, a phenoxybenzoxoborole, is a nonsteroidal topical medication used for the treatment of mild-to-moderate atopic dermatitis in adults and children.

Mechanism of Action

- Crisaborole is a phosphodiesterase-4 inhibitor, mainly acting on phosphodiesterase

4B (PDE4B), which is an intracellular enzyme that degrades cAMP.
- Increasing intracellular cAMP levels activates protein kinase A, leading to enhanced expression of several transcription factors including cAMP-response element binding protein (CREB), while inhibiting others such as nuclear factor kappa B (NF-κB).

Indications

Mild to moderate atopic dermatitis in adult and paediatric patients 3 months of age and older.

Pharmacology

- Crisaborole is 97% bound to human plasma proteins.
- It is metabolized into inactive metabolites which are excreted by renal route.

Dosage

2% ointment to be applied twice daily to affected areas.

Adverse Effects

- Application site pain (burning or stinging)
- Contact urticaria

Contraindication

- Known hypersensitivity to crisaborole or any component of the formulation.
- Application site hypersensitivity reaction.

Pregnancy: No data available regarding use in pregnancy.

Lactation: No data available regarding use in lactation.

Children: Contraindicated below 3 months of age.

Roflumilast

Indications

Approved

Treatment of plaque psoriasis, including intertriginous areas, in patients 12 years of age and older.

Mechanism of Action

It is highly selective PDE-4 inhibitor.

Dosage

Apply 0.3% cream to the affected areas once daily and rub in completely.

Side Effects

- Application site pain
- Diarrhea
- Headache
- Insomnia
- Upper respiratory tract infection
- Urinary tract infection

Contraindication

In patients of Moderate-to-severe liver impairment.

Pregnancy category: No data available regarding use in pregnancy.

Lactation: No data available regarding use in lactation.

Children: Contraindicated below 12 years of age.

Topical JAK Inhibitors

Janus kinase (JAK) is a family of cytoplasmic non-receptor tyrosine kinases that includes four members, namely JAK1, JAK2, JAK3, and TYK2. The JAKs transduce cytokine signalling through the JAK-STAT pathway, which regulates the transcription of several genes involved in inflammatory, immune, and cancer conditions.

Classification

- JAK inhibitors can be divided into two generations. The first-generation acts as non-selective inhibitors of JAKs. On the other hand, second-generation drugs have selective inhibitory activity against JAKs. This difference in the selectivity of the two generations is associated with some differences in their safety and efficacy.
- JAK inhibitors may also be classified based on their binding mode and the type of interactions with the amino acids in JAKs into reversible (competitive) and irreversible (covalent) inhibitors.
- **Reversible inhibitor:** (a) *ATP-Competitive Inhibitors:* The mechanism of action of these inhibitors depends on their competition with ATP for the catalytic ATP-binding site in JAKs. These inhibitors may also be classified based on the conformation of the kinase domain to which they bind; **Type 1:** These inhibitors bind to the ATP-binding site of the JAKs under the active conformation of the kinase domain; **Type 2:** Type II JAK Inhibitors also bind to the ATP-binding site of the kinase domain in the inactive conformation of JAKs. **(b) Allosteric JAK Inhibitors:** The allosteric JAK inhibitors include small molecule inhibitors that bind to a site other than the ATP-binding site in JAKs.
- **Irreversible inhibitor**: The mechanism of action of these inhibitors depends on the covalent interaction with the unique Cys909 residue in JAK3.
- **Ruxolitinib**: It is a topical JAK1/2 inhibitor, recently approved for treatment of atopic dermatitis.
- **Indication:**
  Approved:1.5% cream twice daily is used in short-term and non-continuous chronic treatment of atopic dermatitis in non-immunocompromised adults and children 12 years of age and older (up to 20% body surface area) whose disease is not well controlled with topical prescription therapies or when those therapies are not recommended.
  - Treatment of nonsegmental vitiligo in adults and children 12 years of age and older (up to 10% body surface area).

Pharmacology

- Plasma protein binding is approximately 97%.
- Elimination the mean terminal half-life of ruxolitinib following topical application is approximately 116 hours.
- Ruxolitinib is primarily metabolized by CYP3A4 and to a lesser extent by CYP2C9.
- Ruxolitinib and its metabolites are primarily excreted by urine (74%) and feces (22%). Less than 1% is excreted as unchanged drug.

Adverse Effects

- **Respiratory**: Running nose, sore throat, bronchitis, nasopharyngitis, ear infection, tonsilitis.
- **GIT**: Diarrhea
- **Skin**: Acne on application site, itching on application site, erythema and swelling around hair pores, folliculitis, urticaria.

Contraindication

- Known hypersensitivity to the drug or to a component of the vehicle.
- Active infection at the site of application
- Pregnancy and lactation.

Pregnancy: Category C

Lactation: Contraindicated

Children: Contraindicated below 12 years of age.

Delgocitinib

- Delgocitinib ointment is a pan JAK inhibitor first approved in Japan for the treatment of atopic dermatitis in children ≥2 years of age.
- It has also been approved by European medical agency for the treatment of Moderate-to-severe chronic hand eczema in adults who cannot use topical corticosteroids or are refractory to topical corticosteroids.

TOPIAL MINOXIDIL

Originally developed as an antihypertensive agent, minoxidil has been known for decades to promote hair growth.

Mechanism of Action

- Minoxidil causes premature termination of the telogen phase, lengthens the anagen phase, and can increase follicle size, particularly of miniaturized follicles.
- Stimulation of vascular endothelial growth factor and prostaglandin synthesis may also play a role.
- Prostaglandins are stimulated by minoxidil in the dermal papillae.

Pharmacology

- Minoxidil does not bind to plasma proteins and does not cross the blood brain barrier.

Indications

Approved

Both 2% and 5% is approved for male-pattern androgenetic alopecia (MPHL); and 2% is approved for female-pattern androgenetic alopecia (FPHL).

Unlicensed

- Alopecia areata, chemotherapy induced alopecia.

Dosage

- Oral: 0.25 to 1.25 mg daily are usually used for FPHL and doses ranging from 2.5 to 5 mg/day for MPHL.

Adverse Effects

Topical minoxidil: Dryness, irritation, and (uncommonly) allergic contact dermatitis, hypertrichosis. Systemic side effects such as headache and peripheral oedema are occasionally observed.

Contraindication

- Hypersensitivity to the product.
- It is not recommended for pregnant or nursing women.

Pregnancy: Category C

Lactation: Not recommended

Children: Not recommended in patients under 18 years old.

SUNSCREEN

Sunscreens are a constantly evolving component of the dermatologist's therapeutic armamentarium. Most broad-spectrum sunscreens provide protection against UVB radiation and short wavelength UVA radiation.

An ideal sunscreen should be:
- Combination of physical and chemical agents.
- Broad spectrum
- Cosmetically elegant
- Non-irritant
- Hypo-allergenic
- Non-comedogenic
- Cost effective.

Classification

Sunscreens may be classified as organic and inorganic, replacing the previously used terms "chemical" and "physical", respectively.

Organic

They are active ingredients that absorb UV radiation within a particular range of wavelengths. Once the UV filter absorbs energy, it moves from a low-energy ground state to a high-energy excited state. From this state, any of the following three processes may occur, depending on the ability of the filter to process the energy it has absorbed:
1. Photostable filter: This type of filter dissipates its absorbed energy to the environment as heat energy, and returns to the ground state. It can subsequently absorb UV energy again.
2. Photo unstable filter: Following UV energy absorption the filter undergoes a change in its chemical structure, or is degraded. It is not capable of absorbing UV energy again.
3. Photoreactive filter: In its excited state, the filter interacts with surrounding molecules, including other ingredients of the sunscreen, oxygen, and skin proteins and lipids. This leads to the production of reactive species, with unwanted biological effects.

Organic sunscreens are further divided into UVB and UVA filters:
- **UVB filters**
  - PABA derivatives-Padimate O
  - Cinnamates-Octinoxate, Cinoxate
  - Salicylates-Octisalate, Homosalate, Trolamine salicylate
  - Octocrylene
  - Ensulizole
- **UVA filters**
  - Benzophenones (UVB and UVA2 absorbers)-Oxybenzone, Sulisobenzone, Dioxybenzone
  - Avobenzone or Parsol 1789 (UVA1 absorber)
  - Meradimate (UVA2 absorber)
- **Newer generation broad spectrum (UVA + UVB) filters/hybrid filters**: Ecamsule (Mexoryl SX), Silatriazole (Mexoryl XL), Bemotrizinol (Tinosorb S), Bisoctrizole (Tinosorb M)

Inorganic Sunscreens

1. Zinc oxide (nanoforms)
2. Titanium dioxide (nanoforms)
3. Others—iron oxide, red veterinary petrolatum, kaolin, calamine, ichthammol, talc

Inorganic agents function by reflecting, scattering or absorbing UV radiation. They are opaque and show a "whitening effect" which may be cosmetically unacceptable. This may be minimized by the use of micronized or ultrafine particles.

Systemic Photoprotective Agents

Oral photoprotectors do not directly protect the skin against the damage induced by high energy photons; therefore, they are not very effective against the erythema and other deleterious effects caused by the sun. These oral photoprotective products usually contain one or more active principles that activate different mechanisms of photoprotection, mainly due to their anti-oxidant actions.

Examples: β-carotene, antimalarials, ascorbic acid, α-tocopherols, retinol, selenium, green tea polyphenols, PABA.

Indications

Approved
- Prevention of sunburn
- Prevention of skin damage, freckling, discoloration and lip damage.
- Prevention of photoaging
- Prevention of sun cancers.

Unlicensed
- Photoallergic or phototoxic drug reactions
- Photosensitive and photo aggravated disorders.

Sunscreen-Related Indices

Sun Protection Factor (SPF)

- Indicates the level of sunburn protection provided by the sunscreen product.
- SPF values mainly indicate sunscreen's protection against UVB induced erythema.

$$\text{UVB sunburn protection factor (SPF)} = \frac{\text{Minimal erythema dose (MED) of photoprotected skin}}{\text{MED of unprotected skin}}$$

Grading system for SPF:
- Low: SPF 2–15
- Medium: SPF 15–30
- High: SPF 30–50
- Highest: SPF >50

A sunscreen with SPF 30 plus provides adequate sun protection.

2. UVA protection indices
   a. Japanese standard
   b. Australian/New Zealand Standard (in vitro method)
   c. European Union guidelines
3. **Immune protection factor (IPF):** Ability of sunscreen products to prevent UV-induced immunosuppression. IPF is assessed by complex methods such as the ability of a sunscreen to inhibit either the sensitization or elicitation arm of contact or delayed-type hypersensitivity reactions to allergens such as dinitrochlorobenzene (DNCB) and nickel, respectively. IPF is considered to correlate better with the UVA-protectiveness of a sunscreen than with its SPF.
4. Clothing indices
5. Sunglass standards

Critical wavelength: The wavelength below which 90% of the sunscreen's UV absorbency occurs.

Broad spectrum sunscreen: Critical wavelength >370 nm AND UVA protection factor > 4.

Water-resistant sunscreen: Maintains the label SPF value after two sequential immersions in water for 20 min (40 min).

Very water-resistant sunscreen: Maintains the label SPF value after four sequential immersions in water for 20 min (80 min).

Water-resistant or very water-resistant, can also be labelled as "sweat resistant."

Recommendations for Sunscreen Application

Sunscreen should be applied properly to all sun exposed areas (in a concentration of 2 mg/cm^2), and allowed to dry completely before sun exposure. It should be reapplied every 2 hours, and after swimming, vigorous activity, excessive perspiration, or towelling.

"Teaspoon rule":

3 mL (slightly more than half a teaspoon)
- for each arm
- for the face and neck

6 mL (slightly more than a teaspoon)
- for each leg
- for the chest
- for the back

Formulations

- **Emulsions:** Containing both oil/water and water/oil phases in a stable system
- **Gels:** 4 forms-aqueous, hydroalcoholic, microemulsion and oil anhydrous formulations
- **Aerosol:** Oil based, expensive
- **Sun sticks:** Oil and oil soluble components through incorporation of petrolatum and waxes, cover very small surface areas like nose, lips and around eyes.

New Sunscreen Technologies

Sunspheres

Sunspheres are styrene/acrylate copolymers that do not absorb UV irradiation but enhance the effectiveness of the active sunscreen ingredients. The Sunsphere polymer beads are filled with water, which migrates out of the particle, leaving behind tiny air-filled spheres, which have a lower refractive index (1.0) than the dried sunscreen film (1.4–1.5). As a result, scattering of UV radiation occurs, increasing the probability of contact with the active UV filters in the sunscreen. Sunspheres, available in a powder form, and can boost SPF by 50-70% making it possible to reduce the concentration of active ingredients.

Microencapsulation

Active sunscreen ingredients are entrapped within a silica shell, as a result of which, allergic or irritant reactions to the active ingredient can be minimized, and incompatible sunscreen ingredients can be safely combined, without loss of efficacy.

Adverse Effects

- Irritation-immediate stinging/burning post application around eyes
- Contact urticaria – both immunologic and nonimmunologic
- Contact dermatitis – ICD and ACD
- Photosensitivity–oxybenzone most common cause
- Acnegenicity – both induction and exacerbation
- Folliculitis
- Comedogenicity

Contraindications

- Hypersensitivity to active ingredient or vehicle.
- Infants less than 6 months of age
- Should not be used as solitary component of photoprotection.

Phototherapy

Phototherapy represents the use of ultraviolet (UV) radiation for the treatment of skin diseases. Currently, phototherapy encompasses irradiation with broadband UVB (290–320 nm), narrowband UVB (311–313 nm), 308 nm excimer laser, UVA1 (340–400 nm), UVA (320–400 nm) plus psoralens (PUVA) or alone, and extracorporeal photochemotherapy (photopheresis).

UVB Therapy

Principles and Mechanisms

- UVB phototherapy refers to the use of artificial UVB radiation without the addition of exogenous photosensitizers. Endogenous chromophores (mainly nuclear DNA) on absorbing UVB induce photochemical reactions mediating a variety of biologic effects, ultimately leading to the therapeutic effects. Absorption of UV by nucleotides causes the formation of DNA photoproducts, primarily pyrimidine dimers with immunosuppressive effects.
- UVB also induces tumor suppressor gene TP53 expression, leading to either cell cycle arrest (giving time for DNA repair) or apoptosis of keratinocytes ("sunburn cells") if the DNA damage is too severe to be repaired.
- NB-UVB leads to a decrease in pro-inflammatory cytokines, a decrease in antigen presentation through inhibition of Langerhans cell activity resulting in suppression of the cutaneous T-cell-mediated immune responses.

Treatment Protocols

Before starting phototherapy, determination of the patient's UV sensitivity via phototesting is frequently recommended, since skin typing by history alone does not always reflect the actual sensitivity of a particular individual. The minimal erythema dose (MED) is defined as the lowest dose that causes a minimally perceptible erythema reaction at 24 hours after irradiation. An initial therapeutic UVB dose equal to 70% of the MED is typically recommended. Treat on Monday, Wednesday, Friday; increase dose by 10% on each treatment day. If erythema occurs:

- Asymptomatic: Hold dose
- Symptomatic but has subsided: Reduce dose by 20%
- Symptomatic and still present: withhold treatment and reduce dose 20% for next treatment. Alternatively, expert consensus groups have come up with standardized initial dosing of 150 to 200 mJ/cm^2 and dose adjustment protocols based on skin phototype, clinical experience, and adverse effects, usually increasing by 100 mJ/cm^2 or 10 to 15% as tolerated.

Indication

Approved
- Psoriasis
- Stable vitiligo.

Unlicensed
- Mycosis fungoides
- Atopic dermatitis
- Seborrheic dermatitis
- Polymorphic light eruption
- Actinic prurigo
- Prurigo nodularis
- Aquagenic urticaria
- Uremic pruritus
- Generalized lichen planus
- Acquired perforating dermatosis
- Disseminated granuloma annulare
- Graft-versus-host disease
- Progressive macular hypomelanosis
- Pigmented purpuric dermatoses.

Adverse Effects

- Short term—erythema, xerosis, blistering (occasional), an increased incidence of recurrent herpes simplex viral infections.
- Long term—photoaging, carcinogenesis.

Contraindications

Absolute
- Pemphigus and pemphigoid
- Lupus erythematosus with photosensitivity
- Xeroderma pigmentosa
- Below 7–10 years

Relative
- History or family history of melanoma
- History of skin cancer or chronic photodamage

UVA Therapy

1. **PUVA SOL** 1 drop of 0.1% 8-MOP is mixed with 20 drops of water/coconut oil and applied over the affected area 30 minutes before sun exposure. Treatment is done 2-3 times/week. In Turban PUVASOL 1 mL of 0.1% 8-MOP is diluted with 2 L of water.
2. **Bath PUVA:** Bath-water delivery of psoralens has become increasingly popular because it provides uniform drug distribution over the skin surface, very low psoralen plasma levels, and a rapid elimination of free psoralens from the skin, thereby reducing the period of photosensitivity. Bath PUVA consists of 15–20 minutes of whole body (or hand and foot) immersion in solutions of 0.5–5.0 mg of 8-MOP per litre of bath water. Irradiation has to be performed immediately thereafter, as photosensitivity decreases rather rapidly.

Targeted phototherapy: It includes excimer laser (308 nm), or lamp (peak: 308 nm). It is approved for plaque psoriasis and is optimally suited for the treatment of body surface area of 10% of less. Difficult to treat localised sites like palm, soles, elbows and knees benefit with excimer laser. Targeted phototherapy with the excimer laser or excimer lamp can be used as a treatment modality for the management of stable vitiligo, granuloma annulare, lichen planus, lichen simplex chronicus, and alopecia areata.

UVA-1 Phototherapy

UVA-1 (340–400 nm) phototherapy is divided into low dose (10–30 J/cm^2 per exposure), medium dose (50–60 J/cm^2), and high dose (130 J/cm^2). The treatment duration for 130/cm^2 is about 40 minutes in a stand-up UVA-1 unit and about twice as long in a lie-down unit. Major indications include Morphea and systemic sclerosis, atopic dermatitis, solar urticaria.

DEPIGMENTING AGENTS

These are used to treat hyperpigmentation of skin.

Classification

Phenolic Compounds	Non-Phenolic Compounds	Combination Formulas
• Hydroquinone • Monobenzyl ether of hydroquinone • 4–methoxyphenol • 4–isopropylcatechol • N-acetyl-4–S-cystaminylphenol • Mequinol	• Azelaic acid • Tretinoin • L-ascorbic acid • Kojic acid • N-acetylcystein	• Kligman's formula • Modified Kligman's formula • Pathak's formula • Westerof's formula

Hydroquinone

Hydroquinone (HQ) benzene is a hydroxyphenolic compound which is used for hypermelanosis.

Indication

Unlicensed

- Melasma
- Chloasma
- Solar lentigines
- Freckles
- Post-inflammatory hyperpigmentation

Mechanism of Action

- Competitive inhibition of tyrosinase (the initial enzyme in melanin biosynthesis)
- Selective damage to melanosomes and melanocytes via production of reactive oxygen radicals.

Dosage

- A thin layer is applied with fingertips and rubbed into the face (or other affected areas) 1 to 2 times a day for 3 to 6 months.
- If there are no results after 2 to 3 months, hydroquinone should be discontinued.

Adverse Effects

- Irritation
- Allergic contact dermatitis
- Erythema
- Inflammation
- Xeroderma
- Stinging
- Exogenous ochronosis

Contraindications

- Allergic reaction or hypersensitivity hydroquinone
- Sun exposure

Pregnancy Category: C

Lactation: Should be avoided

Children: Not established

AZELAIC ACID

Azelaic acid is a naturally occurring, dicarboxylic acid derived from *Pityrosporum ovale*.

Indication

Unlicensed

- Acne vulgaris
- Rosacea
- Perioral dermatitis
- Plaque psoriasis
- Hypermelanosis caused by physical and chemical agents, post-inflammatory hyperpigmentation, melasma, lentigo maligna, and melanoma.

Mechanism of Action

- Dicarboxylic acids are competitive inhibitors of tyrosinase.
- Azelaic acid suppresses ultraviolet-B light-induced expression of interleukin (IL)-1, IL-6, and tumour necrosis factor (TNF)-α messenger RNA through interaction with the peroxisome proliferators-activated receptor-γ (PPAR-γ).

Dosage

To be applied twice daily.

Adverse Effects

Itching, burning, or scaling.

Contraindications

Allergic reaction or hypersensitivity.

Pregnancy category: B

Lactation: Safe

Children: Not recommended below 12 years of age.

KOJIC ACID

It is a naturally occurring hydrophilic fungal derivative derived from certain species of Acetobacter, Aspergillus and Penicillium.

Indications

- Melasma
- post inflammatory hyperpigmentation,
- anti-aging.

Mechanism of Action

- It inhibits tyrosinase enzyme.
- Kojic acid and kojic acid esters also show antioxidant activity that enhances the depigmenting effect.

Dosage

To be applied twice daily.

Adverse Effects

Burning and allergic contact dermatitis.

Contraindication

Allergic reaction or hypersensitivity.

Pregnancy category: Safe

Lactation: Safe

Children: Not recommended below 12 years of age.

MONOBENZYL ETHER OF HYDROQUINONE

Monobenzone, also called monobenzyl ether of hydroquinone (MBEH) is an organic chemical in the phenol family.

Indications

Approved

Depigmentation therapy of extensive vitiligo (greater than 50 percent of body surface area).

Mechanism of Action

- MBEH reacts with tyrosinase.
- MBEH induces cellular oxidative stress in exposed pigmented cells by producing reactive oxygen species (ROS) such as peroxide. ROS generation also results in release of tyrosinase and MART-1 antigen containing exosomes which further contributes to immune response.
- Rapid and persistent innate immune activation also occurs in MBEH-exposed skin. MBEH is a contact-sensitizer inducing a type IV delayed type hypersensitivity response.

Dosage

A thin layer of 20% MBEH cream should be applied and rubbed into the pigmented area two or three times daily up to 4 months.

Adverse Effects

Mild, transient skin irritation and sensitization, including erythematous and eczematous reactions.

Contraindication

In individuals with a history of sensitivity or allergic reactions to this product, or any of its ingredients.

Pregnancy category: C

Lactation: Should be avoided

Children: Not established below 12 years of age.

Combination Formulas

Kligman's Regimen

This formula contains 5% hydroquinone, 0.1% tretinoin, 0.1% dexamethasone, and hydrophilic ointment.

Indications

Melasma, post-inflammatory hyperpigmentation, and ephelides.

Modified Kligman's Regimen

A triple combination of Fluocinolone acetonide 0.01%, hydroquinone 4%, tretinoin 0.05%.

Indications

Approved

Melasma

Pathak's formula

2% HQ and 0.05–0.1% tretinoin

Westerhof's formula

4.7% N-acetylcysteine, 2% HQ and 0.1% triamcinolone acetonide.

MOISTURIZERS

Moisturizers hydrate, smooth skin, and helps improve barrier function both in normal as well as diseased skin. **Humectants, occlusives,** and emollients are the three main types of moisturizing ingredients.

Types of Moisturizers

Emollients

Salient Features

- Saturated and unsaturated hydrocarbons of variable length which help to maintain skin barrier function by filling up intercorneocyte cluster gaps.
- Used for management of skin xerosis, and for routine skin care.
- Can rarely cause irritant contact dermatitis
- Example: Cholesterol, squalene, fatty acids, fatty alcohols

Humectants

Salient Features

- Humectants are low molecular weight hygroscopic substances that improve skin surface hydration by attracting water from dermis and a humid environment into the epidermis.
- Used for xerotic skin conditions, ichthyosis
- Can cause skin irritation
- Examples: Glycerol, propylene glycol, urea, hydroxy acids

Occlusives

Salient Features

- Oils and waxes form an inert layer and physically block transepidermal water loss.
- Indicated for xerotic skin, atopic dermatitis, prevention of contact dermatitis.
- Can cause folliculitis, acneform eruptions, contact dermatitis and are messy to apply.
- Examples: Petrolatum, mineral oil, lanolin, beeswax.

KERATOLYTICS

Salicylic Acid

Salicylic acid or 2-hydroxybenzoic acid is naturally present in willow bark, wintergreen leaves and sweet birch.

Mechanism of Action

- Exactly not known
- Proposed—there is decrease in corneocyte adhesion, solubilizing of intercellular cement thereby loosening and detachment of corneocytes.
- Damage to corneodesmosomes due to changes in nature of membrane crossing glycoproteins causes desmolysis.
- Due to benzene ring's modulation of UV rays to long waves, which are reflected from skin as heat rusulting in sunscreen effects.
- Anti-inflammatory effect between 0.5 and 5% (w/w) concentration by inhibition of prostaglandin biosynthesis.

Indications in Dermatology

Hyperkeratotic Dermatoses
- Calluses
- Corns
- Different types of Ichthyosis
- Keratodermas

Papulosquamous Disorders
- Psoriasis

Dermatitis
- Seborrheic dermatitis
- Cradle cap

Infections
- Fungal – dermatophyte infection
- Viral – verruca, molluscum contagiosum

Miscellaneous
- Acne vulgaris
- Actinic keratoses – in combination with 5-Fluorouracil
- Antipruritic and analgesic
- Hyperhidrosis

Cosmetic Uses
- Chemical peeling – acne, hyperpigmentation, photodamage
- Photoprotection – as component of sunscreens

Dosage and Concentration

- >2 years of age
- Apply locally 1–2 times daily according to indication.
- 2 to 50% concentration used in various disorders.

Monitoring

- Sign and symptom of salicylism.

Adverse Effect

- Cutaneous: Irritation, burning, redness, itching, stinging, dryness and skin peeling, contact sensitization
  Systemic-Systemic absorption-salicylism
- GI: Nausea, vomiting
- Neuropsychiatric: Confusion, dizziness, delirium, psychosis, stupor, coma
- Metabolic: Metabolic alkalosis, hypoglycemia
- Respiratory alkalosis
- Hyperventilation
- Tinnitus

Contraindication

- Hypersensitivity
- Children <2 years of age.

Pregnancy: Category C

Lactation: Do not apply near nipple area.

UREA

Urea is a hygroscopic molecule present in the epidermis as a component of the natural moisturizing factor (NMF) and is necessary for the adequate hydration and integrity of the stratum corneum.

Mechanism of Action

- Increases moisturization of the stratum corneum.
- Regulates epidermal proliferation
- Increases the skin's barrier function and antimicrobial defense.
- Keratolytic action – breaks hydrogen bonds and denatures keratin.
- Increases drug penetration – helps in the transport of antifungals, corticosteroids and hormones through the skin and nails.

Indications

- 10–25% concentration of urea: Xerosis and xerotic dermatitis, atopic dermatitis, keratodermas, keratosis pilaris, ichthyosis, psoriasis.
- 30–50% concentration: Localized hyperkeratosis (psoriasis, keratoderma, callosities or corns), chemical avulsion of dystrophic nails, pretreatment of hyperkeratotic actinic keratoses.

Adverse Effects

- Irritant reaction and maceration (specially if used under occlusion)
- Stinging and irritation if applied over fissured or excoriated skin.

AMMONIUM LACTATE

Lactic acid is an alpha-hydroxy acid. It is a normal constituent of tissues and blood.

Mechanism of Action

- The alpha-hydroxy acids (and their salts) act as humectants when applied to the skin. This property may influence hydration of the stratum corneum.
- Lactic acid, when applied to the skin, may act to decrease corneocyte cohesion.

Indication

- Xerosis
- Ichthyosis Vulgaris

Dosage

12% cream to be applied twice daily.

Adverse Effects

Erythema, irritation and burning/stinging.

Pregnancy category: B

TOPICAL ANTIPRURITIC AGENTS

Topical antipruritic agents may help reduce the urge to scratch, potentially improving the efficacy of skin disease-specific therapies.

Pramoxine

It is an ester anesthetic.

Mechanism of Action

- Blocks transmission of sensory nerve impulses.
- Hypoalgesic effect on cold pain, but not heat pain.
- Duration of effect is 2-4 hours.

Indication

- Uremic pruritus
- Histamine-induced itch
- Pruritus ani
- Notalgia paresthetica
- Nonspecific mild pruritus

Side Effects

Allergic contact dermatitis

Menthol

It is cyclic terpene alcohol derived from plants in the *Mentha* genus.

Mechanism of Action

- Activates TRPM8 cation channels, which also respond to cold thermal stimuli.
- Possible central itch modulation via Aδ fiber and/or κ-opioid receptor activation.

Indication

- Provides a cooling sensation

Side Effects

- Irritation, especially of inflamed or eroded skin
- Allergic contact dermatitis

Capsaicin

It is natural alkaloid derived from Solanaceae family members, including hot chili peppers of the *Capsicum* genus.

Mechanism of Action

- Activates the TRPV1 vanilloid receptor expressed by sensory neurons.
- Repeated release of substance P from C fiber sensory afferent neurons eventually leads to depletion of this neuropeptide and reduced transmission of heat, pain, and itch.

Indication

Approved

Transdermal patch is approved for treatment of postherpetic neuralgia.

Unlicensed

Notalgia paresthetica, Brachioradial pruritus, Renal pruritus, Prurigo nodularis, Psoriatic pruritus, and itch associated with a burning sensation.

Side Effects

Burning, stinging, and/or erythema at the application site.

PHENOL

It is originally a distillation product of coal tar.

Mechanism of Action

Thought to act directly on cold receptors

Indication

Cooling and antipruritic effects.

Side Effects

- Irritation, especially of inflamed or eroded skin.
- Note: Should not be used in pregnant women or infants <6 months of age.

CAMPHOR

It is ketone originally derived from the camphor laurel tree (*Cinnamomum camphora*).

Mechanism of Action

Local anesthetic effect

Indication

Cooling sensation may relieve mild pruritus

Side Effects

Irritation, especially of inflamed or eroded skin

Doxepin

It is a tricyclic compound.

Mechanism of Action

- Potent histamine antagonist (H1 and H2)
- Sedation via anticholinergic properties

Indications

Pruritus associated with
- Atopic dermatitis
- Lichen simplex chronicus
- Nummular eczema

Side Effects

- Drowsiness due to systemic absorption.
- Irritant or (less often) allergic contact dermatitis

Contraindicated

- Patients with untreated narrow angle glaucoma or urinary retention and those receiving MAO inhibitors.
- Use during lactation is not recommended.

HYPOHIDROTIC AGENTS

Aluminum Chloride Hexahydrate

Aluminium chloride hexahydrate is a first-line treatment for excessive sweating.

Indications

Unlicensed
- Palmar hyperhidrosis
- Plantar hyperhidrosis
- Axillary hyperhidrosis
- Hemostasis during surgical procedures

Mechanism of Action

- Aluminum chloride reversibly inhibits eccrine gland secretion by obstructing the eccrine pores and inducing transient secretory cell atrophy.
- It creates a low-grade generation of thrombin, which is followed by activation of the platelet-dependent clotting factor XI to XIa.

Dosage

- Apply 20% solution to completely dry affected area once daily at bedtime.
- After 6–8 hours (usually the following morning), remove garments and/or plastic wrap; to prevent irritation, wash treatment area(s) thoroughly with soap and water or shampoo.

Adverse Effects

Irritant contact dermatitis, burning, or a prickling sensation.

Iontophoresis

Iontophoresis (Greek—introduction of ions) is defined as the introduction, by means of an electric current, of ions of soluble salts into the tissues of the body for therapeutic purposes.

Indications

Unlicensed
- Palmoplantar hyperhidrosis
- Hyperkeratosis of palm and sole
- Scleroderma
- Lymphedema
- Lichen planus

Mechanism of Action

- Ion-electric field interaction provides an additional force that drives ions through the skin.

- The flow of electric current increases the permeability of the skin.
- Electro-osmosis produces bulk motion of solvent that carries ions or neutral species with the solvent stream.

BARRIER CREAM

- A barrier cream is a product applied directly to the skin surface to help maintain the skin's physical barrier, providing protection from irritants and preventing the skin from drying out.
- These are used in treatment of hand dermatitis, napkin dermatitis, stoma dermatitis, pressure sore and very dry skin.
- They contain occlusives and humectants.
- Occlusive include petroleum jelly, silicone/dimethicone and zinc oxide.
- Humectants increase the skin's ability to hold onto water. They include glycerine, sorbitol, urea, seaweed extract, hyaluronic acid and alpha hydroxy acids.

LOCAL ANESTHETIC AGENT

Lignocaine Injection

Lidocaine or lignocaine is by far the most common local anesthetic in use today.

Indications

Approved
- Infiltrative anesthesia
- Regional nerve blocks
- Topical anesthesia

Unlicensed
- Tumescent anesthesia
- Postherpetic neuralgia
- Pruritus

Mechanism of Action

It blocks conduction in nerves by minimizing or preventing the influx of sodium ions, thereby preventing depolarization.

Pharmacology

- Without epinephrine, the approximate duration of action of lidocaine is 30–60 minutes. With epinephrine, this duration can be extended to approximately 120–360 minutes.
- Lidocaine is 60–80% protein-bound and has an elimination half-life of 1.5–2.0 hours.
- Lidocaine is specifically metabolized by hepatic microsomal enzymes of the cytochrome P-450 (CYP) 3A4 system.

Dose

1% of lignocaine to be injected @ 3 mg/kg/dose.

Adverse Effects

- Allergic reaction
- Toxic effects depending on blood level: Increased anxiety, Talkativeness, Tinnitus, Circumoral numbness, Nausea and vomiting, Metallic taste, Diplopia, Nystagmus, Cardiopulmonary depression

Contraindications

Absolute

Hypersensitivity to lidocaine or preservatives

Relative
- Hypersensitivity to amide naesthetics
- Significant hepatic impairment
- Significant cardiac impairment
- Myasthenia gravis
- Hyperthyroidism

Pregnancy category—category B

Lactation: Safe

Children: Safe

EMLA

It consists of eutectic mixture of lignocaine 2.5% and prilocaine 2.5%.

Indication

- Topical analgesia of intact skin in connection: Needle insertion, vaccination with only the following vaccines that does not interact with EMLA in MMR, DPTP; Haemophilus influenzae b and Hepatitis B, superficial surgical procedures, e.g., removal of molluscum contagiosum, split skin grafting, electrocautery, laser treatment for superficial skin surgeries, such as treatment of telangiectasia, port wine stains, warts, moles, skin nodules, and scar tissue.
- Topical analgesia of genital mucosa: Local infiltration anesthesia; surgical procedures lasting not longer than 10 minutes on small superficial localized lesions, e.g., removal of condyloma by laser or cautery, and biopsies.
- Topical analgesia of leg ulcers: Mechanical/sharp cleansing/debridement, e.g., the removal of necrotic tissue and debris by curettes, scissors etc.

Contraindication

- Patients who are hypersensitive to local anesthetics of the amide type or to any ingredients in the formulation.
- Patients with congenital or idiopathic methemoglobinemia;
- Procedures requiring large amounts of EMLA over a large body area.

Topical Vitamins

Vitamin E

- Vitamin E is an essential lipophilic nutrient with antioxidant properties capable of preventing lipid peroxidation. Tocopherols are saturated forms of vitamin E, while tocotrienols are unsaturated agents.
- α tocopherol is the most commonly used topical form of vitamin E.

Mechanism of Action

Vitamin E scavenges lipid peroxyl radicals and acts as an antioxidant. It accelerates wound healing by promoting epithelialization, angiogenesis, granulation tissue, and collagen production. It has UV absorptive properties, too.

Indication

Unlicensed

- Photoprotection and skin rejuvenation
- Surgical scars
- Granuloma annulare
- Radiation dermatitis
- Management of ulcers in systemic sclerosis
- Melasma

Side Effects

- Irritant and allergic contact dermatitis, erythema multiforme-like eruption, contact urticaria and xanthomatous reaction following contact dermatitis.
- Since vitamin E can inhibit clotting, so topical application on open healing wounds is better avoided.
- As both tocopherol and alkyl esters are oils, so higher doses can make the formulations greasy and sticky, thus causing a negative aesthetic effect.

Vitamin K

Vitamin K is a fat-soluble vitamin that plays a vital role in the blood coagulation cascade. Naturally occurring vitamin K is found in two forms: Vitamin K1 or phylloquinone/phytonadione and vitamin K2, collectively known as menaquinones.

Mechanism of Action

The mechanism of action for topically applied phytonadione(K1) is unknown.

Indications

- Treatment of periorbital hyperpigmentation
- Resolution of post-laser bruising
- Treatment of steroid-induced rosacea

Adverse Effects

- Immediate hypersensitivity following cutaneous application can occur.
- Due to their quinone structure, some compounds of vitamin K undergo photodegradation and are phototoxic when applied to the skin.

Note: Ester prodrugs of menahydroquinone with higher photostability have been evaluated for topical application

VITAMIN B COMPLEX

Vitamin B complex comprises of B1 (Thiamine), B2 (Riboflavin), B3 (Niacin), B5 (Pantothenic acid), B6 (Pyridoxine), B7 (Biotin), B9 (Folic acid) and B12 (Cobalamin). Among these, niacin and pantothenic acid have been well-studied for topical usage.

Vitamin B3

It is the most widely used topical agent among B complex vitamins. Niacin is the acid isotype of vitamin B3, and niacinamide is the amide isotype. For topical applications, it is available as niacinamide (nicotinamide), nicotinic acid and nicotinate esters.

Mechanism of Action

- It inhibits PARP-1 {poly-(adenosine) diphosphate-ribose polymerase-1} which is involved in NFκB (Nuclear factor-kB)-mediated transcription. This leads to dysregulation of adhesion factors (such as intracellular adhesion molecule – 1), thereby altering leukocyte chemotaxis.
- It also reduces interleukin 1 (IL-1), interleukin 12 (IL-12), tumor necrosis factor-alpha (TNF-α), major histocompatibility complex II (MHC-II) and macrophage migration inhibitor factor-1 and is anti-inflammatory.
- It reduces sebum production, improves the skin barrier, and has antiaging and UV protective effects.
- It inhibits melanosome transfer from melanocytes to the keratinocytes.

Indications

Disorders of sebaceous glands

- Acne: It is used at a concentration of 2–4% either as a monotherapy or combined with clindamycin 1% gel.
- Rosacea: 0.25% of 1-methyl nicotinamide (a metabolite of nicotinamide) applied twice daily for four weeks.

Papulosquamous disorders: Psoriasis

Dermatitis: Atopic dermatitis

Autoimmune connective tissue disorders: Discoid lupus erythematosus (DLE)

Pigmentary disorders: Melasma

Premalignant disorders: Actinic keratosis

Photoaging: Anti-aging

Cosmetic uses as a moisturizer, anti-aging agent and sunscreen

Side Effects

- Nicotinamide, on hydrolysis, can be converted to nicotinic acid, which can cause skin redness or even an intense flushing response.
- Under cold and dry conditions, flushing may lead to burning, stinging, and itching.

Vitamin B5 (Pantothenic Acid)

Panthenol, or provitamin B5, is converted to form the active compound pantothenic acid.

Dexpanthenol, the D optical isomer and stable alcoholic analog of panthenol is the most commonly used form. Dexpanthenol is also absorbed from the skin more than pantothenic acid, which forms the basis of its topical usage.

Mechanism of Action

Dexpanthenol is hygroscopic and increases lipid synthesis and fibroblast proliferation. This results in a moisturizing effect, improved skin barrier, accelerated wound re-epithelization, and healing.

Indications

- **Dermatitis**
  - *Atopic dermatitis*
  - *Diaper dermatitis*
  - *Contact dermatitis*
  - *Cheilitis and acute radiation dermatitis*
- Management of minor wounds and scars
- **Cosmetic uses**: Hair conditioners, sunscreens, and fragrances.

Side Effects

- Allergic contact dermatitis is rarely seen.
- High-concentration (>1%) products of topical vitamin B5 have a greasy appearance, so they are not cosmetically appealing and unsuitable for application over the face.

Vitamin C

Vitamin C is a naturally occurring water-soluble vitamin. Following oral administration, it is minimally absorbed in the intestine, leading to decreased bioavailability. L-ascorbic acid is the biologically active form of vitamin C, and its topical application achieves a higher concentration in the skin, resulting in multiple therapeutic benefits.

Mechanism of Action

Topical vitamin C is a potent antioxidant and neutralizes the oxidative stress and subsequent cellular damage caused by environmental pollution and UV radiation. It also helps in regenerating the oxidative form of the lipophilic antioxidant vitamin E. Vitamin C stimulates collagen synthesis, and has depigmenting and anti-inflammatory action also.

Indications

- Anti-aging agent and prevention of photoaging
- Photoprotection
- Depigmenting agent
- Basal cell carcinoma
- Post-laser erythema reduction
- Wound healing

Side Effects

- Stinging, erythema, and xerosis.
- It can cause yellowish discoloration of the skin, hypopigmentation of hair, and staining of clothes due to oxidative changes.
- Urticaria, erythema multiforme and allergic contact dermatitis.

SUGGESTED READINGS

1. Paśko P, Rodacki T, Domagała-Rodacka R, Palimonka K, Marcinkowska M, Owczarek D. Second generation H1–antihistamines interaction with food and alcohol-A systematic review. Biomed Pharmacother. 2017; 93:27-39.
2. Hsieh CY, Tsai TF. Use of H-1 Antihistamine in Dermatology: More than Itch and Urticaria Control: A Systematic Review. Dermatol Ther (Heidelb). 2021;11(3):719-32.
3. Wolverton SE (Ed.). Comprehensive Dermatologic Drug Therapy. 4th edition Philadelphia: Elsevier; 2021.
4. Kang S (Ed.). Fitzpatrick's Dermatology. 9th edition New York: McGraw-Hill Education; 2019.
5. Griffiths C (Ed.). Rook's Textbook of Dermatology. 10th edition Chichester, West Sussex, United Kingdom: Wiley – Blackwell; 2024.
6. Bolognia JL (Ed.). Dermatology 5th edition Philadelphia: Elsevier; 2025.
7. Wakelin SH (Ed.). Handbook of Systemic Drug Treatment in Dermatology. 3rd edition Boca Raton, Florida: Taylor & Francis; 2023
8. Patel AA, Swerlick RA, McCall CO. Azathioprine in dermatology: The past, the present, and the future. J Am Acad Dermatol. 2006;55(3): 369-89.
9. Downing HJ, Pirmohamed M, Beresford MW, Smyth RL. Paediatric use of mycophenolate mofetil. Br J Clin Pharmacol. 2013;75(1): 45-59.
10. Bik L, Sangers T, Greveling K, Prens E, Haedersdal M, van Doorn M. Efficacy and tolerability of intralesional bleomycin in dermatology: A systematic review. J Am Acad Dermatol. 2020;83(3):888-903.
11. Beccari MV, Mogle BT, Sidman EF, Mastro KA, Asiago-Reddy E, Kufel WD. Ibalizumab, a Novel Monoclonal Antibody for the Management of Multidrug-Resistant HIV-1 Infection. Antimicrob Agents Chemother. 2019;63(6):e00110-9.
12. Padda IS, Bhatt R, Parmar M. Golimumab In: StatPearls. Treasure Island, FL: StatPearls Publishing; 2024.
13. Adışen E. Interleukin-23 Inhibitors. Turkderm-Turk Arch Dermatol Venereol. 2022;56(50): 61-6.
14. Ghazawi FM, Mahmood F, Kircik L, Poulin Y, Bourcier M, Vender R, et al. A Review of the Efficacy and Safety for Biologic Agents Targeting IL-23 in Treating Psoriasis With the Focus on Tildrakizumab. Front Med (Lausanne). 2021;8:702-76.
15. Ratnarajah K, Le M, Muntyanu A, Mathieu S, Nigen S, Litvinov IV, et al. Inhibition of IL-13: A New Pathway for Atopic Dermatitis. J Cutan Med Surg. 2021;25(3):315-28.
16. Keam SJ. Nemolizumab: First Approval. Drugs. 2022 ;82(10):1143-50.
17. Bubna AK. Leukotriene Antagonists in Dermatology. Indian J Dermatol. 2021;66(5):575.
18. Centers for Disease Control and Prevention. Treatment regimens for latent TB infection [Internet]. 2020 [cited 2024 Dec 24].Available from:https://www.cdc.gov/tb/topic/treatment/ltbi.htm.
19. Gunawan H, Banjarnahor ID, Achdiat PA. Oral Albendazole as an Alternative Treatment for Moderate Crusted Scabies Along with 5% Permethrin and 5% Salicylic Acid. Int Med Case Rep J. 2022;15:193-9
20. Risadini MW, Mochtar M, Danarti R. Comparison of albendazole tablets with 5% permethrin cream for scabies treatment at AL muayyad Islamic boarding school surakarta [translated title]. Media Dermato Venereologica Indonesiana. 2017;44(3):108-12.
21. Douri T, Shawaf AZ. Treatment of crusted scabies with albendazole: A case report. Derm Online J. 2009;15(2):117-26.
22. Piquero-Casals J, Morgado-Carrasco D, Granger C, Trullàs C, Jesús-Silva A, Krutmann J. Urea in Dermatology: A Review of its Emollient, Moisturizing, Keratolytic, Skin Barrier Enhancing and Antimicrobial Properties. Dermatol Ther (Heidelb). 2021;11(6):1905-15.
23. Hamzavi IH, Ganesan AK, Mahmoud BH, et al. Effective and durable repigmentation for stable vitiligo: A randomized within-subject controlled trial assessing treatment with autologous skin cell suspension transplantation. J Am Acad Dermatol. 2024;91(6):1104-12.
24. Jeong Ju H, Bae JM, Lee RW. Surgical Interventions for Patients with Vitiligo: A Systematic Review and Meta-analysis. JAMA Dermatol. 2021;157(3):307-16.
25. Attria E. Atrophic postacne scar treatment: Narrative Review JMIR Dermatol. 2024

Index

A

Abacavir 117, 118
Abatacept 36
Abdominal discomfort 161
Abrocitinib 157, 160
Acanthosis nigricans 2
Acitretin 131
   monitoring for 132
Acne
   scar 3
   vulgaris 2, 166
      mild to moderate 193
Acnegenicity 227
Acrodermatitis
   continua of Hallopeau 151
   enteropathica 4
Actinic dermatitis, chronic 15, 74
Actinic keratoses 4
Actinic prurigo 5
Actinomycetoma 36
Actinomycosis 5
   therapy 5
Acyclovir 100, 102
Adalimumab 137
Adapalene 2, 213
Agranulocytosis 112
Albendazole 16, 104
Alcohol 190
Alitretinoin 130, 213
Alkylamine 82, 83
Allopurinol 17
Allosteric jak inhibitors 157
Allylamines 194, 198
Alopecia
   areata 7, 163, 221
      natural evolution of 7
   universalis 163
Alpha-hydroxy acids 233
Aluminum chloride hexahydrate 235
Amikacin injection 36
Amlexanox 12
Ammonium lactate 2, 233
Amorolfine 200
Amoxycillin 5

Amputation 36
Anaerobes 87
Anakinra 152
Androgenetic alopecia 8, 166
Angular cheilitis 8
Anthralin 221
   topical 44
Antiacne drugs, topical 191
Antiandrogen 2, 164
Antibacterial indications 87
Antibacterials drugs, topical 8, 186
Antibiotic 2
Antibody origin 135
Anti-cell surface receptor antibodies 135
Anticonvulsants 104
Antidepressants, tricyclic 170
Antifungal agents 96
   topical 8, 194
Antihistamines 81
   first generation 81
Antihuman herpes virus 100
Anti-IgE antibodies 153
Anti-inflammatory 134
   effect 68, 209
   properties 92
Antileprotics 107
Antileukotrienes 85
Antimalarial 126
Antimicrobial spectrum 87
Antimitotic-binds 134
Antiparasitic 103
   agents, topical 205
Anti-proliferative effects 209
Antipruritic agents, topical 233
Antiretroviral drugs 100, 114
Antiseptic 189
   cleansers 17
Antitubercular drugs 111
Antivirals agent, topical 200
Anxiety
   chronic 168
   drugs used for 167
Aphthous stomatitis, recurrent 9

Apremilast 155
Arbutin 34
Ascariasis 105
Atazanavir 120, 121, 123
Atopic dermatitis 9, 163
   mild to moderate 222
   moderate-to-severe 150
Autoimmune
   bullous dermatoses 62, 209
   bullous disorders 78
   connective tissue disorders 62, 67, 71, 73, 76, 78, 134, 209, 216, 238
Azahiprine 39
Azathioprine 15, 46, 57, 73
Azelaic acid 2, 34, 192, 230
Azelastine 83
Azithromycin 34, 89, 90
Azole 17, 195
   antifungals 13, 110

B

B lymphocyte stimulator specific inhibitor 154
Bacteroides spp 94
Baricitinib 157, 159
Barrier cream 236
Bartonella
   henselae 109
   infection 109
Basal cell carcinoma 11
Behçet's disease 11, 62
Belimumab 154
Benzoxaborole 194
Benzoyl peroxide 2, 191
Benzylamines 194, 198
Berdazimer sodium 205
Beta-blockers 174
Beta-lactamase inhibitor 89
Bexarotene 132, 214
Bictegravir 125
Biological therapy 135
Bleaching 27
Bleomycin 79

Blister grafting 59
Blood 130
Botulinum toxin 181
Bowen's disease 202
Brentuximab vedotin 37
Broad spectrum sunscreen 226
Brodalumab 141
   bioavailability of 142
Bullous
   dermatoses 134
   disorders 71
   pemphigoid 12
Bupropion 169
Burrow's solution 42
   wet-dressing with 28
Buspirone 169
Butenafine 199

C

Cabotegravir 125
Calaminol, topical coolant like 35
Calcineurin inhibitor
   tacrolimus 43
   topical 42, 215
Calcinosis cutis 49
Calcipotriene 218
   ointment, topical 44
Camphor 234
Candidal antigen 203
Candidiasis 13
Cantharidin 204
Capnocytophaga canimorsus 94
Capsaicin 234
Capsid inhibitors 114
Carbamazepine 104
Carbapenems 87
Ceftriaxone 5, 23
Cell wall synthesis inhibitors 89
Cellulitis 13
Central nervous system 156
Cephalosporins 87, 88
Certolizumab pegol 139
Cetirizine 83
Chancroid 14
Chemical cautery 57
Chemical peeling 3
Chickenpox 101
Chilblains 14
Chlamydia, cotreatment for 23
Chlorhexidine 190
   gluconate 12
Cholestyramine 43
Ciclopirox olamine 194, 199
Cidofovir 100, 202

Cimetidine 104, 161
Ciprofloxacin 91
Clarithromycin 31, 89
Classical depigmentary agents 34
Clindamycin 94, 191
Clofazimine 12, 31, 110, 111
Clostridium
   botulinum produces 181
   perfringens 94
Clotrimazole 8, 195
Colchicine 9, 12, 18, 21, 134
Colchicum autumnale 134
Comedogenicity 227
Comedonal 2
   mixed 2
Complete blood count 154, 159, 161
Condyloma acuminata 15
Conglobate 3
Contact dermatitis 62
Contact sensitizer 219
Corticosteroids 9
   mid-potent topical 17
   topical 42, 44
Cosmetic uses 232
Cotrimoxazole 38, 93
Creeping eruption 16
Crisaborole 221, 222
Critical wavelength 226
Crohn disease 163
Crotamiton 206
Cryotherapy 17, 44
   immediate prior intralesional injection 29
Cultured melanocyte transplantation 59
Cutaneous amyloidosis 16
Cutaneous larva migrans 16
Cutaneous leishmaniasis 17
Cutaneous sarcoidosis 48
Cutaneous sclerosis 49
Cutaneous tuberculosis 109
Cutibacterium acnes 4
Cyclophosphamide 39, 57, 77, 79
   levels 79
Cyclosporine 9, 40, 44, 51, 55, 57, 71
CYP2C19 inhibitors 161
CYP3A4 inducers 110, 111
Cyproterone acetate 26
Cytodestructive drugs 204
Cytokine 135
   receptor blocking agents 135
Cytomegalovirus 103
Cytotoxic effects 68

D

Dalbavancin 89
Dapsone 9, 12, 18, 21, 31, 107, 193
Darier's disease 17
Darunavir 121, 122, 123
Delgocitinib 224
Demyelinating disorders 140
Depigmenting agents 229
Depilatory creams 26
Depilatory process 26
Depression 169
Dermatitis 62, 67, 74, 180, 232
   herpetiformis 18
Dermatology
   indication in 171, 232
   vaccines in 182
Dermatomyositis 18, 73
Desloratadine 83
Deucravacitinib 157, 163
Diaper dermatitis 19
Dibenzoxepins, tricyclic 82
Dihydrofolate reductase inhibitor 93
Diphencyprone 7
Diphenylcyclopropenone 219
Discoid eczema 19
Discoid lupus erythematosus 20, 163
Dobutamine 95
Dolutegravir 125
Dopamine 95
Doravirine 119, 120
Doxepin 235
Doxycycline 25, 34, 47
Dupilumab 148

E

Ebastine 83
Econazole 196
Eczematous change 35
Efavirenz 119, 120
Efinaconazole 198
Eflornithine hydrochloride 27
Electrolysis 26
Electrothermolysis 26
Elvitegravir 125
EMLA 236
Emtricitabine 117, 118
Enfuvirtide 115
Epidermophyton 195
Epilatory process 26
Epinephrine 95

Erosive oral lichen planus 163
Erysipelas 13
Erythema
    multiforme 21
    nodosum 21
Erythrasma 22
Erythrodermic stage 41
Erythromycin 25, 89, 192
Etanercept 51, 136
Ethambutol 54, 113
Ethylenediamine 83
Etravirine 119, 120
Etretinate 131
Exanthematous pustulosis, acute generalized 6
Exfoliative dermatitis syndrome 22
Exfoliative erythroderma 62
Extensive area 58
Extracellular oxygen free radicals, generation of 221
Eye care 51

F

Famcilovir 102
Familial mediterranean fever 134
Famotidine 84
Fetal risk 43
Fexofenadine 83
Fidaxomicin 89
Finasteride 26, 164
Fluconazole 8, 13, 17, 53, 98
Fluoroquinolones 91
Fluorouracil 204
Fluoxetine 161
Foliaceous 39
Foscarnet 100, 103
Furunculosis 23
    recurrent 23
Fusidic acid 8, 186
Fusion inhibitors 115

G

GABA agonists gabapentin 171
Ganciclovir 100
Generalized pustular psoriasis 141
Genital ulcer, risk of 16
Gentamycin 188
Gentian violet 189
Glucocorticoid 62
    receptor 209
    topical 207
    toxicity, high risk for 66

Gluten-free diet 18
Glycopeptides 89
Golimumab 138
Gonorrhea 23
Gout 134
Gram-negative
    cocci 87
    folliculitis 192
Gram-positive cocci 87
Granuloma inguinale 24
Granulomatous
    cheilitis 110, 137
    dermatoses 137
    disorders 76, 127
Grenz-rays 42
Griseofulvin 53, 99
Guselkumab 144

H

H1 antihistamines 82, 84
    classification of
        first-generation 81
        second-generation 82
    second generation 82
Haemophilus influenzae
    prophylaxis 109
Hailey-Hailey disease 68
Hair follicle tumour, benign 217
Harsh cosmetic ingredients like camphor 47
Heart failure, congestive 140
Heat exposure 35
Hedgehog pathway inhibitors 172
Hematologic 65
Hemodynamic equilibrium 50
Hemolytic 112
Hepatic impairment 105
Hepatotoxicity, developing 69
Herpes genitalis 24
Herpes simplex 24, 102
    infection 102
    subsets of 102
Herpes zoster 24, 101, 162, 183
Hidradenitis suppurativa 25, 129, 137
Hirsutism 25, 166
Hookworm infestation 105
HSV infection, recurrent 101
Human immunodeficiency virus
    associated dermatoses 177
    testing 54
Humectants 231, 232
Hydrocolloid dressing 18
Hydrogen peroxide 190, 205

Hydroquinone 34, 229, 230
Hydroxychloroquine 15, 21, 57
Hydroxypyridone 194
Hyperhidrosis 27
Hyperkeratotic dermatoses 232
Hyperlipidaemia 162
Hypersensitivity 79, 105, 111, 153
    reactions 112
Hypertension 161
Hypertrophic and keloidal scars 3
Hypohidrotic agents 235
Hypothalamic-pituitary-adrenal
    axis suppression 62
    and corticosteroid tapering 66

I

Ichthyosis 27
Ichthyosis vulgaris 233
Idiopathic urticaria, chronic 71
Idiosyncratic 108, 127
Imidazoles 194
Imiquimod 220
Immune
    enhancing drugs 202
    protection factor 226
Immuno-biologics 135
Immunobullous disorders 67
Immunomodulators 215
    topical 215
Immunosuppressive effects 68, 209
Impetigo 28
    herpetiformis 43
Indomethacin 21, 161
Infantile hemangiomas 28
Infection 109
    prevention of 51
    uncomplicated 23
Inflammatory bowel disease 163
Inflammatory dermatoses 129, 131
Inflammatory disorders 216
Infliximab 137, 140
Inorganic sunscreens 225
Insect bite hypersensitivity 29
Integrase inhibitors 114, 123
Integrase strand transfer
    inhibitors 114, 123
Interleukin 12/23 inhibitors 143
Interleukin-1 antagonists 152
Interleukin-13 inhibitors 149
Interleukin-17 inhibitors 140, 142, 144
    contraindications of 142
    monitoring of 142

Interleukin-31 receptor antagonist 150
Interleukin-36 receptor antagonist 151
Intralesional corticosteroid 29
Intralesional immunotherapy 203
Intralesional injections indications 63
Intralesional therapy 66
Intralesional triamcinolone 25
Intralesional triamcinolone remains 29
Intramuscular corticosteroid indications 63
Intramuscular therapy 66
Iontophoresis 235
Irreversible inhibitor 157, 223
Irritant contact dermatitis 6
Irritation 221
Isoniazid 54, 111
Isotretinoin 47
Isotretinoin, monitoring for 132
Isoxazolylpenicillins 87
Itch
　control of 16
　night-time 33
Itraconazole 13, 17, 51, 53, 97
Ivermectin 16, 106, 206
Ixekizumab 141

J

JAK inhibitors 156, 157
　classification of 156
　topical 222

K

Keloid 29
Keratinization, disorders of 129, 131
Keratoacanthoma 68
Keratolytic 57, 232
　emollients 17
　mild 27
Keratosis pilaris 30
Ketoconazole 17, 50, 196
Kligman's regimen, modified 231
Kojic acid 34, 230

L

Labor, early induction of 43
Lactation 110, 184
　category 220

Lactic acid 205, 233
Lamivudine 117, 118
Langerhans cell histiocytosis 68
Lansoprazole 161
Lebrikizumab 149
Leishmania recidivans 17
Leishmaniasis 203
Lenalidomide 179
Leprosy 109
　reaction 31, 62
Levocetirizine 83
Levofloxacin 31, 91
Lichen
　nitidus 32
　planus 32
　sclerosus 33
　simplex chronicus 33
Lichenoid amyloidosis 16
Lignocaine injection 236
Like Sezary syndrome 37
Lincosamides 94
Lindane 207
Linezolid 95
Liposomal amphotericin B 17
Lobomycosis 110
Local anesthetic agent 236
Lopinavir 121, 123
Loratadine 83
Luliconazole 197
Lupus
　erythematosus 31
　nephritis 163
Lymphocytic infiltrates 127, 177
Lymphocytic infiltrates, benign disorders with 127
Lymphogranuloma venereum 34
Lymphoproliferative disorders 67

M

Maceration and foul smell 53
Macrolides 89
Macular amyloidosis 16
Malathion 206
Malignancy 158, 160, 161
　chemoprevention of 129, 131
Maraviroc 116
Maternal complications 43
Measles, mumps, rubella vaccine 203
Meglumine antimoniate 17
Melanocyte keratinocyte transplant procedure 59
Melanoma metastases 203

Melasma 34
Menthol 33234
Metabolic and endocrine 112
Metabolism 117, 119, 120, 123
Metformin 26
Methicillin-resistant *Staphylococcus aureus* 93
Methicillin-sensitive *Staphylococcus aureus* infections 109
Methotrexate 9, 44, 57, 67, 69
Methoxsalen 181
Metronidazole 193
Miconazole 8, 195
Microencapsulation 227
Microsporum species 195
Miliaria 35
Miltefosine 17
Mineralocorticoid potency 62
Minocycline 25, 31, 47
Minoxidil 175
　topial 224
Mirtazapine 169
Mitochondrial respiration, inhibition of 221
Mizolastine 83
Mohs micrographic surgery 11
Moist dressing 18
Moisturizers 231
　types of 231
Molluscum contagiosum 35
Monobactams 87
Monobenzyl ether 230
Montelukast 85
Morphea 36, 209
Morpholine derivatives 194
Mouth and genital care 51
Mucous membrane pemphigoid 73
Multidrug resistance tuberculosis 54
Multiple matrix metalloproteinases, inhibition of 92
Mupirocin 8
Mycetoma 36
Mycobacterial infection 109
　atypical 109
Mycobacterial skin infection, atypical 10
Mycobacterium
　fortuitum infection, treatment of 11
　marinum, treatment of 10, 109
　tuberculosis 109, 111

Index

Mycophenolate mofetil 39, 46, 57, 75
Mycoplasma pneumoniae 193
Mycosis fungoides 36

N

Nadifloxacin 189
Nail psoriasis 163
Naproxen 21
Neck 182
Necrobiosis lipoidica 68
Neisseria meningitidis 109
Nelfinavir 121, 122, 123
Nemolizumab 150
Neomycin 188
Neuromuscular function
   inhibition of 182
   recovery of 182
Neuromuscular toxicity 127
Neuropsychiatric 65
Neutrophilic dermatoses 62, 67, 76, 78, 134, 177
Nevirapine 119, 120
Niacinamide 18, 34, 176
Nizatidine 84
Nodular amyloidosis 16
Non-hydroquinone products 34
Nonnucleoside reverse transcriptase inhibitors 114, 118
Nonsedating second generation H1 antihistamines 83
Nonsteroidal topical anti-inflammatory agents 33
Non-tuberculous mycobacterial 10
Norepinephrine 95
NRTI/NtRTIs, pharmacology and dosage of 117
Nucleoside and nucleotide reverse transcriptase inhibitors 116
Nummular eczema 19
Nystatin 195

O

Ocular subset 47
Oculotoxicity 127
Ofloxacin 31, 91
Omalizumab 55, 153
   binds 153
Omeprazole 161

Onychomycosis, treatment of 53
Opportunistic infections 158
Oral contraceptive pill 26
Oritavancin 89
Oxazolidinones 95
   inhibit protein synthesis 95
Oxiconazole 196
Ozenoxacin 187

P

Palmoplantar pustulosis 37
Pantoprazole 161
Pantothenic acid 238
Papular dermatitis of Spangler 43
Papulopustular 2
   mild 2
   subset 47
Papulosquamous 180
   dermatoses 134
   disease 209
   disorders 62, 67, 74, 76, 177, 216, 217, 232, 238
Parapsoriasis 37
Paronychia 38
   acute 38
   chronic 38
Pathak's formula 231
Paucibacillary 31
PDE4 inhibitor 155
Pediculosis 38
   capitis 205
Pemphigoid gestationis 43
Pemphigus vulgaris 39, 73
Penicillin 5, 87
Pentamidine 103
Pentavalent antimonials 17
Permethrin 38, 205
Persistent asthma, moderate-to-severe 153
Phenol 234
Phenothiazine 82, 83
Phenytoin 104
Phosphodiesterase-4 inhibitors, topical 221
Photoaging 238
Photodermatitis 62
Photodermatoses 74
Photosensitive disorders 127
Photosensitivity dermatoses 180
Photosensitizing agents 111
Phototherapy 42, 227
   particularly 43
Phototoxic reactions 181

Phthalazinones 82
Phymatous subset 47
Pigmentary disorders 216, 238
Pilosebaceous unit, disorder of 216
Pimecrolimus 15, 42, 44, 216
Pimozide 103, 171
Piperazine 82, 83
Piperidines 82, 83
Pityriasis lichenoides
   chronica 40
   et varioliformis acuta 40
Pityriasis rosea 40
Pityriasis rubra pilaris 40, 137
Pityriasis versicolor 41
Plaque psoriasis, moderate-to-severe 145
Plasma
   half-life 62
   protein binding 123
Plasmapheresis 57
Polyenes 13, 194, 195
Polymicrobial infection 5
Polymorphous light eruption 41, 74
Pompholyx 42
Posaconazole 100
Post-exposure prophylaxis 125
   regimen 125
Postinflammatory
   hyperpigmentation 3
Potassium
   hydroxide 204
   iodide 21, 51, 80
      saturated solution of 80
Potent topical steroid 33
Povidone-iodine 190
Pralatrexate 37
Pramoxine 33, 234
Prednisolone 9
Pre-exposure prophylaxis 126
Pregabalin 171
Pregnancy 84, 110, 118, 123, 125
   atopic eruption of 42
   category 120, 222
   cholestasis of 43
   dermatoses 42
      with fetal risk 43
      without fetal risk 43
   monitoring guidelines 133
   polymorphic eruption of 42
   pruritic folliculitis of 43
Premalignant disorders 238
Pressure, removal of 17

Propranolol 174
Propylene glycol 27
Protease inhibitors 114, 120
Protein binding 117, 119, 120
Prurigo nodularis 43, 68, 148
   treatment of 43
Pruritus 43
Pseudoephedrine 95
Pseudofolliculitis barbae 45
Pseudogout 134
Pseudomembranous colitis 192
Psoriasis 44
Psoriatic arthritis 141, 163
Psoriatic erythroderma 141
Psychosis 171
Psychotropic agents 167
Punch grafting 59
Pyoderma gangrenosum 46, 62, 151
Pyrazinamide 54, 112
Pyridoxine deficiency 112

R

Rabeprazole 161
Radiotherapy 29
Raltegravir 125
Rational skin therapy 1
Raynaud's phenomenon 48
Reactions 31
Reactive oxygen species 231
Receptor binding affinity 211
Refractory cases 43
Reiter disease 68
Resiquimod 220, 221
Retapamulin 187
Retinoic acid metabolism blocking agents 133
Retinoid 2, 211
   second-generation 131
   third-generation 132
   topical 2, 211
Reversible inhibitor 157, 223
Rheumatoid arthritis protocol 146
Rifabutin 108
Rifampicin 31, 54
Rifampin 108
Rifamycins 108
Rifapentin 108
Rilpivirine 119, 120
Risankizumab 145
Risperidone 171

Ritlecitinib 7, 157, 162
Ritonavir 121, 123
Rituximab 39, 146
Roflumilast 222
Romidepsin 37
Rosacea 47, 129
Rotational therapy 45
Roxithromycin 89
Ruxolitinib 36, 223

S

Salicylic acid 205, 232
Saquinavir 121, 122, 123
Sarcoidosis 48, 62, 68
Scabies 48, 205
   indication 207
Scalp
   application 207
   dissecting cellulitis of 129
   psoriasis, moderate-to-severe 163
Scleredema diabeticorum 68
Scratching, role of 33
Sebaceous glands, disorders of 238
Seborrheic blepharitis 49, 50
Seborrheic otitis externa 50
Secukinumab 140
Sedating first-generation H_1 antihistamines 83
Selective serotonin
   norepinephrine reuptake inhibitor 169
   reuptake inhibitors 34
Selenium sulfide 194, 199
Sequential therapy 45
Sertaconazole 197
Serum uric acid 112
Sexual partner 34
Sexually transmitted diseases 87
Shaving 26
Shingles, vaccination for prevention of 183
Shingrix 183
Silver sulfadiazine 189
Sinecatechin 205
Sirolimus 217
Skin
   and soft tissue infection, treatment of 89
   grafting 46
   hydration 27

   involvement, mild-to-moderate 44
   lesion, specific 31
Sodium
   stibogluconate 17
   sulfacetamide 194
Sonidegib 173
Spesolimab 151
Spinosad 207
Spironolactone 26, 166
Split thickness grafting 59
Sporotrichosis 51, 80
Squaric acid dibutyl ester 220
Staphylococci 109
Steroids, classification of topical 208
Stevens-Johnson syndrome 50
Streptomyces
   hydroscepicus var ascomyceticus 216
   mediterranei 108
Strongyloidiasis 105
Sulconazole 196
Sulfapyridine 18
Sun-protection, art of 34
Sunscreen application 226
Surgery, types of 59
Surgical excision 29
Sweat resistant 226
Sweet syndrome 62
Synthetic retinoids 129
Syphilis 52
Systemic antibacterial agents 87
Systemic antifungal 96
Systemic antiviral agents 100
Systemic corticosteroid 26, 51, 57, 62
   classification 62
   indications 62
   mechanism of action 63
Systemic drugs 61
Systemic immunosuppressive and immunomodulatory agents 67
Systemic lupus erythematosus 163
Systemic photoprotective agents 225
Systemic retinoids 48, 128
Systemic sarcoidosis 48
Systemic sclerosis, cutaneous management 48
Systemic vasculitis 137

T

T cell lymphoma 203
Tacrolimus 12, 15, 42, 215
　topical 44
Tavaborole 194, 200
Tazarotene 2, 214
Teaspoon rule 226
Teicoplanin 89
Telavancin 89
Temperature regulation 50
Tenofovir 118
　disoproxil fumarate 117
Terbinafine 51, 53, 96, 198
Tetracycline 12, 18, 92
　moderate-to-severe flushing
　　oral 47
Thalidomide 12, 43, 176
Thiabandazole 16, 105
Thiocarbamates 194
Thrombocytopenia 154
Tildrakizumab 145
Tinea
　cruris, treatment of 53
　infection 52
　manuum, treatment of 53
　pedis, treatment of 53
Titration schedule dose 156
Tofacitinib 15, 36, 157
Toxic epidermal necrolysis 50
Tralokinumab 150
Tretinoin 2, 34, 212
Trichinosis 105
Trichloroacetic acid 204
Trichophyton 195
　skin antigen 203
Trichuriasis 105
Triclosan 191
Trifarotene 215
Trimethoprim sulfamethoxazole 93
Tuberculosis 54
　infection evaluation 159
　screening 152
Tubulin, dimers of 134

Tumor necrosis factor inhibitors, classification 136

U

Ulcer
　arterial 30
　cutaneous 49
　decubitus 17
　leg 30
　venous 30
Ulcerative colitis 163
Ultraviolet
　A phototherapy 229
　A therapy 228
　B therapy 227
Upadacitinib 157, 161
Upper abdominal pain 161
Upper face 182
Upper respiratory tract infection 161, 162
Urea 233
Ureaplasma urealyticum 193
Urinary tract infections 159, 162
Urticaria 54
　refractory to antihistamines 56
　totally refractory to antihistamines 56
　treatment
　　algorithm for 55
　　of acute 54
　　of chronic 54

V

Vaccine series 183
Valacyclovir 102
Vancomycin 89
Vancomycin-resistant
　Staphylococcus aureus 95
Varicella-Zoster infections 102
Vascular lasers 47
Vasculitis 57, 62, 67, 76, 74, 78, 134

Verruca plana 202
Vesiculobullous disorders 177, 216
Viral warts 57
Viricidal drugs 201
Visceral larva migrans 105
Vismodegib 172
Vitamin 176
　A 211
　B complex 238
　B3 238
　B5 238
　C 239
　D analogues 218
　D3 analogue calcipotriene 43
　E 237
　K 237
　topical 237
Vitiligo 58
　surgery 58
Voriconazole 99

W

Water-resistant sunscreen 226
Weinstein frost regimen 68
Westerhof's formula 231
Wet dressing 42
Whitfield ointment 194
Wound 51
　care 50
　healing 211
　swab 18

X

Xerosis 233

Z

Zafirlukast 85, 86
Zidovudine 117, 118
Zinc 176
　sulfate 4
　supplementation 4